Kingdom
of the Sick

D1557595

Kingdom of the Sick

A History of Leprosy and Japan

Susan L. Burns

University of Hawai'i Press
Honolulu

Library of Congress Cataloging-in-Publication Data

Names: Burns, Susan L., author.
Title: Kingdom of the sick : a history of leprosy and Japan / Susan L. Burns.
Description: Honolulu : University of Hawai'i Press, [2019] | Includes
    bibliographical references and index.
Identifiers: LCCN 2018043547 | ISBN 9780824879013 (cloth ; alk. paper)
Subjects: LCSH: Leprosy—Japan—History—20th century. |
    Leprosy—Patients—Japan—History—20th century. | Leprosy—Government
    policy—Japan—History—20th century.
Classification: LCC RC154.7.J3 B87 2019 | DDC 616.99/800952—dc23
LC record available at https://lccn.loc.gov/2018043547

ISBN: 9780824892388 (paperback)

Cover art: Utagawa Kuniyoshi, from *The Sixty-Nine Stations of the Kisokaidō*, 1852
(Museum of Fine Arts, Boston). This print, numbered fifty-seven for the town of
Akasaka-juku, evokes the famous story of Empress Kōmyō washing a *rai* sufferer.

Contents

Acknowledgments

IN THE MANY YEARS it has taken me to complete this project, I have had the good fortune to receive a series of fellowships and grants to support my research. Fellowships from the National Endowment for the Humanities and the Japan Society for the Promotion of Science allowed me to carry out the first stage of research for this project in Japan. Additional research was accomplished with the support of the International Research Center for Japanese Studies and a Fulbright-Hays fellowship. Research support from the Division of the Social Sciences of the University of Chicago and the Japan Committee of the University of Chicago's Center for East Asian Studies funded targeted research trips to Bergen, Norway; London; Austin, Texas; Washington, DC; and Honolulu.

I am profoundly grateful to the residents and staff of Tama Zenshōen, Nagashima Aiseien, Kuryū Rakusen'en, and Kikuchi Keifūen and the curators, guides, and staff of the former Takamatsu no Miya Kinen Hansenbyō Shiryōkan, the National Hansen's Disease Museum of Japan, and the Jyu-kanbo National Museum of Detention for Hansen's Disease Patients. Special thanks to Tamura Tomohisa, the curator of Aiseien's museum, Kitahara Makoto of the Jyu-kanbo National Museum, and Sigurd Sandmo of the Lepramuseet (Bergen, Norway), who shared their insights about the public history of leprosy with me. I have learned a great deal from the work of Angela Leung, Jane Kim, Hirokawa Waka, Kathryn Tanaka, Jo Robertson, and Kerri Inglis, all scholars of the history of leprosy. David Howell, Daniel Botsman, Sally Hastings, Amanda Seaman, Nancy Stalker, Jim Huffman, Daniel Trambaiolo, Ken Ito, and the late Barbara Brooks all offered encouragement and advice at crucial points in this project. The extended and thoughtful comments of Kuriyama Shigehisa and William Johnston aided me tremendously in making the final revisions to this work.

I have also benefited from the vibrant and supportive community of East Asian scholars at the University of Chicago. Thanks to Michael Bourdaghs, Reggie Jackson, and Nobuko Toyosawa for reading parts of the work and to Hoyt Long for inspiring me to think "digitally." Watching Johanna Ransmeier complete her book was inspiring; so, too, was Ken Pomeranz's exemplary combination of productivity and collegiality. Thanks to my "sensei" Aratake Ken'ichiro and to Hiroyoshi Noto and the other members of the University of Chicago's Kuzushiji reading group and the Kuzushiji summer workshop, all of whom helped me learn to read manuscript texts. The Japanese librarians of the University of Chicago, the late Okuizumi Eizaburō and Ayako Yoshimura, both aided me greatly in securing the materials I needed. Thanks to my graduate students, past and present, including Tanya Maus, Patti Kameya, Maki Fukuoka, Tomoko Seto, Wei-ti Chen, Tadashi Ishikawa, Jessa Dahl, and Kyle Pan. In different ways, their projects have informed my own. I am grateful as well for the hard work of my research assistants, Abigail Kim, Eigen Aoki, and Angela Zhao.

Some portions of chapter 3 were published earlier in "Rethinking 'Leprosy Prevention': Entrepreneurial Doctors, the Meiji Press, and the Civic Origins of Biopolitics," *Journal of Japanese Studies* 38, no. 2 (summer 2012): 297–323, while parts of chapter 6 previously appeared in "Making Illness Identity: Writing 'Leprosy Literature' in Modern Japan," *Japan Review* 16 (2004): 191–211. I thank both journals for granting permission to reuse this work. Thanks as well to the Aomori Kenshi Hensan Group for kindly granting permission to use figure 5.1 and to the National Hansen's Disease Museum of Japan for permission to use figure 5.2. I am grateful to Pat Crosby and Stephanie Chun of the University of Hawai'i Press for their patience and for making the publication process go smoothly and to Eileen G. Chetti for her careful copyediting.

Finally, I want to express my deep appreciation to my much-loved and much-missed father, the late Frank H. Burns, who died in 2013. A lover of history himself and a devoted father who was always my safety net, he had been urging me to "hurry up and finish your book" for many years. I only wish I had been faster, so that he could have seen this project come to fruition. And thanks, as always, to my daughter, Hannah. This project was the background of her childhood, and although she may have tired of changing countries, schools, and friends to accommodate my research, she bore it all without complaint, embracing our peripatetic life as an adventure. She was my partner on this journey and enriched it with her presence.

Introduction

Over the course of the first half of the twentieth century, the Japanese government constructed one of the largest sustained programs of medical quarantine in modern history. The object of this effort was leprosy, or Hansen's disease as some now prefer to call it, a chronic infectious disease caused by the bacillus *Mycobacterium leprae*. Between 1907 and 1945, the government oversaw the construction of thirteen leprosy sanitaria around the country, from Aomori in far northern Honshū to Miyakojima, an island in Okinawa Prefecture. The number of those in quarantine peaked in 1955 when the national sanitaria housed more than twelve thousand people. This date is significant. While Japan's prewar system of quarantine reflected international norms of the time, its expansion in the postwar era did not. In the wake of the discovery that sulfone drugs were effective in treating leprosy, outpatient treatment became the preferred response to the disease around the world. Nonetheless, in 1953, the Japanese Diet revised the 1931 law that had authorized the confinement of leprosy sufferers and preserved the requirement for quarantine. The postwar law was not repealed until 1996, even though the number of new cases of leprosy declined dramatically from the 1960s. Even today more than thirteen hundred former patients, now referred to as "residents" (*nyūjosha*), continue to live within the sanitaria. Their average age is well over eighty and some have lived six or more decades within these institutions.[1]

This book explores the history of leprosy in Japan and the rise of this system of quarantine by taking an approach that is *longue durée*, interdisciplinary, and international in its focus. I argue that leprosy was a profoundly stigmatized disease in Japan in the period before modernity and that this stigma was accompanied by forms of social and spatial exclusion. In the

1

Name	Type	Dates	Prefecture
Ihaien	Mission (Protestant)	1894–1942	Tokyo
St. Barnabas Mission	Mission (Protestant)	1915–1941	Gunma
Fukusei Hospital	Mission (Roman Catholic)	1889–present	Shizuoka
Kaishun Hospital	Mission (Protestant)	1898–2013	Kumamoto
Tairōin	Mission (Roman Catholic)	1898–2013	Kumamoto
Jinkyōen	Private (Buddhist)	1906–1992	Yamagata
Matsuoka Hoyōen (Northern Area Rest Home)	Public → National	1909–present	Aomori
Zenshōen (Zensei Hospital)	Public → National	1909–present	Tokyo
Seishōen (Ōshima Sanitarium)	Public → National	1909–present	Kagawa
Keifūen (Kyūshū Rest Home)	Public → National	1909–present	Kumamoto
Komyoen (Sotojima Rest Home)	Public → National	1909–present	Osaka→Okayama
Aiseien	National	1930–present	Okayama
Nanseien	Public → National	1931–present	Okinawa
Rakusen'en	National	1932–present	Gunma
Keiaien	National	1935–present	Kagoshima
Shinseien	Public → National	1938–present	Miyagi
Airakuen	National	1938–present	Okinawa
Wakōen	National	1943–present	Kagoshima
Suruga Ryōyōjō	National	1945–present	Shizuoka

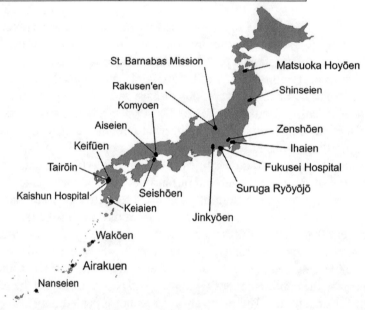

MAP 1.   Private, public, and national leprosy sanitaria.

late nineteenth century, new ideas about causality and curability and a new international debate about how to control leprosy transformed a familiar disease into a social and political issue. From the 1880s through the 1930s, physicians, bureaucrats, politicians, journalists, local communities, and leprosy sufferers themselves grappled with the question of how to respond to the disease and the place of those infected within the body politic. At stake in both issues were still-evolving conceptions of individual rights, government responsibility, and the delicate balance between care and control. The turn towards coerced quarantine came only in the late 1930s as mobilization for total war transformed Japanese society. The postwar policy, I argue, represents not a simple continuation of the prewar approach but a new moment of contestation in an ongoing citizenship project, a term I borrow from Nikolas Rose and Carlos Nova.[2]

In approaching the history of leprosy in Japan this way, I am departing from and seeking to cast critical light on the politicized terrain of the history of leprosy as it has come to be written in Japan in the last two and half decades. While studies of disease, public health policy, and medical institutions might seem to be a genre of historical writing that appeals primarily to historians of medicine and social welfare and perhaps some scholarly inclined physicians, in Japan leprosy has been the object of intense public interest and considerable activism for more than a decade and a half. The history of Japan's leprosy policy has been the topic of television documentaries and feature films and an extraordinary flood of publications that include a twenty-volume collection of historical sources, a ten-volume collection of patient writing, and even a scholarly journal published annually. Since 2000, more than seven hundred books on leprosy have been published in Japan.[3] The official websites of many of the Japanese prefectures have a page on leprosy, and there are now five publicly funded museums devoted to the history of the quarantine policy.[4]

The Politics of Leprosy History

The books, films, and reportage on leprosy reflect a powerful narrative that first emerged in the 1990s. Until that point, the history of leprosy, to the extent that it was written at all, took the form of a Whiggish celebration of Japan's success in responding to a terrible disease. Authored primarily by those working within or connected to the public health bureaucracy, it made heroes of physicians such as Mitsuda Kensuke, one of the architects of the quarantine system, and Ogawa Masako, whose account of her efforts to convince leprosy sufferers to enter a sanitarium in the early 1930s became a best-selling book and then a popular film.[5] In contrast, the new literature on leprosy casts a harsh light on Japan's leprosy policy, the state that enacted it, and the physicians and others who implemented it. This new critical history unfolded at an important moment: in the early 1990s a new wave of activism had begun in the sanitaria. Residents not only organized to call for the repeal of the 1953 law; they also began to craft the public history of their own experience. In 1991, a group of residents became involved in raising funds to establish a museum on the grounds of Tama Zenshōen, a sanitarium located outside of Tokyo, that was to be devoted to the history of leprosy. It opened two years later.[6]

Against this backdrop, three monographs on the history of leprosy were published in rapid succession: Yamamoto Shun'ichi's *A History of Leprosy in Japan* (*Nihon raishi*), Sawano Masaki's *Life as a Leper: As a Requirement for Civilization and Enlightenment* (*Raisha no sei: Bunmei kaika no jōken toshite no*), and Fujino Yutaka's *Japanese Fascism and Medicine: An Empirical Study of Hansen's Disease* (*Nihon fashizumu to iryō: Hansenbyō wo meguru jisshōteki kenkyū*).[7] Of these three authors, only Yamamoto had previously published on medical history and public health policy. A physician by training, he had written on the history of cholera and venereal disease policy. While *A History of Leprosy in Japan* is almost chronicle-like in form, with minimal argumentation, its excavation of new information about the formation of the national sanitaria and their operation cast Japan's modern policy of leprosy prevention in new and critical light.

However, the heightened rhetoric of Fujino Yutaka and to a lesser degree Sawano Masaki proved more influential than Yamamoto's dry description. Sawano is one of the generation of scholars who came of age during the so-called cultural turn. Taking a Foucauldian approach, he argued that the stigmatized figure of the leper (*raisha*) was a form of modern subjectivity produced by the Japanese state's policy towards leprosy. In contrast to Sawano's theoretically informed approach, Fujino's work is typical of an earlier generation of progressive activist scholars. Before he turned to the issue of leprosy, he had worked primarily on *buraku* history, the study of Japan's best-known "minority," the descendants of stigmatized status groups of the early modern period who continue to face social discrimination even up to the present. Although he would go on to write on other topics, Fujino's career has largely been defined by his work on leprosy. After *Japanese Fascism and Medicine*, he published another four monographs on the disease, including one on leprosy during the war era and two on the postwar period.

Hirokawa Waka, one of a handful of scholars in Japan who have begun to revise the powerful narrative that Fujino put forth, has termed his work "denunciatory history" (*kyūdan no rekishi*), a phrase that neatly conveys the palpable sense of outrage that animates it.[8] In Fujino's view, from the passage of the first law that addressed leprosy in 1907, policy towards the disease was the tool of a fascist state in the making, and he likens the prewar leprosy laws to the eugenicist policies of Nazi Germany. Evoking the image of the Holocaust, Fujino argues that "leprosy prevention" was in reality a campaign to eradicate its sufferers for purposes of "racial purity."[9] This is history written in black and white, with clearly delineated heroes and villains. Mitsuda Kensuke, who had been celebrated for leading the fight against leprosy, was now cast as villain in chief. Fujino made support for quarantine a kind of ethical litmus test and celebrated men such as Ogasahara Tōru, a previously obscure member of the faculty of medicine at Kyoto University who had spoken out against the need for quarantine in the 1930s. This view ignores the fact that Ogasahara was by no means an unproblematic figure: for one, he promoted scientifically baseless theories of the disease.[10]

It would be easy to dismiss Fujino's work on scholarly grounds. The analogy with Nazi Germany that frames *Japanese Fascism and Medicine* ignores a substantial historical literature on the question of whether 1930s Japan can rightly be termed fascist, and Fujino cherry-picks evidence, reads sources in an arbitrary manner, and is guilty of frequent interpretive sleights of hand. But such an evaluation would ignore the powerful contribution he made in the context of the early 1990s, when Japan, like other countries, was still grappling with the HIV/AIDS epidemic. *Japanese Fascism and Medicine* compelled its readers to critically scrutinize seemingly benevolent public health policies and to consider the damage done to individuals in the name of the social good. It brought new attention to the national sanitaria and to those who remained within them and thus played a role in rallying support for the belated repeal of the 1953 law.

Subsequent events, however, have transformed the "denunciatory history" from a politically oriented revisionist history into a body of historical "facts" no longer open to question. In 1998, a group of thirteen recovered leprosy sufferers, all longtime residents of one of the national sanitaria, filed suit against the Japanese government in Kumamoto District Court with the support of a group of lawyers that took the name the Hansen's Disease Legal Committee for State Compensation for Constitutional Violations (Hansenbyō Iken Kokubai Soshō Bengodan).[11] The plaintiffs, whose number grew to include more than 589 people, charged that the requirement for quarantine had been in violation of Japan's constitution and that the Ministry of Health and Welfare had allowed the systematic infringement of the patients' human and civil rights by authorizing policies that included forced sterilization and abortion, coerced labor, and arbitrary punishment without due process. The following year, two similar suits were filed in Tokyo District Court (126 plaintiffs) and in Okayama District Court (64 plaintiffs). Together, the plaintiffs in the three cases represented about 20 percent of the total number of sanitarium residents at the time.[12]

As the legal process unfolded at the snail's pace typical of the courts in Japan, the plaintiffs' counsel in the Kumamoto court relied heavily upon the testimony of their clients to make their case. They submitted 127 written plaintiff statements and called twenty-four witnesses to address the court directly. One was Ueno Masako, who had entered the sanitarium in her early teens and lived there for half a century. She testified that when she married a fellow patient at the age of nineteen, she still hoped that she would recover enough to "return to society" (*shakai fukki*) and have a family. She was shocked, then, when she learned that her new husband had complied with sanitarium policy and undergone a vasectomy. Another witness was Shimamura Yasushi, who had entered the sanitarium at age sixteen in 1948. He testified that when the woman he married in the sanitarium became pregnant she was scheduled for an abortion by the staff "as though it was the normal course of things." Others told the court of the rejection of family members, the burden of the stigma of the disease, and the frustrations, restrictions, and loneliness of institutional life.[13]

The ruling, when it finally came on May 11, 2001, was both unexpected and carefully delimited. Although the Kumamoto court affirmed both the harsh assessment of the sanitaria offered by plaintiffs and their claim that the leprosy prevention laws had fostered a culture of stigma, its judgment on the legality of the leprosy policy focused specifically on the postwar era. It ruled that by 1960 "at the latest" quarantine was no longer justifiable on medical or public health grounds and that the ministry and the Diet had violated the rights of the patients when they had failed to repeal the 1953 law in a timely manner. The court ordered the payment of compensation to 127 of the plaintiffs in the amount of 1,823,800,000 yen (approximately 15 million US dollars at the time), a little more than a tenth of the amount requested by the former patients.[14]

Although the judgment and award fell short of what the plaintiffs had requested, both were hailed as "epochal" (*kakkiteki*) and "historical" (*rekishiteki*) by jurists, journalists, activists, and others. In the 1990s, Japanese courts had been flooded with cases that sought apology and compensation from the Japanese government. Plaintiffs included the so-called comfort women, Korean and Chinese forced laborers, American and Australian POWs, non-Japanese A-bomb survivors, and the Chinese victims of biological warfare. These cases had met with little success. The Japanese government defended itself based upon the principle of sovereign immunity, the statute of limitations, and other issues of law, thereby avoiding the question of the factuality of the plaintiffs' claims.[15] Thus, the outcome of the leprosy case broke new legal ground. It was the first time the Japanese government was ordered to pay compensation to victims of its policies. As a result, the court's decision was celebrated by a wide swath of groups and individuals concerned with issues of social justice and critical of the Japanese state's record on human and civil rights.

Only two weeks after the Kumamoto court issued its ruling, Prime Minister Koizumi Jun'ichirō announced that his government would not appeal. The unprecedented decision to allow the lower court's order to stand was interpreted as an acknowledgment of the aptness of the judgment, but it was also politically strategic. It positioned the Japanese government as sensitive to civil rights in relation to an issue where the stakes may have seemed small. The public health threat posed by leprosy had long been resolved, and most of the remaining residents of the leprosy sanitaria were, after all, Japanese citizens. Elderly and in many cases disabled, they evoked considerable sympathy from the public. In a matter of weeks, the Diet passed a law that extended compensation to all residents of the sanitaria. Apologies in this case came quickly, first from Koizumi himself, then from the Diet and the Supreme Court, and then from a series of prefectural governors. Sakaguchi Chikara, minister of health, labor, and welfare, soon undertook an apology tour, visiting each of the national sanitaria in turn to make a formal apology, bowing deeply before the patients—and the cameras.[16]

The political calculation behind the ritual of apology and the offer of compensation proved to be deeply flawed. In the years that followed, former patients of Japan's two colonial-era sanitaria in Korea and Taiwan also sued the Japanese government asking for compensation, and they, too, prevailed. In Japan, plaintiffs and their advocates soon pressed for more than compensation and expressions of regret. They called for "the restoration of the honor" (*meiyo kaifuku*) and "the restoration of the humanity" (*ningen kaifuku*) of Japan's leprosy sufferers. These phrases came to mean that the government must take full responsibility not only for the policy of quarantine and the abuses that occurred within the sanitaria but also for the stigma of the disease itself. Soon after the May decision, the Kumamoto plaintiffs, their lawyers, and representatives of the National Conference of Sanitarium Residents joined together to create a new organization, the United Negotiation Committee, to pursue further concessions from the Japanese government.

In December 2001, the two sides announced an agreement. The lengthy document later produced committed the government to a number of new concessions, including the payment of compensation to "nonresidents" (leprosy patients who had not been confined) and to family members of patients, but it also included a section called "Inquiry into Truth" that directly addressed the history of leprosy in Japan. The government agreed that it would (1) "verify in a multidisciplinary manner . . . the history and real conditions of the Hansen's disease policy with the aim of making suggestions to forestall a reoccurrence of such a policy"; (2) "strive to open to the public and preserve historical materials and buildings related to Hansen's disease policy"; and (3) "strive to expand as much as possible the budget, facilities, and human resources devoted to the Hansen's Disease Museum."[17]

The terms of the "Inquiry into Truth" authorized the transformation of the denunciatory history of leprosy into an official history. Two sites are particularly illuminative of this process. The first is the two-volume work called *The Final Report of the Verification Committee on the Hansen's Disease Problem* (hereafter *The Final Report*). The term "verification" here is important; the committee was tasked with fulfilling the government's promise to "verify . . . the history and real conditions of the Hansen's Disease policy." Published in 2005 under the auspices of an organization called the Japan Law Foundation, *The Final Report* was the product of research and writing undertaken by a committee not of historians but of lawyers. The introduction makes clear the significance of the project for committee members: "The Hansen's disease problem is not at all extraordinary. It is simply the best reflection of the nature of the Japanese nation and our society. . . . We think that with the promulgation of the postwar constitution the protection of fundamental human rights has progressed since the prewar period. However, that is something of a myth."[18] This assertion of the representational value of the leprosy policy for the nature of modern Japanese state and society informs the whole of *The Final Report*. It devotes little time to the long history of leprosy before modernity, and little attention is paid to the international context within which it unfolded. Instead, the work traces a straight line of growing oppression from the law of 1907 to that of 1953. Given its origins in litigation for compensation, it is unsurprising that the organizing theme of the work as a whole is "responsibility" (*sekinin*) and the apportionment of blame. While the state is held primarily responsible for the policy of quarantine, the authors also find fault with the medical establishment, religious institutions, social welfare authorities, the media, and their fellow jurists, all of whom are declared to have been complicit with the state. This focus on institutional power over individual agency is by no means new. In fact, it reflects the cultural logic of the dominant postwar narrative of state / civil society relations in Japan that has at its center the issue of war responsibility and that has long held that the Japanese people were victims of the prewar and wartime state.[19]

If *The Final Report* sought to confirm the denunciatory history, the purpose of a second site, this one material rather than discursive, was to publicize it. The National Hansen's Disease Museum opened on March 31, 2007, fulfilling the government's promise of five years before to "strive to expand as much as possible the budget, facilities, and human resources devoted to the Hansen's Disease Museum" by nationalizing the small museum at Tama Zenshōen that had opened in 1993. The process of designing the new museum was lengthy and deliberate, and it involved patient representatives, civil rights lawyers, academics, and disability rights advocates.[20]

When it reopened, the new museum had three galleries, each with its own theme. The first, described as a "historical display," provides a timeline of the history of leprosy in Japan from ancient to modern times, ending with the Kumamoto legal victory, through a series of panels that combine texts and illustrations, with a small number of artifacts arranged in glass cases below them. The second gallery, entitled "The Leprosy Sanitaria: Exclusion with No Exit," features the re-creation of a patient room from the 1930s and exhibits that illustrate human rights abuses in the sanitaria, including the reliance on patient labor, restrictions on marriage, the use of sterilization and abortion, and the sanitarium jails. The third gallery, entitled "Proof of Survival," depicts the history of patient activism, literary and cultural activities within the sanitaria, and the impact of effective treatments. It also includes a "testimony corner" that allows visitors to listen to curated audio recordings of interviews with residents.

To the dismay of those involved in its planning, the national museum met with criticism from the moment it opened. The opening ceremony was presided over by Yanagisawa Hakuo, then minister of health, labor, and welfare in Abe Shinzō's first government. In his greeting to an audience comprised of journalists, officials, activists, physicians, and some former patients, Yanagisawa stated that he hoped that the museum "would become a core institution in the dissolution of prejudice and discrimination." Yanagisawa was followed by Miyasato Mitsuo, the head of the National Conference of Sanitarium Residents. He seized the opportunity to express his dissatisfaction with the new museum, declaring that "the exhibits are entirely inadequate and conceal the shadow of the patients' own testimony that is like blood spewing forth."[21]

Miyasato's comment set off a storm of criticism in the weeks and months that followed. Newspapers published negative reviews of the museum, while some visitors took to the new blogosphere to publicize their reactions, often with biting contempt.[22] Much of the criticism was directed towards the first exhibit, which began with a description of the stigma of leprosy in the premodern era. This, it was claimed, was nothing more than an attempt to diminish state responsibility for the discrimination suffered by leprosy patients in the modern era. The space dedicated to cultural activities within the sanitaria, from brass bands to poetry circles, was another target, with critics arguing that the display belied the real harshness of institutional life. In the same vein, critics charged that the groundbreaking victory in the Kumamoto suit was not given enough coverage; that figures like Mitsuda Kensuke were treated too generously; and that iconic cases of abuse within the sanitaria went unmentioned.

Leprosy and Biological Citizenship

Prasenjit Duara has written of the need to "rescue history from the nation," arguing that the linear histories of the rise of the nation-state, the dominant mode of history writing since the Enlightenment, required the repression of other contesting narratives, personal, local, and transnational.[23] The denunciatory history is similarly problematic, the appeal of its seemingly progressive politics notwithstanding. My early work on leprosy, written around the time of the Kumamoto judgment, was very much in the mode of denunciation, although it gave some weight to the premodern forms of exclusion.[24] But a chance encounter in the summer of 2002 prompted a long period of research and reflection. I was visiting the sanitarium in Kumamoto, known as Kikuchi Keifūen, where I spoke with members of the Self-Government Committee (Jichikai), who shared photographs and stories. Several of those with whom I spoke had been plaintiffs in the case settled only the year before, and they were thrilled with its outcome. At one point, however, I found myself talking with a lively woman who looked to be in her sixties, as she guided me from one building to another. The only visible sign that she had once suffered from leprosy was the paralysis of several fingers on one hand. When I asked her if she, too, had been a plaintiff, she paused for a moment before stating that she had not, because "I wasn't forced to stay here. I chose to. My life was here."

In the decade and a half since that meeting, I have thought often of that statement and the dignity and even defiance with which it was spoken. My attempt to make sense of it in this book reflects my debt to Adriana Petryna, Nikolas Rose and Carlos Nova, and others who have complicated the Foucauldian notion of biopolitics by what they term "biological citizenship." Foucault, of course, used "biopolitics" to describe the array of "technologies of power"—from sanitary regulations and public health policies to discourses on nutrition, exercise, and hygiene—that are deployed in modern societies to regulate, monitor, and organize human beings so that they are both productive and docile. In contrast, the concept of biological citizenship draws our attention away from the disciplinary regimes imposed from "above" and asserts that the biological needs of individual bodies, particularly those that are sick or disabled, can prompt the formation of new kinds of alliances, collective action, and conceptions of rights from "below."[25]

Petryna initially coined the term "biological citizenship" in her study of the aftermath of the 1986 Chernobyl disaster.[26] She argued that the tens of thousands of victims of radiation, both ethnic Russians and Ukrainians, were forced to negotiate for their social and economic survival within the fragile post-Soviet Ukrainian state founded only four years later. Individually and together, they attempted to lay claim to welfare benefits and medical care as their right as citizens of the new democratic state of Ukraine. Radiation exposure thus became the basis for the formation of a new political alliance that challenged and to a degree overcame distinctions of language and ethnicity. Petryna argues that this biologically defined citizenship shaped the Ukrainian state by propelling the establishment of multiple medical and scientific institutions and complex bureaucratic practices, the role of which is not only to weigh competing claims for aid but also to demonstrate the legitimacy of the state.

Ukraine in the 1990s and Japan in the late nineteenth century were very different places, and leprosy and radiation-related diseases are different as well. But I argue that leprosy first became an issue when Japan, too, was still a nation under construction and that the debates that surrounded it played a role in shaping the nature of the nation-state it became. There is a large and growing literature that explores how compulsory education, linguistic and legal reform, new social sites, and cultural practices were implicated in the process of nation making in Japan, but little attention has been paid to what Rose calls the "politics of life," the question of the place and value of sick and disabled bodies within and for specific societies.[27] In the case of Japan, leprosy policy was, to be sure, part of a larger public health regime, the construction of which began soon after the revolution of 1868, but leprosy was also a special disease, marked by a long history of stigma. Thus, while tuberculosis infected many more people and the mentally ill were also the objects of considerable concern, it was leprosy that gave rise to a network of state-supported institutions, national campaigns, and public displays of imperial philanthropy. Attempts to define leprosy policy resulted in decades of debate, experimentation, and contestation about the government's responsibility towards its vulnerable citizens but also their rights and obligations as citizens.

Leprosy sufferers, I argue, were part of this process, not merely the passive victims of the state and its allies. To explore their "participation," as I will term it, I draw upon a large and diverse body of patient-authored writings. Beginning in the 1920s, public health authorities, sanitarium staff, and their fellow patients began to encourage sanitaria residents to write prose, poetry, and fiction. This body of work has been largely ignored within the denunciatory history of leprosy because it suggests that at least some patients within the sanitaria embraced confinement and were no less nationalistic and supportive of the Japanese state than their fellow citizens outside the walls of the sanitaria. Fujino Yutaka, for example, mined patient writing for any criticism of the sanitaria but otherwise ignored it. Others reject outright the notion that patient writing can tell us anything about the agency of leprosy sufferers. A case in point is Arai Yūki, the author of a recent study of patient-authored fiction. He argued that while literature was a powerful mode of self-expression in the postwar sanitaria, works written before the 1950s reveal only the oppression of the patients, who were so effectively disciplined that "even the words of the individuals clearly express normative national values."[28]

The approaches of Fujino and Arai reflect a similar evaluation of prewar patient writing: in contrast to the authentic "testimony" (shōgen, katari) of leprosy sufferers in the postwar era, the stories and essays authored in the sanitaria before 1945 were written under conditions of coercion that render them useless for understanding the perspective of patients. My position is that the "testimony" voiced in the courts, interviews, and the proliferation of oral histories and memoirs published in recent years is no less mediated, no less "managed" than the patient-authored works of the earlier period.[29] I interrogate both, not to elicit "facts" but to explore the perspective of patients on the experience of quarantine, government policy, and their place within Japanese society. Needless to say, there is no stable subject position that can be labeled "leprosy sufferer" or "sanitarium resident"; a shared disease does not preclude different choices, views, and experiences. The critical reading of patient writings brings into sharp focus the divergent position of patients in relation to policies such as abortion and sterilization. Today the use of reproductive controls in the sanitaria has come to be understood as evidence of the state's concern for eugenics and racial purity. In contrast, I argue that many patients were deeply concerned about their biological responsibility towards their offspring and thus embraced sterilization and abortion as offering reproductive choice, something unavailable to those outside the sanitaria until the postwar era.

The concept of biological citizenship also compels new consideration of the sanitaria themselves, both as materially defined places and as spaces that allowed for new kinds of social relationships. Giorgio Agamben famously characterized "the camp" as the "biological paradigm of the modern." He argued that as modern societies made the collective bodies of people the source of wealth and political power, they began to exclude those regarded as weak or defective, a process that culminated in the Nazi concentration camps.[30] In contrast, Rose and Nova have emphasized the power of "biosociality," a term they adopt from anthropologist Paul Rabinow, to create new forms of community among those with sick or imperfect bodies. I explore the sanitaria in light of these opposing positions and argue that they were complex social sites that gave rise to divergent views on their purpose and significance. Moreover, as we shall see, patient activism in the 1950s sought not to bring an end to the sanitaria but to reform them, and many patients opposed any discussion of their dismantlement.

The sanitaria were important not only for their residents but also for those who lived beyond the walls, hedges, and gates that denoted their borders. This work explores as well the place of leprosy and quarantine in the public imagination. My title, *Kingdom of the Sick*, comes from Susan Sontag's powerful work on illness and metaphor. She wrote, "Everyone who is born holds dual citizenship, in the kingdom of the well and in the kingdom of the sick. Although we all prefer to use only the good passport, sooner or later each of us is obliged, at least for a spell, to identify ourselves as citizens of that other place."[31] The discourse that surrounded the sanitaria reveals that many in Japan did indeed identify with the "citizens of that other place," in terms that both reflected and contested contemporary social and political discourse on biological citizenship.

The Disease in Question

Bruno Latour, the sociologist of science, has provocatively declared that microbes, too, have agency and that we must consider how they interact with human beings, from the scientists who study them to those whose bodies they inhabit.[32] Although this book is primarily concerned with the human realm, we cannot ignore the role of *Mycobacterium leprae* in shaping policy in Japan and elsewhere. A bacterium of ancient origin, *M. leprae* is now believed to have originated in either East Africa or Asia and then spread around the world following paths of human migration and transported within human bodies. Its preferred mode of travel seems to be via nasal discharge or sputum, although speculation about other vehicles, including breast milk, continues. The earliest textual evidence of *M. leprae*'s clinical manifestations comes from a Sanskrit text from the sixth century BCE and Chinese works from the third century BCE, but there are Egyptian mummies more than five thousand years old that have skeletal deformities associated with its effects. In contrast, *M. leprae* arrived in the Americas only in the eighteenth century, and it did not reach Australasia and Polynesia until the 1800s.[33]

As it moved around the world, *M. leprae*'s legacy has been a number of epidemiological puzzles. Europe is a case in point. Although it was widely held that *M. leprae* was transmitted to the Mediterranean by Greek soldiers returning from Alexander the Great's invasion of India in 327 BCE, recent genetic research suggests that the strain of *M. leprae* responsible for leprosy in Europe may have originated instead in the areas that are now Iran and Turkey.[34] While clinical, or "true," leprosy, defined by the presence of *M. leprae*, was endemic in Western Europe by the thirteenth century, estimates of its prevalence vary dramatically, from 1 percent in Normandy to a tenth of that number in Britain, just across the channel.[35] There are, to be sure, a host of methodological issues involved in such estimates, but they are indicative of ongoing debates about the virulence of *M. leprae* and the ability of human hosts to resist it. Equally mysterious is the disappearance of the disease from Western Europe. One theory holds that segregation eventually controlled its spread, another that the black plague killed off those who were infected, eliminating *M. leprae* at the same time. More recently, some scientists have argued that Europeans may have developed immunity to the infection.[36]

M. leprae was discovered in 1873 by Gerhard Armauer Hansen of Norway, making it the first disease-causing bacterium to be identified. Hansen's research was driven by more than just scientific curiosity. In the mid-nineteenth century, Norway had remarkably high rates of leprosy. For the country as a whole, prevalence was 11 cases per 10,000 in 1852, but in some western districts, that figure was an astounding 700 per 10,000.[37] As a point of comparison, according to a World Health Organization (WHO) study published in 1966, the prevalence rate of leprosy in India and China, considered leprosy hot spots at the time, was 5.56 per 10,000 and 3.42 per 10,000, respectively.[38] Today the WHO considers a prevalence rate of 2 or more per 10,000 "a high burden."

Although this was the heyday of germ theory, Hansen's discovery of *M. leprae* did not settle the issue of leprosy's etiology. In fact, it raised new questions. *M. leprae* did not behave according to the newly defined rules of bacteriology. For one, it proved impossible to culture, making it difficult to investigate paths of transmission. Nor was it clear why its incubation period (up to twenty years) was so prolonged and why some people became infected while others, even those who had intimate and sustained contact with an infected person, did not. Perplexing, too, were the different ways the disease progressed. Some patients developed what became known as lepromatous leprosy, the most disabling and disfiguring form of the disease, in which *M. leprae* proliferates, causing damage to joints, bones, and internal organs and producing numerous external lesions and often significant disfigurement; others developed what is termed tuberculoid leprosy, a milder form of the disease characterized by hypopigmented anesthetic patches of skin. As a result, physicians and scientists continued to debate for decades after 1873 whether something other than *M. leprae*—an environmental factor, a parasite, heredity, or a metabolic abnormality—might be involved in the process of infection and the progress of the disease.

In the last two decades, the sequencing of both the human genome and *M. leprae* has provided some answers to the questions about leprosy's etiology and progression. We now know that *M. leprae* is capable of only limited metabolic activity, the result of a long process of reductive evolution that has rendered half of its genes dead or decayed. It is in essence an intercellular parasite that cannot exist outside a host. This explains the difficulty in culturing *M. leprae* and its slow rate of reproduction. Scientists now believe that the genetic makeup of the host plays a crucial role in determining both vulnerability to infection by *M. leprae* and the subsequent course of the disease. Genetic analysis suggests that one group of genes governs susceptibility or resistance to infection, while a second group controls the host's immune response. It is the robustness of the immune response that determines whether the infected person develops a full-blown case of lepromatous leprosy or a milder form of the disease.[39]

Of course, none of this was known to physicians, researchers, and policy makers in Japan (or elsewhere) during the period that saw the establishment and expansion of forms of quarantine worldwide. Leprosy, for them, was a poorly understood disease that was both all too common and seemingly intractable. Through the 1940s, Japanese physicians, like those around the world, relied primarily on chaulmoogra oil to treat the disease. A substance produced from the seeds of a tree in the Archariaceae family native to Southeast Asia, chaulmoogra oil was used topically, orally, and eventually intramuscularly, and with prolonged and continuing use it did reduce the symptoms of the disease in some patients.[40] But although chaulmoogra oil is now known to have antimicrobial properties, *M. leprae* proved to be remarkably resilient, and the effects of the oil declined over time. The first truly effective treatment came in the form of the two drugs known as Promin and dapsone, which were first tested in the 1940s in the US national sanitarium at Carville, Louisiana. Both were bacteriostatic in nature: that is, they did not kill *M. leprae* but stopped it from reproducing, giving the host's immune system a chance to do its work. This took time. Treatment by Promin required frequent injections for a period of as long as three or more years. Dapsone was less expensive and could be used orally, but because of its low bacteriostatic effect, it had to be taken daily for many years, and some patients, particularly those who suffered from lepromatous leprosy, required lifetime treatment to keep *M. leprae* under control. Both drugs were associated with debilitating side effects, including anemia and anorexia. Stopping treatment too early or poor adherence to the drug regime (a common problem when treatment is prolonged) led to relapse and the reappearance of symptoms and also propelled the emergence of resistant strains of *M. leprae*, which first appeared in the 1960s.[41]

Since the 1980s physicians worldwide have adopted multidrug therapy (MDT) that combines dapsone with two other drugs, rifampicin, the first bactericidal treatment for leprosy, and clofazimine, which inhibits the growth of mycobacteria. Although there are reports that strains of *M. leprae* resistant to rifampicin have developed, today even advanced cases of leprosy can generally be treated effectively within two years. The WHO's program of providing free treatment for leprosy, which began in 1995, has had a dramatic effect. Globally the prevalence of the disease has fallen below 1 per 10,000. Officially, then, leprosy has been eliminated as an international public health problem. However, in many parts of the world, *M. leprae* continues to thrive. There are about 200,000 new cases of leprosy diagnosed each year, mostly in Indonesia, India, and Brazil.[42]

Throughout this work I use the term "leprosy" rather than "Hansen's disease" in deference to its continued use in medical discourse and in the historical literature outside of Japan. It should be noted, however, that the Japanese terms for the disease, *rai* and *raibyō*, are now considered discriminatory by many, and Hansen's disease (*Hansenbyō*) is the preferred term. In this work, however, I use *rai* intentionally to distinguish premodern conceptions of the disease from clinical leprosy defined by the presence of *M. leprae*. Before the late nineteenth century, *rai* referred to an undifferentiated group of skin diseases that included but was not limited to true leprosy. I use "leper," an offensive term that reduces an individual to his or her disease, only as a translation for the terms *raisha* and *raibyōsha* as they appear in historical sources. At the risk of some awkwardness, those with the disease are referred to by terms such as "people with leprosy," "leprosy sufferers," or "leprosy patients," with the latter term reserved for instances when sufferers became the object of medical discourse, treatment, and authority. In contrast, "sanitarium residents" and "former patients" are used to capture the ambivalent social position of those who, while they have recovered from the disease, nonetheless continue to be identified with it.

Leprosy as Lens

This work is divided into three sections. Chapters 1 and 2 explore the long history of *rai* before modernity. This "prehistory" of leprosy policy is important because the understanding of the disease that made its sufferers "outcasts" in the early modern period did not simply disappear with the formation of the modern state. It continued to shape attitudes towards the disease and its sufferers for decades to come. Chapters 3 to 5 focus on the period from the 1870s to the 1910s, which saw the newly biomedically defined disease become an object of international concern, with the result that governments around the world began to create institutions of confinement. I argue that in Japan it was civic actors, such as physicians, pharmaceutical manufacturers, journalists, and foreign missionaries, who took the lead in rendering leprosy a national concern and in pushing the government to define a leprosy policy, initiating the process that led to the establishment of the first public sanitaria. Chapters 6 to 8 explore the ongoing debates about the place of leprosy sufferers in Japan's body politic in the period from the 1920s through the 1960s, a period of intense political change, war, defeat, occupation, and recovery. In this section, I am concerned with exploring the engagement of patients with state policy and their place in the debates that surrounded it.

By taking an approach that interrogates the contemporary politics of leprosy, this work seeks to complicate our understanding of the modern Japanese state and its biopolitics. While the denunciatory narrative of leprosy has portrayed the state as a unitary and powerful agent that oversaw a progressively oppressive set of policies towards leprosy sufferers (and the sick generally), *Kingdom of the Sick* exposes a different kind of state, one shaped by contesting interests, multiple and competing agendas, and lacunae of power, one in which individual politicians and bureaucrats to varying degrees were shaped by but also sought to confront the long-standing prejudice towards the disease and its sufferers. It is undeniable that Japan's approach to leprosy prevention resulted in flawed policies that harmed people in real and enduring ways. Seeking to understand how and why that happened is in no way a denial of that historical fact.

Chapter 1
The Geography of Exclusion

Rai in Premodern Japan

In a quiet neighborhood in the ancient city of Nara, about a twenty-minute walk from one of the most visited tourist sites in Japan, the temple Tōdaiji and the giant statue of the Buddha it houses, there stands another less famous historical structure on a quiet street in a residential area. Known as the Kitayama Jūhachikenko (literally "Kitayama Hall of Eighteen Rooms"), it is a long, narrow building divided into eighteen small, windowless rooms (figure 1.1). A sign posted just inside the fence that surrounds the building alerts the passerby to its significance. It relates that the hall was founded in the thirteenth century by the monk Ninshō, who established it as a hostel for leprosy sufferers on the site of what is termed a "village" called Kitayama-juku. The text of the sign concludes, "As a precursor to our country's leprosy relief efforts and as a means for thinking about human rights, it is a valuable part of our historical heritage." What the sign leaves unmentioned is that the Kitayama Hall is the only surviving material artifact of the many communities of those called *raisha* (people with *rai*) that dotted Japan well into the nineteenth century. Known by terms such as *"rai* hostels" and *"rai* villages," they became a feature of both urban and rural life in the early modern period and disappeared only with the establishment of the modern state.

This chapter explores the social exclusion of sufferers of *rai* over the course of the long premodern period. I argue that any superficial resemblance to modern quarantine facilities notwithstanding, the "huts" and "villages" in which those with *rai* lived were not established to prevent infection or to provide care for the sick and disabled. Rather, they reflected Buddhist and Confucian conceptions of immorality and its consequences, evolving ideas about status and social order, and the ideologies

19

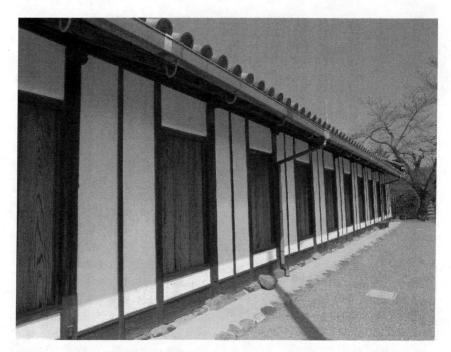

FIGURE 1.1.   The reconstructed Kitayama Hall of Eighteen Rooms, 2016. Photograph by the author.

that emanated from a succession of premodern states. In the period before modernity, *rai* was more than just a disease. Profoundly marked by social, political, and religious meanings, it stigmatized its victims but also singled them out for particular forms of charity, albeit ones that do not mesh easily with the modern conceptions of social welfare or philanthropy.

Karma, Pollution, and Sites of Exclusion

The Japanese term *rai* derives from the Chinese *lai* and was introduced to Japan as texts and technology from the continent began to flow to the archipelago in the mid-part of the first millennium CE. We find it in some of the earliest Japanese texts, including the early eighth-century *Chronicles of Japan* (*Nihon shoki*), where it is used in reference to a migrant from the Korean peninsula, and the ninth-century legal commentary *Ryōgige*, where it names a disease that disqualifies one from assuming the role of family headship. But the limited and fragmented textual record that survives makes it impossible to know whether *rai* renamed a disease category already recognized, propelled a new understanding of a familiar set of symptoms, or described a new disease that was unknown before this time.

Six centuries later the meanings attached to *rai* begin to come into sharper focus. Among the more than one thousand stories that make up the collection *Konjaku monogatari* (Tales of Times Now Past, ca. late twelfth–early thirteen century) there are several in which *rai* figures centrally. One appears in a section of the text called "Buddhist Law in this Kingdom," a title that illuminates the thematic thread that organizes the *Konjaku monogatari*, that is, the tracing of the influence of Buddhism as it was transferred from India to China and Japan. The story in question tells of a monk named Shinkai who served the provincial governor of Minō. The governor was a minor member of the nobility, and this relationship gave Shinkai an inflated sense of his own importance. As a result, when another priest was given the honor of performing a religious ritual at the famous temple complex on Mount Hiei, a resentful Shinkai disrupted the ceremony in a fit of pique at the perceived slight. Not long after, he became ill with *rai*, a development that is explained as the result of "karmic retribution in this present life" for his sin of envy. According to the narrator of the tale, with the appearance of the disease, "even his old nurse who had vowed to be a parent to him thought him unclean (*kegare*) and would not let him come near. With nowhere else to go, he took refuge in a hut among the beggars at Kiyomizu at the foot of the slope. Even there, among the crippled and deformed (*katawamono*), he was held in abomination; and after three months he died."[1]

The simple parable, all of six pages in the heavily annotated modern edition of the *Konjaku monogatari*, is a window into how *rai* was understood in the environs of the imperial capital at the end of the twelfth century.[2] The disease was the result of the workings of karma, a punishment for those who went against Buddhist law. Its sufferers were considered "polluted" (*kegare, fujō*) and were rejected even by their closest kin. They took refuge along the sloping path that led to Kiyomizu Temple, among other marginalized people. What the story leaves unexplained is how and why this understanding of the disease and the forms of exclusion that accompanied it emerged.

To interrogate the story, we can begin with the problem of pollution. Although the concept of pollution—the result of contact with the dead, the sick, and bodily fluids—had long been a concern within indigenous ritual practices, it became the object of intense anxiety in the imperial capital of Kyoto beginning in the eleventh century. This concern for pollution was new. Scrutiny of the family registers suggests that until the tenth century, the sick and dying were not abandoned but continued to reside at home, and in some cases sufferers of *rai* even held the family headship, although the legal codes issued by the newly formed imperial state in the seventh century explicitly forbade this.[3] As fear of pollution grew, families stopped burying their dead close to home and instead dispatched them to newly designated sites on the periphery of the capital. Similarly, the execution grounds and the officially funded hospices (*hiden'in*) for the sick were removed from the center of the capital.[4]

Concern for pollution coincided with another development, the appearance of people designated as *hinin*, a term that literally means "nonhuman" but is generally translated as "outcast" in the English language historiography. By the fourteenth century, a variety of groups and individuals were designated as *hinin*, including some kinds of entertainers, gardeners, well diggers, fishermen, roof thatchers, and leatherworkers.[5] However, the term originally seems to have been applied more narrowly to those who removed human corpses and animal carcasses from the streets and homes of Kyoto and those who survived by begging. The origin of the *hinin* has long been one of the most contested issues in the historiography of medieval Japan, the object of ongoing research since the late nineteenth century. One theory was that these people were the descendants of the "base" (*sen*), or unfree, people created by laws of the seventh-century state; another held that their ancestors were migrants from the continent or members of minority ethnic groups on the archipelago. Historians in the 1970s and 1980s, however, rejected these theories, which sought an explanation for discrimination in the "difference" of those who were its object, and asserted instead that *hinin* were the product of the medieval social order itself.

Amino Yoshihiko was one of the first historians to argue that *hinin* emerged in relation to the concern about pollution in the capital. He characterized them as professional "purifiers" (*kiyome*), who served the major religious institutions, and argued that they were regarded with respect because they performed the crucial social work of purification.[6] Other scholars disagreed. Kuroda Toshio described the *hinin* as those who were "outside of status." That is, a "nonhuman" was someone without ties to the institutions that conveyed "personhood," the imperial state, the aristocratic nobility, and Buddhist and Shinto institutions. Described as "freakish and aberrant" in medieval sources, *hinin* were people who did not engage in agrarian work and thus did not pay the taxes or rents that supported these great landholding institutions and families. Kuroda asserted that those who did the stigmatized work of dealing with pollution did so because they were already marginalized in relation to this conception of "personhood." He noted as well that for the medieval people of the capital, the image of the *hinin* was not that of a "purifier" but of a sufferer of *rai* begging on the streets.[7]

Neither Amino nor Kuroda addressed the heightened concern for pollution that produced the need for "purifiers," so Niunoya Tetsuichi broke new ground when he demonstrated that the imperial court actively fostered concern about pollution, deploying a new "pollution ideology" to maintain its authority over the people and space of the capital. Fear of pollution was cultivated primarily through the actions of the capital police force, known as the *kebiishi*, who patrolled the center of the capital looking for evidence of pollution on temple and shrine grounds and in the vicinity of the palace. When they found it, they would compel the removal of its source, by ordering the disposing of corpses and the transfer of the sick and dying from the center of the city. When religious rites or festivals occurred, they ordered that signs be posted on the streets, warning those in a state of pollution, such as menstruating women, not to pass near the sacred site. And when someone was rumored to have breached the taboos regarding pollution, they investigated and sometimes punished the transgressor.[8]

A crucial aspect of the new "pollution ideology" was the assertion that it was the emperor who safeguarded the capital and its residents through his performance of and support for rituals of purification and expiation. A case in point was the Great Purification Ceremony, one of the most important imperial rites. It had originally been a semiannual observance, but in the medieval period it began to be performed whenever pollution was thought to have intruded on the sacred space of the palace. As Thomas Kierstead has noted, "Pollution emerged as a special, political principle as the medieval court defined itself."[9] It was in relation to this new political principle that sufferers of *rai* began to be expelled by their families and the organized *hinin* groups took form. These were under the control of a "boss" (*chōri*) who, while a *hinin* himself, was also a subordinate of the *kebiishi* and religious institutions.

A 1275 document, authored by a priest called Eison (also known as Eizon, 1201–1290) and addressed to a *hinin* boss in Kyoto, describes the process by which sufferers of *rai* became *hinin*:

> When someone who has contracted *rai* is to be taken [into the group], the messenger [of the *hinin* boss] who is sent to explain the details must convince that person and others, such as the members of his household. Since

in the case of this serious disease, in the end you cannot allow the afflicted person to continue living at home, he should agree to come, but do not be too persistent. And if he will not agree, then he must make a settlement and thereafter you must stop bothering him. You must stop those who go against this principle and try to gain an excessive amount by sending many *hinin* to make recriminations and cast insult upon the family.[10]

As this suggests, the belief that sufferers of *rai* should join the ranks of the *hinin* seems to have been taken for granted by this time. Eison's concern was the use of threats and extortion to achieve this, and thus he used his moral authority to urge the *hinin* boss to wait until the afflicted person and his family had resigned themselves to this fate. Elsewhere in this document, Eison also acknowledged the right of the *hinin* to seize *rai* sufferers who were begging on the streets—but only in the central part of the city, the symbolically charged area where the palace and the mansions of the nobility lay. Those found in the "upper and lower neighborhoods" could be left alone.[11]

The story of Shinkai reveals a second important aspect of the medieval conception of *rai*, the fusion of concern for pollution with another new idea, that illness was the consequence of one's own bad acts. In his seminal 1975 essay, the historian Yokoi Kiyoshi argued that the growing cultural influence of the Buddhist concept of karma was "the mechanism of discrimination" (*sabetsu no shikumi*) that propelled the identification of *rai* with wrongdoing and retribution.[12] Buddhism had been introduced from the continent to the archipelago as early as the third century CE, and the imperial state later embraced it, with the result that members of the imperial family and the aristocracy filled the ranks of the clergy and became patrons of temples, monasteries, and convents. Even so, the influence of Buddhism outside of elite circles was muted until the aftermath of the devastating civil conflict known as the Gempei War of 1180–1185, which resulted in the death of the emperor and the systematic extinguishment by the victors of one of the most powerful noble families in the land. The conflict ushered in the new political and economic power of the warriors and brought considerable suffering to ordinary people. Yokoi suggests that in this time of turmoil the concept of karma found a newly receptive audience, because it provided a way to make sense of the new divisions of wealth and power and the changing fortunes of the powerful.[13]

In the new Buddhism of this period, the Lotus Sutra (Skt. *Saddharma puṇḍarīka sūtra*; J. *Myōhō renge kyō*) became an object of particular and intense veneration. It had long had an important place within the esoteric (and monastic) Tendai sect, but now new faith-based sects, like that founded by the priest Nichiren (1222–1282), and practice-based sects like Zen valorized it as well. Many sutras of Indian origin expressed the idea that illness resulted from karmic retribution for bad acts, but the Lotus Sutra advanced a particularly powerful claim: *rai* was a form of karmic retribution that occurred in this life, offering immediate bodily and therefore visible evidence of the consequence of wrongdoing.[14] Those who read, chanted, or listened to sermons on the Lotus Sutra would have heard several descriptions of the horrors of *rai*. Typical was this one, which described the fate of anyone who attacks a faithful Buddhist: "In existence after existence, he will have teeth that are missing or spaced far apart, ugly lips, a flat nose, hands and feet that are gnarled or deformed, and eyes that are squinty. His body will have a foul odor, with evil sores that run puss and blood."[15]

The documents known as *kishōmon* offer evidence of the influence that the concept of *rai* as karmic retribution came to exercise at every level of medieval society. *Kishōmon* were written to record an oath, a pledge, or a contract and were utilized to formalize a wide range of agreements, economic and other, as well as to validate claims of truthfulness in relation to charges of criminal acts. Typically, they have two distinct sections. The first relates the promise to perform or refrain from some act or a pledge of truthfulness or loyalty, while the latter puts forth the punishment that will result if the signatory breaks his promise or his pledge. Punishments cited included the wrath of the deities as well as poverty, death, and descent into hell, but most often *rai*, which by the early fourteenth century had come to be evoked in the majority of *kishōmon*.[16]

An example of the use of *rai* in *kishōmon* is the oath offered by the warrior Kikuchi Takemochi to the emperor Go-Daigo in the aftermath of the latter's abortive effort to reestablish imperial authority, an event known as the Kemmu Restoration. Composed in 1338, this document elaborated on Kikuchi's vow of loyalty to the imperial institution and ended with the words "If I should break this pledge, . . . let me suffer from white *rai* and black *rai* in this life and be denied the grace of Buddhist law for seven incarnations."[17] The terms "white *rai*" and "black *rai*," which appear in the Lotus Sutra, would be used throughout the premodern period and were something of a stock phrase in *kishōmon*. The former term referred to an illness characterized primarily by patches of depigmented skin, and the latter to one marked by the proliferation of deep purplish lesions. In the second half of the sixteenth century, *kishōmon* were written to record the oaths of fealty extracted from vassals by new regional warlords. In 1566, for example, a warrior named Saigusa Shūjirō pledged that no matter what kind of reward he was offered, he would not plot against the warlord Takeda Shingen. The pledge ended with the words "If there is an untruthfulness in this oath, let me incur the wrath [of the gods], be struck down with *rai*, and dwell in hell for all eternity."[18]

Although the use of *kishōmon* declined after 1600, there is some evidence of their use, with the usual threat of punishment by *rai*, into the seventeenth century. Suzuki Shōsan's *Tales of Karmic Justice* (*Inga monogatari*, pub. 1661) is a case in point. Suzuki was a Zen priest, and *Tales of Karmic Justice* is a collection of stories that reveal the working of karma in everyday life. Filled with stories of the strange and nefarious and illustrated with images showing the unhappy fate that awaited wrongdoers, it proved immensely popular. One of Suzuki's stories concerned several villages in the province of Ōmi that were locked in a dispute over their boundaries in 1648. Unable to reconcile their positions, the representatives of the villages decided to write a *kishōmon* in which each swore to the accuracy of their community's position. This document concluded with the statement that *rai* would be the punishment for bad faith. According to Suzuki, the following year every member of one of the villages was struck down with *rai*, clear evidence that this village had provided false evidence.[19] While this story is surely apocryphal, it suggests both the longevity of the concept of "karmic retribution disease" and its utility in social life.

Together with pollution and karmic retribution, the third important element of the story of Shinkai was the reference to the sloping path that led to Kiyomizu Temple, where he found refuge among the beggars and disabled. That Shinkai ended up at Kiyomizu-zaka, as this path was known, was not a random occurrence. Kiyomizu-zaka was the location of a *shuku* (literally "lodging"), the name given to the sites of organized communities of *hinin*. According to thirteenth-century sources, there were thirteen *shuku* in the two provinces of Yamato and Yamashiro and together they may have housed several thousand people. Seven were in Yamato, where the old imperial capital of Nara was located, and six in Yamashiro, where Kyoto was located. The two most important *shuku* were at Kiyomizu-zaka and Nara-zaka, and they seem to have exercised some degree of authority over the others.[20] The sign that stands outside of the Kitayama Hall today notes that it was established on the site of Kitayama-juku (*juku* is the same word as *shuku*, pronounced differently as a result of consonant mutation), but it terms this simply a "village," concealing its relationship with those called *hinin*.

The formation of the *shuku* at Kiyomizu-zaka and Nara-zaka is a window into the social geography of exclusion that emerged in relation to the "pollution ideology." Established in 778, Kiyomizu Temple was located halfway up Mount Otowa and well outside the densely inhabited parts of the capital until the 1600s, when the growing city expanded to the foothills. The path known as Kiyomizu-zaka was, however, well traveled by the eleventh century, when the temple became a popular pilgrimage site for nobles in the capital, who came to worship at its statue of the Bodhisattva Kannon. There was an economic logic at work in the formation of the *shuku* here. The many pilgrims traveling to Kiyomizu Temple would have been a reliable source of alms for beggars.

Begging was, however, not the only means of support for those who gathered at Kiyomizu-zaka, and the formation of the *shuku* here reflected more than simple economic expediency. The path that followed the incline of Kiyomizu-zaka led not only to the temple but also to the area known as Toribeno, one of three sites outside the city proper where the dead of the capital were discarded (figure 1.2). Today, Toribeno looks like a typical Japanese cemetery with many closely packed tombs decorated by flowers, cups of sake, and wooden memorial boards, but in the medieval period it would have presented a very different sight. Then, it functioned primarily as a charnel ground, where corpses were often simply discarded to decay, although those of the wealthy might be buried or cremated. The *shuku* was located nearby for a reason: when someone died within the city, the *hinin* at Kiyomizu-zaka were called upon to transfer the corpse to Toribeno. Thus, Kiyomizu-zaka was a liminal space that lay between the sacred grounds of the temple and the polluted realm of Toribeno, the world of the dead and the world of the living, the release of salvation and the cycle of rebirths, and the *hinin* who inhabited this space traversed the divide between pollution and purity, life and death.[21]

Nara-zaka was similarly placed, situated just outside the old imperial capital of Nara, a city by this time given over to powerful temple and shrine complexes.[22] It, too, was a sloping path, a topographical indication of liminality, and like the community at Kiyomizu-zaka, the *hinin* here were responsible for removing pollution from the sacred sites in the city, a task that included disposing of the carcasses of the sacred deer that, then as now, wander the grounds of the Kasuga Shrine. Part of a road that stretched from the old to the new capital, Nara-zaka, too, thronged with people and thus was well situated to facilitate the collection of alms. Finally, like their counterparts in Kyoto, the *hinin* at Nara-zaka sometimes adopted aggressive tactics to bring *rai* sufferers into their ranks. For example, in 1473, when a high-ranking priest at the temple Kōfukuji in Nara developed *rai*, the *hinin* gathered outside the temple and pressed for his removal, prompting him to flee to the monastic establishment at Mount Kōya, ninety kilometers away, to escape them.[23]

The Economy of Salvation

The flight of this priest and the evidence that some sufferers of *rai* in Kyoto chose to pay off the *hinin* boss rather than join the *shuku* suggest that the symptoms of *rai* did not automatically or immediately render one a *hinin*. Was it only those who lacked financial resources or connections to the powerful who suffered this fate, or was it perhaps only those whose condition was so advanced as to be disabling? These questions cannot be answered, but what is clear is that sufferers of *rai* came to be embedded in an economy of salvation that required their visibility. The famous medieval legend of the eighth-century empress Kōmyō expresses the principle at the center of this economy. According to the version of the story included in an early fourteenth-century collection of biographies of iconic Buddhists, one day Kōmyō offered to personally bathe one thousand people, a pledge that reflects the medieval practice of opening medicinal baths on temple grounds. This was not an act of charity in the modern sense of that term. It was instead a merit-making activity intended to reduce the karmic burden of its sponsor. According to the story, the thousandth person who presented himself to the empress was a sufferer of *rai* whose body was covered with open oozing sores. The empress hesitated for a moment but then proceeded to wash him with care and even used her mouth to suck pus from the lesions

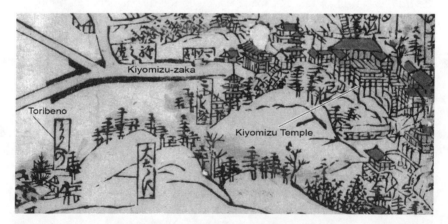

FIGURE 1.2.   The environs of Kiyomizu Temple. Detail from *Shinpan Heianjo tōzai nanboku machi narabi ni rakugai no zu*, 1654. University of British Columbia Library.

on his body. When she was finished, the *rai* sufferer emanated a bright light and was revealed to be the Bodhisattva Ashuku.[24]

Stories such as this one reveal the ambivalence that surrounded the sufferers of *rai* in medieval culture. Although they were regarded as marked by the physical manifestation of their own misdeeds, those afflicted by *rai* were not just the object of fear, disdain, or pity. They were also regarded as a particularly potent means to gain merit and thereby to improve one's own chance of salvation. It is this understanding of the sufferer of *rai* that motivated the priest Eison and his follower Ninshō (1217–1303) to become involved with the various *shuku* in the Kinai region. Both men were leading figures in the so-called Ritsu, or Precepts, sect of Shingon Buddhism, which promoted the revival of monastic discipline in an age when new faith-based sects were gaining popularity among laypeople. Eison and his disciples venerated the Mañjúsrī (J. Monju) Bodhisattva, who was said to have taken a vow to aid the poor, disabled, and sick. Reverence for Mañjúsrī inspired them to undertake what Janet Goodwin has somewhat misleadingly described as "charity and public service," building shelters and distributing food to the poor, the disabled, abandoned children, and the elderly, preaching against the killing of animals, and praying for Japan's deliverance from Mongol invaders, activities that won them the support of both courtiers and powerful warriors.[25]

Eison and Ninshō's involvement with the *hinin shuku* began in the 1240s and continued for four decades. Towards the end of this period, the rites they organized were attracting huge crowds of *hinin*. One held at Kiyomizu-zaka in 1275 is said to have been attended by 3,335 *hinin*, while another held in Yamato Province in 1282 reportedly had more than 1,700 participants. The former event took place after the boss of the *shuku* agreed to sign the document composed by Eison that was quoted earlier, in which he criticized the forcible removal of *rai* sufferers from their homes and other similar acts.[26] It seems then that Eison used the promise to perform religious rites to extract concessions from the *hinin* boss, perhaps at the behest of elites within the city who were alarmed by behavior they considered overly aggressive.

Eison and Ninshō's sponsorship of such events and their establishment of Kitayama Hall at Nara-zaka and similar institutions at Kamakura and elsewhere must be understood in light of this economy of salvation.[27] Although some have characterized the religious rites they held, which included the distribution of food and other goods, as charitable in nature and the hostels as precursors to the modern institutions such as the hospital, hospice, and sanitarium, this framing is problematic.[28] The primary purpose of both the religious rites and the hostels was not to provide care for the *hinin* but rather to encourage them to engage in penitence and prayer, with the hope that this would facilitate both their salvation and that of their benefactors.[29] A famous story about Ninshō's work at the Kitayama Hall provides evidence of his aims. Recorded in *Genkō shakusho*, a fourteenth-century history of Buddhism, it relates that when a man with *rai* became so infirm that he could no longer walk to the road to beg for alms, Ninshō began to carry him there each morning, returning to retrieve him each evening. Needless to say, the point of this exercise was not to aid the *rai* sufferer. Rather, by positioning him in a public site, Ninshō made the afflicted person into a visible display of the workings of karma in order to encourage reflection on the part of others.[30]

The concern for visibility explains the characteristic clothing worn by people with *rai*, specifically "persimmon-colored" robes of a distinctive yellowish brown and white headcloths wrapped to conceal their faces.[31] The persimmon-colored robe figures prominently in a story from the handscroll *The Illustrated History of Ishiyama Temple* (*Ishiyamadera engi ekotoba*), a collection of miraculous stories about the temple. It tells of the daughter of a wealthy man from Ise who developed a terrible case of *rai*. In desperation, her father took her to the temple to pray for forgiveness. While sleeping there, he had a dream in which an elderly monk appeared and instructed him to tell his daughter to discard her persimmon-colored robe. When he awoke and did as he was told, the daughter was miraculously healed.[32] There is other evidence as well. Kuroda Hideo, the medieval historian who pioneered the use of visual sources, points to the thirteenth-century handscroll on the life of the itinerant priest Ippen (1234–1289), who like Eison and Ninshō became well known for his charitable work among the *hinin*. Known as the *Illustrated Biography of the Priest Ippen* (*Ippen shōnin eden*), it includes several depictions of religious ceremonies in which Ippen participated. Figure 1.3 is a detail from one such scene. It shows *rai* sufferers, clothed in orange-brown robes and with their faces concealed by white headcloths, among other *hinin*, including some who are disabled.[33]

Religious art continued to "display" *rai* sufferers even into the sixteenth century. *The Mandala of a Pilgrimage to Yasaka Hōkanji Stupa* (*Yasaka Hōkanji tō sankei mandara*) depicts a beggar, his face marked by the distinctive red blotches that became part of the iconography of *rai*, sitting near the entrance to Kiyomizu-zaka, begging bowl in hand, as a pilgrim passes by (figure 1.4).[34] In images like this one, sufferers of *rai* were depicted as part of the sacred landscape of the temple environs and the

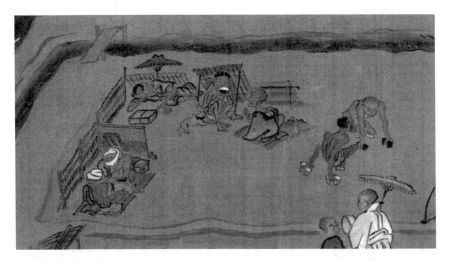

FIGURE 1.3.   *Rai* sufferers and other *hinin*. Detail from *Ippen shōnin eden*, Tokyo National Museum. Reproduced from Komatsu Shigemi, ed., *Nihon no emaki*, vol. 20, *Ippen shōnin eden* (Tokyo: Heibonsha, 1988), 196.

journey towards salvation. Writing on medieval Europe, Caroline Walker Bynum noted, "There is something profoundly alien to modern sensibilities about the role of [the] body in medieval piety."[35] Her statement holds true for attempts to understand Buddhist piety in medieval Japan as well. The body of the *rai* sufferer was simultaneously the object of both reverence and fear, a corporal embodiment of pollution, the power of karma, and the possibility of salvation.

Rai and the Geography of Status in Early Modern Japan

The conception of *rai* as the "bad karma disease" proved to be remarkably durable, as did the relegation of many of its sufferers to begging communities. This arrangement caught the attention of the Portuguese missionaries who arrived in Japan in the late sixteenth century. In the dictionary they compiled and published in Nagasaki in 1603–1604, known as *Nippo jiten* (Vocabulário da Língua do Japão; Japanese-Portuguese Dictionary), *kojiki* (romanized as *cojiqi*), a word that later came to mean "beggar," is explained as "a person with leprosy," while *chōri*, or "boss," is defined as "the person who has the right to control those who suffer from leprosy."[36] But as the new state headed by the Tokugawa shoguns took form in the seventeenth century, *rai* sufferers came to be reconceptualized within the

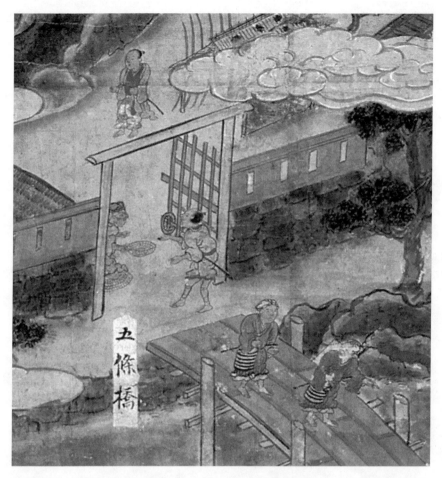

FIGURE 1.4.   A *rai* sufferer begging at the entrance to Kiyomizu-zaka. Detail from *Yasaka Hōkanji tō sankei mandara*, Hōkanji Temple. Reproduced from Osaka Shiritsu Hakubutsu-kan, ed., *Shaji sankei mandara* (Tokyo: Heibonsha, 1986), plate 32.

emergent early modern system of status. They were newly understood as part of a larger status group comprised of so-called base people (*senmin*), a heterogeneous mix of marginalized social groups that constituted one of the major status categories of this period, together with "villager," "war-rior," "townsperson," "noble," and "cleric." In contrast to the medieval era, conceptions of status were now institutionalized via laws and administra-tive procedures and policed by local, domainal, and shogunal authorities, making status, in the words of historian David Howell, the "universal con-struct" that bound people together in a new form of political community.[37]

Of the many kinds of "base people," the largest groups were those described as *eta* and *hinin*, although there was a great deal of local variation in the work they performed and their rights and duties. Generally, the *eta* were involved in various kinds of stigmatized work, which included not only slaughtering animals and working with leather but also official duties performed under the authority of samurai officials, such as the execution of criminals and the policing of festivals, markets, and highways. The term *hinin* survived into the early modern period, but it now referred to groups of officially recognized beggars, who were allowed to collect alms on specific occasions, although they, too, could be called upon to perform official tasks, such as carrying out fire watches and disposing of animal carcasses. While *eta* status was generally determined by birth, one could become a *hinin*. It was one form of punishment in the Tokugawa system of justice, and as we shall see, sickness and disability too could lead to this status.

There were many other kinds of "base people" as well, including certain kinds of mendicant priests and performers, graveyard workers, sandal makers, and in some localities, midwives. The prostitutes in the celebrated "pleasure quarters" of the early modern cities too were considered "base"— but only for the term of their indentures. Some of those termed "base" were itinerant, and this may have been one of the reasons they were marginalized. Officials in this period had an intense suspicion of those not rooted to a particular place and developed multiple bureaucratic procedures designed to hinder the movement of the populace. People belonging to base groups were often relegated to specific sites: so-called *eta* villages typically stood adjacent to (and under the control of) officially recognized communities of those with "villager" status. In spite of the legal abolition of the status system in 1871, this kind of spatial segregation continued and the former outcast communities came to be known generically as *buraku* (literally "hamlets"), and those who lived within them as "*buraku* people," designations that allowed social discrimination to continue, even up to the present.

The recognition that sufferers of *rai* were regarded as a distinctive status group marked as "base" came in the late 1950s when Kobayashi Keiichirō (1919–2009), a historian of the Tokugawa period with a strong interest in local history, began to explore the history of Zenkōji, an important and influential Buddhist temple in Nagano that gave rise to a thriving "temple town," with many inns, eateries, and amusements that catered to pilgrims. While examining documents in the temple archive, he discovered materials that described the activities of "people with *rai*" (*raisha*) on temple grounds.[38] In an article published in 1958, Kobayashi described the relationship between the temple and the *rai* sufferers: in addition to being allowed to collect dues (*ichiyaku*) from those who sold their goods at temple markets, members of what Kobayashi described as a "*raisha buraku*" were also allowed to beg within the confines of the temple. In return, they had the responsibility of caring for those who fell ill on temple grounds and for disposing of the bodies of those who died there.[39]

Kobayashi's research initially attracted little attention outside the then relatively small circle of historians working within the new historical subfield called *buraku* history, which focused on the early modern "base people." In 1967, he published a revised version of his previous work that introduced both documentary and oral history evidence to describe the *raisha buraku*, and two years later a slightly revised version of this article was included as one chapter in Kobayashi's massive eight-hundred-page study of Zenkōji.[40] Then in 1980, twelve years after the publication of this book and twenty-two years after the publication of the original article, Kobayashi became the object of a campaign by the members of the Nagano city chapter of the Buraku Liberation League, a national organization founded to address the ongoing social discrimination against *buraku* people that was well known for its militancy. They charged him with "preserving and abetting" discrimination and eventually took their case to the Nagano Prefectural Board of Education, which responded by ordering libraries and schools in the prefecture to remove Kobayashi's book from open shelves and to allow patrons access only after a registration process.[41]

The campaign by the Buraku Liberation League focused on a single line that summarized the organization of the "base people" of Zenkōji. It stated, "In the town of Zenkōji, [these] groups were of the following types: 1) *eta* 2) *hinin* 3) *raisha*."[42] The Buraku Liberation League charged that Kobayashi conflated *raisha* with the *eta* and *hinin* and thus encouraged discrimination against its constituents. According to the editor of the monthly newsletter *Buraku Education* (*Buraku kyōiku*), "It is really terrible that he has said that people with leprosy were among the roots of the discriminated *buraku*," and Kobayashi would later recall that in his initial meeting with members of the editorial board of *Buraku Education* one of them berated him in similar terms, stating that it was "outrageous" that he included leprosy sufferers among the other "outcasts."[43] In response to the league's protest, the Nagano Prefectural Board of Education eventually released a public statement that "there were no *raisha* among the ancestors of the [people of the] *buraku* of today."[44]

The controversy over Kobayashi's work reveals the profound discrimination that leprosy sufferers faced even in 1980—and even at the hands of members of the Buraku Liberation League, whose supposed mission was social justice. Ironically, Kobayashi, who was labeled a bigot and had his work censored, was one of the few who recognized the irony of the league's position. Referencing its famous slogan, he wrote that its desire to dissociate "*buraku* people" from leprosy sufferers "departed greatly from the stance that 'no form of discrimination is permissible.'"[45] But the campaign is significant as well for its impact on scholarship. Academic historians and others quickly stepped forward to denounce the campaign against Kobayashi as an attack on intellectual freedom, and they defended his work as an empirically based examination of past forms of discrimination. Nonetheless, this event had a chilling effect on further research on *rai* and status. Even as the disease became an important topic within the historiography of medieval Japan, there was no similar trend among historians of the early modern period.

It was not until 1991 that the new research on *rai* in the early modern period finally appeared, when Yokota Noriko, a young historian who later became well known for her work on the social history of medicine, published a carefully researched study of a "*raisha* village" in Kyoto in an influential historical journal.[46] She was careful, however, to distance herself from the controversy that surrounded Kobayashi's work on Zenkōji. He is relegated to a footnote, and while she notes that the medievalists had taken up leprosy as a problem of outcast status, she defines her goal in carefully delimited terms, stating that "for the present, it is essential to clarify the real conditions of early modern *raisha*."[47]

Its carefully couched language notwithstanding, Yokota's work is important. She demonstrates that between the mid-sixteenth and early seventeenth centuries, the *shuku* at Kiyomizu-zaka disappeared and a community of *rai* sufferers came to be based in a location situated between the Kamo River and Kenninji, an important Zen temple. The relationship between the two communities is unclear, but aspects of the new location are intriguing. Seventeenth-century maps of Kyoto suggest that the new "village," as it was called, was located near a crematorium.[48] Although there is no evidence that its members engaged in funerary work, the association of *rai* with death seemed to have been maintained into the early modern period. In other ways, the new site differed from the medieval *shuku*. The latter had housed the sufferers of *rai*, but it had not confined them. Instead, they had spilled out into the streets, roads, and temple grounds. In contrast, at some point the "village," which came to be associated with a temple called Seienji in the eighteenth century, was surrounded by a deep ditch.[49] The point was not to limit the movement of the residents. Rather, the "moat" was one of the new material signs of demarcation associated with communities of "base people" in this period. The so-called pleasure quarters, where licensed brothels were located in Japan's major cities, too were surrounded by ditches and walls, as were the villages of leather workers in and around Kyoto and Osaka.[50]

In the twenty-five years since the publication of Yokota's work, studies of *rai* communities have gradually appeared, most authored by historians carrying out delimited local studies on marginal status that avoid any engagement with the contemporary politics of leprosy. This research includes studies of Hirosaki (now southwest Aomori Prefecture), Yonezawa (now southern Yamagata Prefecture), Miharu (now the southern part of Fukushima Prefecture), Sendai (present-day Miyagi Prefecture), and Aizu (now the western part of Fukushima Prefecture) in the Tōhoku region; Matsushiro (now part of Nagano Prefecture) in central Honshū; Kagoshima and Takanabe on the island of Kyūshū; and Takamatsu on Shikoku, as well as the communities at Nara and Kyoto. Taken together, they reveal that in the early modern period the equation of *rai* with "baseness" and the exclusion of those afflicted was a "national" phenomenon.

These communities took different forms and were known by different names. Like the *raisha* village in Kyoto, some clearly had their origins in the medieval *shuku*. A case in point is the community at Nara-zaka, which survived the upheavals of the sixteenth century, although the Kitayama Hall was destroyed in a fire in 1567. Sometime between 1661 and 1673, the hall was rebuilt in a new location, albeit one not far from the original site. The reconstruction was apparently carried out with funds from Kōfukuji, an influential temple in Nara that was given authority over the *hinin* of Nara by the Tokugawa shogunate, which in turn granted it a yearly stipend of twenty-one thousand *koku* of rice, an amount on par with the annual stipend of a minor shogunal vassal.[51] The new location shows intriguing similarities to the spatial arrangement of the "village" in Kyoto. In the many "picture maps" (*ezu*) of Nara produced over the course of the eighteenth and nineteenth centuries for tourists, the hall is depicted as a long one-story structure that bears a striking resemblance to the Kitayama Hall today.[52] On the maps, the building was labeled in various ways including "*raisha*," "Kitayama," "eighteen-room hall," and often "Ashuku Temple," evoking the famous legend of Empress Kōmyō. Significantly, in several maps, including *Nanto machijūki* (1837) and *Washū Nara no ezu* (1844), the hall stands adjacent to a crematorium, more evidence that the association of *rai* sufferers with funerary work persisted long into the early modern period (figure 1.5).[53]

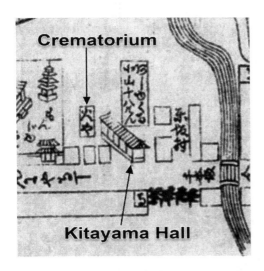

FIGURE 1.5. The Kitayama Hall in a tourist map of Nara. Detail from *Washū Nara no ezu*, 1844. Nara Prefectural Library and Information Center.

Another medieval *shuku* that became a *raisha* village in the early modern period was located southwest of the city of Nara, less than nine kilometers from Nara-zaka. Known as Nishiyama ("western mountain," in contrast to Kitayama, "northern mountain") it was one of the seven *shuku* in Yamato at the end of the thirteenth century. At some point, the community came under the authority of the temple Yakushiji, and the *rai* sufferers were housed in a subtemple known as Kōmyōin, obviously named in homage to Empress Kōmyō. However, in the early Tokugawa period, a new arrangement took form. The shogunate gave control over this area to one of its vassals, and cadastral records for Kōriyama domain, as it was known, reveal that Rokujo village, which had a population of 418 people, had authority over an outcast hamlet consisting of five households and twenty-five people. This outcast hamlet included among its members the *rai* sufferers who were housed in the Kōmyōin.[54]

The arrangement at Rokujo village, where *rai* sufferers were placed under the authority of other "base people," was replicated elsewhere in Japan. In many places, those afflicted with the disease were housed in officially authorized hostels known as *raisha* huts reflecting an approach taken towards others with *hinin* status, who were required to dwell in what were known as "*hinin* huts" (*hinin koya*). Miharu, for example, had four *raisha* hostels in place by 1689, although they housed only about twenty people in total. Located outside the castle town, the hostels were under the authority of the *eta* headman, an indication of the hierarchy of status that functioned even among those deemed "base." The situation in neighboring Aizu and Sendai was similar, although in these domains the *raisha* huts were established within the castle towns in the so-called *eta* wards (*eta chō*; *kawahara chō*), areas of the town reserved for "base" people. In a nineteenth-century map of Wakamatsu, the castle town of the Aizu lord, the *raisha* hut is located immediately adjacent to the *eta* ward.[55] These arrangements reflect the typical organization of early modern towns, where the spatial order reflected status distinctions.

Outside the castle towns, communities of *rai* sufferers were typically organized into "villages." In Kagoshima and Takanabe on the island of Kyūshū, distinctive villages that were associated with those identified as suffering from *seirai* (literally "green *rai*," a term of unclear origin and meaning), were in place by the early seventeenth century.[56] A similar arrangement existed in Kaga, where each district seems to have had at least one designated *raisha* village.[57] In Takamatsu, a specific village located near the castle town was designated for "*raisha* containment" (*raijin azukari*).[58] The emergence of these kinds of sites is not the only evidence that *raisha* had become a distinctive form of base status. Tokugawa policy required temples to maintain registries of their parishioners (*shūmon ninbetsu aratame chō*) that recorded basic demographic information on each household unit. In domains as regionally diverse as Miharu, Takamatsu, and Kagoshima, *raisha* were removed from the ordinary registries and listed within special registries of base people, with *raisha* designated as their status.[59]

As David Howell has noted, status in early modern Japan was required to be visible, and so, unsurprisingly, many domains had rules governing the appearance of people with *rai*.[60] In Miharu in the early seventeenth century, sufferers of *rai* were ordered not only to wear a wooden tag engraved with the character *hi* (for *hinin*) but also to shave their heads as a mark of their low status, and they were explicitly forbidden from wearing a headcloth to hide their shaved heads. In 1646, the residents of the *raisha* huts responded with a petition to domainal officials arguing that it was unreasonable to force them to adopt a hairstyle otherwise reserved for criminals and prisoners, which invited abuse at the hands of commoners (*heimin*). They cited the requirements of neighboring domains as examples of reasonable practice. In Sōma, *raisha* were required to shave their hair but were not prohibited from then covering their heads, while in eight other nearby domains, they were required only to adopt a specific hairstyle, that known as *chasen-gami*, a short ponytail worn high on the head. In response,

Miharu authorities agreed to make *chasen-gami* the required hairstyle, but they continued to forbid the use of concealing headcloths.[61]

Whether they lived in huts or villages, the organized communities of *rai* sufferers had specific begging rights. In Miharu, where the four *raisha* huts were apparently in close proximity to one another—and where officials seemed to have had a particular passion for bureaucratic oversight—each hut was assigned specific villages (as many as forty in one case) where they were allowed to canvass for alms. In addition, specific dates were designated in each month, apparently to ensure that *raisha* did not come calling too often.[62] In Kaga, begging occurred in conjunction with celebratory occasions, including the five seasonal holidays (*sekku*) that fell on the first day of the first month, the third day of the third month, the fifth day of the fifth month, the seventh day of the seventh month, and the ninth day of the ninth month.[63] In Sendai, *raisha* were allowed to beg at private celebrations and religious observances, including weddings, funerals, and Buddhist memorial services, although a domainal edict required them to refrain from "pestering" (*nedari*) participants.[64]

As with other forms of status, that of *raisha* carried with it specific privileges and obligations and duties, which served the larger social interest but also functioned as a public demonstration of "baseness." The pattern that Kobayashi Keiichirō identified at Zenkōji, where *raisha* were allowed to canvass for alms but also required to engage in forms of stigmatized work, was the norm. In Sendai, for example, where those within the *raisha* huts were under the authority of the *eta*, domainal policy required them to take responsibility for removing the skins from dead horses and other animals left at designated "animal dumps" and then to dispose of the remains. The skins were then sold to neighboring *eta*, who monopolized the lucrative leather trade.[65] In other domains, too, *raisha* were involved in the disposal of animal carcasses and the corpses of executed criminals and indigent travelers, as well as the performance of guardhouse duty, policing activities, and fire watches, unsavory but necessary forms of public service that officials typically relegated to outcasts. Those not incorporated into huts, as in Takamatsu, Kagoshima, and Kaga, engaged in cultivation, although they, too, were subject to service requirements.

The village in Kyoto seems to have been unique in that it was apparently unburdened by the performance of stigmatized labor as public service. Although its members farmed and made and sold straw sandals, its main source of support seems to have been the officially authorized gathering of alms. In fact, the residents were known as *monoyoshi*, a term that means "felicitations" or "good luck."[66] This term apparently derived from the greeting they used to announce their presence when they canvassed for alms from house to house. The *Illustrations of Various Workers* (*Jinrin kinmō zui*, printed 1690), a work that might be best viewed as an attempt to make sense of new forms of status in relation to occupation, includes an illustration of *monoyoshi* depicted in the act of begging (figure 1.6). Their faces are marked with the lesions that signified *rai* in this period, and they have begging bowls in their hands and baskets on their backs. Over time the alms-gathering work of the Kyoto community expanded. Initially, it was limited to central Kyoto and took place twice a year, at the time of the lunar New Year and during the religious holiday known as O-bon, both auspicious occasions. But by the early nineteenth century, canvassing took place as many as seven times a year and involved carefully planned routes that extended as far as the neighboring province of Tamba, evidence perhaps that people were becoming less generous.[67]

The performance of stigmatized work became an issue of considerable contention for the *rai* sufferers based at Nara-zaka. As in Kyoto, the sufferers at Kitayama Hall (and at Nishiyama as well) were known as *monoyoshi*, suggesting that they, too, were primarily associated with the gathering of alms. But unlike their Kyoto brethren, those at Kitayama also engaged in work associated with "baseness." In the second half of the seventeenth century, they were still involved in removing the carcasses of the sacred deer—albeit unwillingly. According to the procedure then in place, Kōfukuji was notified by the town magistrate when a dead deer was discovered, and the temple then alerted both the *eta* (who were based at a site known as the Eastern Hill, or Higashi no Saka) and those at Kitayama. After the former removed the valuable hide, the *raisha* were charged with the disposal of the remains. However, they repeatedly complained about this requirement, until in 1710 Kōfukuji relieved itself of what was apparently a burdensome responsibility by turning authority for the hall over to Tōdaiji. As a result, the removal of the deer carcasses became the responsibility of the *eta*, and like the *monoyoshi* of Kyoto, those at Kitayama came to be primarily a community of alms gatherers.[68]

The process by which those with the disease came to enter the ranks of the "base people" is far from clear. In his analysis of early modern status, Howell argued that as long as a sick or disabled person was cared for within the home, he could retain his original status identity. It was only when someone left home that the "taxonomic principle" of status propelled absorption into a new status group. As evidence, Howell points to the famous example of the guild of the blind, an officially recognized

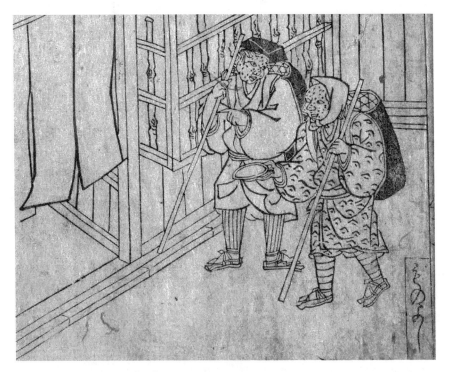

FIGURE 1.6. *Monoyoshi* canvassing for alms. Detail from *Jinrin kunmō zui*, 1690. National
Diet Library, Digital Collection.

organization that had monopolistic control over certain occupations.[69] But
the situation of *rai* sufferers was more complicated than Howell's analysis
suggests. Miyamae Chikako has argued that Sendai required all those with
rai status to submit to *eta* control, regardless of their status by birth or
whether they were residing with their families. As evidence, she points to
an edict from 1686 that stated, "It has previously been ordered that *raisha*
are under the control of the *eta* of Kawaramachi ward. It is now ordered that
all *raisha* throughout the domain are to be under the control of the *eta*."[70]
A similar situation seems to have existed in the nearby domain of Miharu,
which required that cases of *rai* be reported to town officials, after which
the sufferer was required to relocate to one of the domain's huts.[71]

   As in the medieval period, not every sufferer of *rai* readily accepted
his change in status. While Kagoshima and other domains in southwestern
Kyūshū in principle required *raisha*, even those of samurai status, to relocate to the *raisha* villages, some refused to comply. In 1619, a father and

son of samurai birth in Takanabe domain tried to flee the village to which they were consigned after developing the disease. They were apprehended but eventually were allowed to remain within the castle town—but only after they agreed to send two of their servants to the village as proxies.[72] A case from the Kagoshima domain a few decades later is similar. It involved a samurai official who was in charge of the tea ceremonies held within the castle of the Kagoshima lord. After he developed *rai*, the headmen of the local *raisha* village arrived to take possession of him, although they were also apparently willing to accept a financial settlement instead. Conflict emerged when the samurai refused to accept either option and the headman attempted to forcibly remove him. Eventually, the headman was reprimanded as "unreasonable" (*hidō*), but it is unclear what happened to the samurai whose condition sparked the controversy.[73] The use of proxies and the possibility of paying compensation is evidence that the logic of exclusion at work in both cases had nothing to do with fear of transmission but rather reflected a desire to maintain the form (if not the fact) of the status system.

Yokota Noriko has argued that the specific Buddhist associations of *rai* diminished as *raisha* was transformed into a status identity, with the result that the giving of alms that had previously been associated with the accumulation of merit became nothing more than a semirequired act of charity to one's social inferiors.[74] At the same time, the associations with Buddhism never entirely disappeared. For one, there was a distinctly Buddhist cast to many aspects of life in the communities of *rai* sufferers. In addition to the spatial proximity to temples in Kyoto, Nara, and Nagano, in both eastern and western Japan those with *raisha* status abandoned their original names and adopted so-called *amida-gō*, Buddhist names that expressed their removal from secular life. Moreover, social relations reflected a common pattern of hierarchical relations within religious communities, in which newer members were regarded as the "disciples" of those who entered the community before them.[75]

An extraordinary document offers us some evidence of how those designated *raisha* made sense of their place in the world. Authored by residents of Sendai's *raisha* hut and addressed to domainal officials, it was apparently composed to defend their begging rights after repeated admonitions by authorities to curb their aggressive behavior.[76] Their defense took the form of a discourse on the history of their community and the social meaning of their condition. Written in *sōrōbun*, the linguistic style characteristic of official documents, the petition opens with an explanation of the origins of Sendai's *raisha* huts.

The first leader of the *raisha* hut was the second son of the emperor of the Engi era [901–923 CE] who unfortunately began to suffer from this terrible disease. Because of his sickness, the emperor removed the prince from the lineage and, lamenting this, had a residence built for him at the base of the [Kiyomizu] hill and had him moved there. . . . Because of the example of the prince, now in every province in each county outside of the town there are huts for those who suffer from this illness and are removed from their lineages.[77]

This spurious claim of ancient and august origins was by no means unprecedented. In the early modern period, other groups of "base people" composed similar narratives, some of them lengthy and elaborate, that traced their association with the imperial institution, specific deities, or powerful religious institutions in order to counter discriminatory policies and attitudes and seek or retain specific privileges.[78] The Sendai *raisha* followed this pattern, blending fact and fiction, to link their disease, their humble dwelling, and even their removal from their families to an imperially authorized policy of the distant past. This made them part of a country-wide system that extended to "every province."

Having established the origins of their community, the authors of the petition next turned to discuss the significance of their alms gathering. Here, the emphasis is not on the economic value of these activities for themselves but on the benefits they bring to others. By going door-to-door, singing songs of good fortune, and pounding loudly upon a drum, they "remove the fear of this terrible disease," "drive away troubles associated with all the various sicknesses," and "celebrate the production of the five grains and the business of sericulture." As this suggests, the authors of the petition laid claim to a semidivine ability to aid the larger community by warding off illness and thereby encouraging prosperity, presumably through the expiatory power of their own bodies. But this description of the ritual value of alms gathering is no longer specifically linked to Buddhism. The only deity referenced in the petition is Hakusan Daimyōjin, a mountain god of syncretic Buddhist-Shinto origin who was the object of considerable popular devotion in this period. The petition ends by asserting the close links between those within and those outside the *raisha* huts: "We" are not outsiders who have wandered here from other domains; we are *raisha* from your own villages.[79]

The Sendai petition suggests that while the specifically Buddhist associations of the disease with karmic retribution and atonement had indeed diminished, *rai* continued to be a special disease, not least of all for those who suffered from it. But perhaps the most striking evidence of the special nature of *rai* is the fact that not all those categorized as *raisha* may actually have suffered from any disease at all. In his discussion of the *raisha buraku* at Zenkōji, Kobayashi Keiichirō suggested that many of its residents did not seem to have been sick, and he speculated that at some point the *buraku* came to be largely comprised of the healthy descendants of the sufferers who had initially been its members.[80] Similarly, Kujirai Chisato has argued that in Sendai by the mid-eighteenth century, the term *raisha* had become completely detached from the disease and was simply one term among many used to describe marginalized status groups.[81]

Miyamae Chikako, who also works on the Sendai, rejects this as a misguided attempt to detach premodern forms of exclusion from the modern politics of disease. She argues, instead, that in Sendai, Kaga, and elsewhere, *raisha* seems to have been applied to those identified as descendants of *rai* sufferers.[82] Additional evidence that the designation of *raisha* was applied to family members and even perhaps second- and third-generation descendants of sufferers comes from population registries of domains from various parts of the country: in Hyūga and Saga in Kyūshū and Takamatsu in Shikoku, entire families were designated as *raisha*.[83]

This extension of the label of *raisha* to even the healthy is a development that requires further examination. The next chapter explores the rise of a new medical discourse on *rai* that, over the course of the Tokugawa period, transformed it from the "bad karma disease" to a "bad blood disease" that potentially tainted all members of a lineage. But the examination of the forms of social and spatial exclusion associated with the disease has already begun to expose the long and deep history of leprosy. Ideas about *rai* began to coalesce in the twelfth century, propelled by premodern "pollution ideology" as well as the concept of causality known as karma. As the early modern state took form over the course of the seventeenth and eighteenth centuries, *rai* sufferers were absorbed into the "national" culture of status and became subject to distinctive, if variable, patterns of social marginalization. While it is unlikely that all sufferers of *rai* were absorbed into the *raisha* villages and *raisha* huts, this does not negate the significance of these sites. Indeed, there is considerable evidence that even those who were not incorporated into organized communities faced various forms of social exclusion, even in death. In some areas, for example, those who died of *rai* could not be cremated for fear that the smoke would poison the surrounding countryside; elsewhere, it was the practice to inscribe the term "unclean" (*fujo*) upon the wooden tablet that marked their graves.[84]

This long and evolving history of exclusion has been effectively erased from social memory in Japan. This process began in the prewar period, when proponents of the quarantine began to celebrate the *raisha* hostels, casting them as indigenous and prescient precursors to modern public health facilities. Writing in 1902 in a then influential medical journal, one physician described the Kitayama Hall as "something to be proud of before the rest of the world" and stated that he hoped that its history would "arouse the determination of the Japanese people to create new leprosy hospitals."[85] It was this understanding that prompted officials to declare the hall a recognized historical site in 1921, a designation that required its preservation.

By the 1980s the hall had fallen into a state of disrepair. It was reconstructed in 1999–2001 under the direction of the Nara Prefectural Board of Education with funding from the Ministry of Cultural Affairs. The timing of the project is significant: this was the moment when the repeal of the Leprosy Prevention Law and the filing of the suit by the Kumamoto patients were transforming Japan's leprosy policy into a human rights issue. In this context, the Buraku Liberation League now made common cause with activists within and outside the sanitaria, and the Nara branch of the Buraku Liberation League was actively involved in pressing for the reconstruction of the hall.[86] The official opening of the reconstructed Hall took place on May 20, 2001, only nine days after the plaintiffs' victory in the Kumamoto case was announced. However, even though the project was clearly driven by the politicization of leprosy policy, the text of the hall's historical marker left the interpretation of the site ambiguous: while it asserts historical continuity between medieval and modern forms of "leprosy relief," it also calls for reflection on the question of human rights, leaving it unclear whether the hall represents a cautionary tale or is a model to be emulated.

The interpretation of the site became more complicated in the wake of the Kumamoto decision. When the National Hansen's Disease Museum opened in 2007, critics fiercely attacked an exhibit that mentioned the Kitayama Hall, arguing that any reference to premodern practices was nothing more than a tactic to call into question the responsibility of the modern state for the stigma of the disease. In contrast, others have embraced the hall and transformed it into an unlikely symbol of inclusion. While it is not open to the public, local school groups visit it as part of their civics classes, as do participants in so-called Human Rights Tours organized by the local governments in western Japan and by local branches of the Buraku Liberation League.[87] The new understanding of the site is exemplified by a report on a classroom visit by sixth graders at a public school in Nara that is showcased on the Nara Board of Education website. It reveals that the hall was introduced to the children as a "welfare facility" for sufferers of "Hansen's disease" that was supported by "the people of Nara."[88] This is an appealing story to be sure, but one that, as we have seen, has little to do with the historical reality of this and the other sites. In the chapters that follow, I explore the multiple ways in which the premodern practices of exclusion came to be evoked in relation to the modern policy of quarantine.

Chapter 2

From "Bad Karma" to "Bad Blood"

Medicalizing *Rai* in Early Modern Japan

Sometime in the 1790s, Nakagami Kinkei (1744–1833), a well-known physician in the city of Kyoto, took on the care of a very ill man.[1] According to the case notes Nakagami later published, his patient had lost sensation in many parts of his body, had a face that was red and swollen, and was missing his eyebrows. One can imagine that he came to Nakagami in a state of considerable desperation, since his symptoms (particularly the loss of eyebrows, a condition now known as madarosis) were closely associated with *rai*. Nakagami identified this as a case of *raifū* (*rai* wind), adopting the terminology that prevailed in the Chinese medical literature, and the treatment he prescribed was aggressive. He first dosed his patient with a medical compound called "three sage powder" (*sanseisan*), a powerful emetic; then he gave him several "dragon gate pills" (*ryūmongan*), apparently a laxative. Next he took up a lancet-like instrument and bled his patient. Finally, Nakagami supplied yet another herbal compound, a variant of the "rhubarb root and rhizome decoction" (*daiōtō*), to cool and quicken the blood. After the patient successfully endured what must have been a grueling (and no doubt expensive) course of treatment that lasted some weeks, Nakagami pronounced him cured.[2]

The experience of Nakagami's anonymous patient is a window into the medicalization of *rai* over the course of the early modern period, circa 1600–1850s. By medicalization, I mean specifically the erosion of the belief that the disease was the somatic consequence of the sufferer's moral transgressions and the new view that it was somatic in origin and thus amenable to medical treatment. Over the course of two centuries, a growing number of physicians speculated about the etiology of *rai* and experimented with new therapies, and many claimed that the disease could be cured if treated correctly and promptly. Luke Demaitre has traced a similar process in Europe between the thirteenth and seventeenth centuries. He argues that leprosy was gradually "secularized" as doctors began to explain it in terms of the then dominant humoralist system of medicine, rejecting moral and biblical theories of its origin, and this, he suggests, may have contributed to the lessening of its stigma.[3] In contrast, in Japan, the new medical discourse on *rai* had a very different effect. While there was considerable debate on what caused the disease, by the end of the eighteenth century the dominant theory was that *rai* was a disease of "bad blood" that could be passed from parent to child and lurk within a lineage, striking at any time. Unlike the idea of karmic retribution, which stigmatized the afflicted person, the new concept of "bad blood" as a transferable material substance provided justification for the social exclusion of whole families across generations.

Medicalization in Context

Until the seventeenth century, *rai* appeared only sporadically in Japanese medical texts. The earliest mention of the disease is found in the *Ishinpō* (Formulary for the Heart of Medicine, 984 CE), famed as the oldest extant medical text in Japan. Authored by Tanba Yasunori, a physician in service to the imperial court, the *Ishinpō* cites more than one hundred Chinese medical texts from the period between the late sixth and the early tenth centuries. *Rai* is taken up in the discussion of wind diseases, following the classification established in the canonical *Inner Canon of the Yellow Emperor* (*Huangdi neijing*). In the *Inner Canon*, wind is named as one of five atmospheric forces (the others are cold, damp, heat, and dryness) that singularly or in combination cause disease. The disease known as *lifeng* (or *laifeng*; J. *raifū*) was characterized by lesions, changes in skin color, and the collapse of the nose and was the result of wind entering the body through skin and "polluting" *ki* (Ch. *qi*), the vital energy or "ether" that flowed through and animated the human body.[4]

Tanba, however, referenced not the *Inner Canon* but a later Chinese text, the *Zhubing yuanhou lun* (J. *Shobyō genkō ron*; Treatise on Disease Causality, 610 CE), authored by Chao Yuanfang. Following Chao, he characterized *rai* as the result of a combination of both endogenous and exogenous factors: "As for what is called *rai*, all its forms are because of bad wind. If you have contact with something that is forbidden or commit some forbidden act, then because of the harm [that results], you will be

vulnerable to this illness."[5] The reference to "forbidden acts" might lead
to the conclusion that even at this early moment *rai* was already associated
with moral transgressions, but the degree to which the *Ishinpō* reflected or
influenced ideas about disease is difficult to discern, and Tanba may have
simply incorporated the theory that he believed had currency in China. In
any case, upon its completion the *Ishinpō* was presented to the emperor
and disappeared into the imperial library, where it was accessible to only
a very small group of court physicians. It was not published until 1860,
twelve hundred years after its compilation.[6]

The first evidence that physicians were attempting to treat cases of
rai comes from the late thirteenth and early fourteenth centuries, when the
disease began to appear in medical texts produced by elite physicians in the
political centers of Kamakura and Kyoto. Like Japanese physicians before
and after them, medieval doctors, too, drew upon the Chinese medical literature, albeit selectively and with their own set of concerns. Unsurprisingly,
in this period, discussion of *rai*, even in medical texts, was invariably mediated by the theory of karmic retribution. A case in point is the description of
the disease in the *Idanshō* (A Compendium of Medical Talks, ca. thirteenth
century) by Koremune Tomotoshi, a court physician.[7] Koremune characterized *rai* as a fatal disease (*shibyō*), although he acknowledged that some
Chinese physicians, such as the famous Sun Simiao (?–682 CE), believed
that some cases could be successfully treated. Koremune disagreed and
suggested that attempting to treat *rai* was dangerous—for the physician.
As evidence, he pointed to a passage in the eleventh-century formulary *Su
Shen liang fang* (Beneficial Formulas of Su and Shen), compiled by Shen
Kuo (1031–1095), which described the experience of a certain physician
who was attempting to treat a patient afflicted with *rai*. In the midst of this
endeavor, the physician had a dream in which a mysterious voice told him,
"This is a disease that is caused by heaven. If you try to treat a disease
caused by the retribution of heaven, you too may become sick."[8]

The anecdote ends with the physician abandoning his efforts, and
this, it seems, was Koremune's advice to any of his colleagues who might
be tempted to treat the disease. The reference to "heaven" in Shen Kuo's
story is significant, revealing the flexibility and pervasiveness of the idea
that the disease resulted from immorality. Over the course of the medieval
period, texts associated with Song Confucianism began to be introduced
to Japan, often brought by Buddhist priests traveling between China and
Japan. Within Confucian discourse, "heaven" referred to the natural moral
order of the cosmos that worked to reward good and punish evil in the

human realm, and in Japan, the diffusion of Confucian texts led to the popularization of the term *tenkeibyō* (heavenly retribution disease) as another way to refer to *rai*.

But not every medieval doctor shared Koremune's belief that the disease could not be treated. Kajiwara Seizen (1265–1337) was a Buddhist priest and physician associated for several decades with Gokurakuji, a temple in Kamakura of the Ritsu sect, whose members included Eison and Ninshō, the two priests discussed in chapter 1. Andrew Goble has described the temple as "the most comprehensive medical facility constructed in Japan to this time," noting that it included a clinic, a hostel for *rai* sufferers, a dispensary, a medicinal bathhouse, and even a veterinary clinic specifically for horses (a valuable asset for the warrior elite of Kamakura).[9] Sometime between 1302 and 1304, Kajiwara completed a medical text he called *Jottings on Medicine* (*Ton'ishō*) that summarized and organized new Chinese medical knowledge from the Song period. In the chapter he devoted to *rai* (one of fifty in total), Kajiwara was primarily concerned with categorizing what he regarded as different types of the disease, based upon clusters of symptoms, etiology, and prognosis. He identified twelve in all, three of which he believed were responsive to treatment, and for these he provided recipes for medicinal compounds. In contrast, the other nine were described as the result of "punishment from the gods because of bad karma from a previous incarnation," and Kajiwara suggested that sufferers had no recourse but to "practice every kind of meritorious act, atone for bad acts, and strive for goodness" in the hope of divine relief.[10]

While *Jottings on Medicine* suggests a new and intriguing willingness to interrogate the theory of karmic retribution and to deconstruct the disease category of *rai*, its limited circulation, like that of all texts in this era, meant that its impact was probably muted. That situation changed dramatically after 1600. The period of sustained peace and economic growth that followed the establishment of the Tokugawa shogunate saw a tremendous expansion of medical practice with growing numbers of physicians and a booming market for all manner of medical texts that made medicine an important part of the new print and reading culture. While self-identified doctors had widely disparate levels of training and expertise and were in competition with a variety of other kinds of healers, from priests to medicine peddlers, they were nonetheless increasingly influential in shaping ideas about sickness and health. By the early eighteenth century, medical care at the hands of a physician was widely available in major cities, and by the end of the century, doctors had become a feature of life in towns and villages as well.[11]

As the number of practicing physicians increased, the scope of the "medical" expanded as well. Some physicians began to treat illnesses heretofore regarded as divine in origin, and temples and shrines began to sell medical compounds, blurring the line between the medical and the sacred. There was simultaneously a new trend towards specialization. Physicians who became known for their skill in treating particular disorders founded so-called schools (*ryū*), medical lineages that offered their (fee-paying) students exclusive access to their techniques and treatments, control of which was maintained by their descendants. A famous example of such a medical lineage was the Kagawa School, founded by Kagawa Gen'etsu, who pioneered new obstetrical techniques to aid women experiencing difficult childbirth. Central to the new schools were so-called secret teachings (*hiden*), a feature of many forms of scholarly practice in this era that allowed scholars and others to enhance the value of the knowledge they held by monopolizing it.[12]

The case of smallpox is illuminative of the process of medicalization in this period. Endemic to Japan since ancient times, smallpox was popularly attributed to the smallpox deity, and a variety of charms and amulets were deployed to either keep him at bay or appease him. In times when smallpox was epidemic, whole communities would come together to perform rituals meant to convince the deity to leave.[13] But while such practices continued, over the course of the eighteenth century, the so-called Ikeda School of physicians rose to prominence for its expertise in treating smallpox. The secret at the heart of the Ikeda School was its technique of tongue and lip diagnosis, information that was supposedly conveyed to its founder by Dai Mangong, a Chinese scholar who had fled to Japan after the Ming dynasty. This information supposedly allowed for the more effective treatment of smallpox. The claim to have singular access to specialized knowledge may well have been spurious, but even so it was a source of legitimacy for the Ikeda physicians. By the end of the eighteenth century, the school had almost three hundred members, and Ikeda Kinkyō, its head, was so well known for his skill that he was invited to join the shogunate's medical institute, the Igakukan, as its first smallpox specialist.[14]

Rai, however, departs from this pattern of increasing specialization. Although the disease was the object of extended discussion by physicians who debated its etiology and the efficacy of various treatments in medical treatises, compendia of case notes, and formularies, it never became the province of a specific school. This is especially puzzling because the disease was the topic of a specialist medical literature in which "secret teachings" figured. The *Union Catalogue of Early Japanese Books*, the most comprehensive guide to premodern print and manuscript materials, includes the titles of more than fifty medical texts devoted to *rai*, most of which date from the period after 1725, and with one notable exception these survive only in manuscript form. These manuscript materials have titles such as *Secret Notes on Rai* (*Reifū hiroku*), *Secret Prescriptions for Rai* (*Raisō hihō*), and *Miraculous Medicines for Rai Secretly Transmitted* (*Hiden raifū myōyaku*).

There is no definitive answer to the question of why the treatment of *rai* did not give rise to a specific "school," the proliferation of "secret teachings" notwithstanding. But one possibility is that the treatments advocated by different physicians simply failed to produce the kind of reliable results necessary to found and sustain a medical lineage, since ultimately it was the claim to superior efficacy that brought both patients and students. Without the monopolizing structure of a medical lineage, the "secret teachings" concerning *rai* circulated widely in manuscript form. A work called *A New Method of Treating Rai* (*Raibyō chiryō shinpō*) is a case in point. Attributed to a physician named Satake Kūjuku and dated to 1618, like Koremune's *Jottings on Medicine*, it, too, attempted to schematize the different forms of *rai* but with a new emphasis on the visual representation of symptoms. Each form of the disease is described in brief blocks of text that are accompanied by a simple line drawing that attempts to illustrate it (figure 2.1). One kind of *rai*, for example, is described as "a disease that arises from the heart and causes bones to dissolve and flesh to rot," while another is characterized by edema ("the flesh swells with water") and lack of sensation in the hands and feet.[15]

There was a new focus on treatment as well. One section of the work is devoted to so-called southern barbarian treatments and takes the form of a collection of recipes for medicinal compounds. The term "southern barbarian" was used to refer in this period to "European," but the substances that appear in the "treatments"—chaulmoogra seeds (*daifūshi*), *Coptis chinensis* (*ōren*), and *Bupleurum chinense* (*saiko*), for example—were a part of Chinese, not European, pharmacology. Given that goods from Southeast Asia and China were often transported to Japan on European ships, the use of "southern barbarian" may reflect confusion about the origin of new formulas, although it is also possible that Satake referenced "southern barbarians" as a means to authorize the "new treatments" he offered. As we saw in the case of the Ikeda School, the evocation of an exclusive source of new information was common practice among medical lineages.

A New Method of Treating Rai was never published, but this does not seem to have limited its influence within the new medical discourse

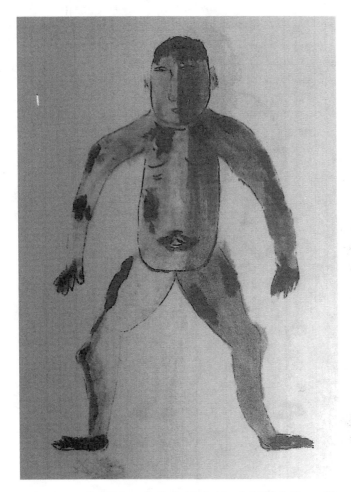

FIGURE 2.1. Detail from *Raibyō chiryō shinpō*, 1618. Fujikawa Yū Bunkō, Kyoto University Library.

on leprosy. A tattered copy of a manuscript on *rai* labeled "secret" was among the possessions of a village doctor who worked in Kawaba village in what is now Gunma Prefecture in the early nineteenth century.[16] This work clearly derives from *A New Method of Treating Rai*, but it shows evidence of considerable revision as well. For example, while the textual descriptions of the six types of *rai* seem to be drawn directly from Satake's work, the illustrations are more elaborate, vividly depicting the skin lesions associated with *rai*. In addition, new information is incorporated—specifically, the appropriate spots to bleed the patient are indicated on some illustrations, reflecting the new technique with bloodletting that began in the late eighteenth century, a development explored further in this chapter (figure 2.2). As this suggests, manuscript texts had wide circulation, and those who encountered them felt free to edit, revise, and reorganize. With this in mind, in the discussion that follows, I explore the unfolding of the medical discourse on *rai*, drawing on both print and manuscript materials by both famous and obscure physicians. What emerged over the course of the Tokugawa period is not a systematic development of a coherent disease

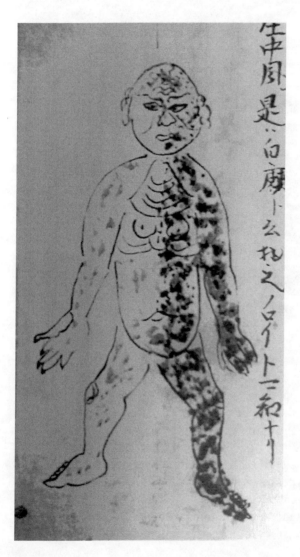

FIGURE 2.2.   Detail from "Sanbyō gorai wazurai no ken." Kobayashi Kyōichi Household Papers, Archives of Gunma Prefecture.

theory but a set of competing ideas that came to converge around the concept of "bad blood," an idea that reflected the intersection of ideological concerns and medical discourse.

Theorizing Causality

Sometime in the early decades of the eighteenth century, a student of medicine posed a question to his teacher, Katsuki Gyūzan (1656–1740). Katsuki was a well-known physician in Kyoto at the time, a defender of the tradition of so-called Rishu medicine that drew upon Song-era medical knowledge against the rising popularity of the new "ancient formulas" school. The latter rejected the abstract theorizing based upon Confucian concepts advocated by Song physicians in favor of an empirically based approach to treatment. The student's question, however, had little to do with the intricacies of medical theory or internecine strife; rather it reflected an observation that many were beginning to make at the time. Why was it, he asked, that when a man who suffered from *rai* married and had a child, that child would later develop the disease but it was never transmitted to the wife? Katsuki replied that *rai* was unlike any other disease. It was the result of heavenly retribution, which could extend even to one's descendants. As a result, it was important to choose one's marriage partner carefully, since the children or grandchildren of a sufferer, while appearing healthy, could carry the disease. Moreover, since *rai* reflected the workings of heaven, it could not be cured—although it could be managed. Eating the meat of animals or oily foods and exposing oneself to the damp air of deep mountains could worsen its symptoms, while the use of emetics and laxatives to cleanse the body of the "poison" of *rai* together with the avoidance of sex and specific foods could bring improvement. In serious cases, one could also use a needle to disperse and remove "bad blood."[17]

Katsuki's response to his student is a window into the evolving conceptions of *rai* in this era, as new ideas about etiology, transmission, and treatment led many to question the concept of karmic retribution. Even Katsuki, who clung to the theory of retribution—and in fact extended it to the lineage—eschewed many of its rhetorical trappings. He made no mention of the immorality of those afflicted and no recommendations for prayer, penitence, or the necessity of good works. Other doctors went further and dismissed the concept of retribution outright. Writing in the late eighteenth century, the physician Minamisono Ishin, who practiced in the area around Sendai in northeast Honshū, commented that "ordinary people think this disease is punishment from the gods or Buddha or the result of

karma, and so they just pay priests to pray over them and do not seek treatment and, thinking their disease is fatal, just wait for death. . . . There is
nothing more ridiculous than this. *Rai* is just one disease among many."[18]
Writing a few decades later, the physician Okamura Wajun, who practiced
in Sasayama in what is now Hyōgo Prefecture, openly mocked the theory
of heavenly retribution, which he attributed to "Confucianists." He noted
that while the city of Osaka had few sufferers, the disease was known to
be prevalent in some villages; should one conclude then that the villages
were filled with evildoers and those in the city were all sages who followed
the will of heaven?[19] Physicians who rejected the idea of divine retribution
also took note of the impact it had upon those who were afflicted. In the
preface he provided for a treatise on treating *rai* authored by his father, a
physician called Tatebe Yudō commented on the human suffering that was
the result of the theory of retribution: "Because people think that this is
heaven's punishment, they reject [those who are sick] and make no efforts
to treat them."[20]

To be sure, not every doctor was as unequivocal as Okamura and
Tatebe. Katakura Kakuryō (1751–1822) was a famous physician in Edo and
the author of *Bairai shinsho* (A New Work on Syphilis and *Rai*, pub. 1786),
the only published medical text devoted primarily to *rai*. He suggested
that some cases might indeed be caused by divine retribution; these were
the ones that did not respond to his treatments.[21] While this might seem to
be just an expedient way for a renowned doctor to excuse his failures, it
also reflects the changing nuance of the term "heavenly retribution." By
the end of the eighteenth century it began to be used metaphorically to
describe a disease that was difficult to treat. Hanaoka Seishū (1760–1835),
the pioneering Japanese surgeon known for developing general anesthesia,
was one of those who used "heavenly retribution" in this way. Among his
many unpublished works is one called "Tenkei hiroku" (Secret Notes on
the Heavenly Retribution Disease), which treats the disease in thoroughly
medicalized terms.[22]

While a growing number of physicians rejected the explanation of
divine retribution, there was considerable disagreement over what did,
then, cause the disease. Some accepted the orthodox designation of *rai*
as the result of wind and endogenous factors. This was the position taken
by Ashikawa Keishū, an entrepreneurial scholar cum physician based in
Hikone, not far from Kyoto, who published a medical reference book called
Byōmei ikai (Explaining the Names of Diseases, pub. 1686). *Byōmei ikai*
was a kind of dictionary of diseases that summarized the Chinese medical
literature in simple Japanese. Since the convention was that medical texts

should be written in classical Chinese, *Byōmei ikai* may have been intended as an aid for relatively uneducated doctors. Ashikawa referenced the *Yixue rumen* (Introduction to Medicine; J. *Igaku nyūmon*, 1575) by Li Chan to offer up this theory of the disease: *rai* erupted when wind entered the body of someone already suffering from "heat poison," the result of overexertion during sex or too much rich food and drink. The result was that blood was adversely affected, and the patient developed purplish lesions, swelling of the extremities, and patches of white skin. As the disease progressed, the symptoms worsened. The voice became hoarse, eyebrows disappeared, flesh rotted from the hands and feet, and the nose collapsed. Once the disease reached this stage, it was incurable, although it could be successfully treated early on.[23]

But while many physicians continued to use the term "*rai* wind," the idea of wind was subject to considerable revision as doctors attempted to account for the fact that the disease seemed to be common in some locales and rare in others—a pattern that would later be borne out when the first national survey of prevalence was conducted in the late nineteenth century. Okamura Wajun was one of many who pondered the distribution of the disease. He concluded that it must be environmental in nature and used the term *fūdobyō* (that is, a disease that resulted from the wind and soil of specific places) to describe it. Tatebe Seian (1712–1782), who authored the work for which his son Yudō provided the preface, was another proponent of the environmental theory. A physician who worked in Ichinoseki (now in Iwate Prefecture) in northern Honshū, Tatebe ridiculed Katsuki Gyūzan's defense of the idea of heavenly retribution. The disease was known to be common among those who lived in mountain valleys and along rivers, but "why would heaven's wrath fall mainly on those who live [in such places] and why would heaven fail to punish those who live along the shore or in temperate places?"[24]

As the idea that cases of *rai* were associated with particular kinds of places gained adherents, many physicians began to view it as the result of "bad air" (*akki*), a term that is probably better translated as "miasma." In a work published in 1846, a doctor named Yamashita Genmon, a resident of Kyoto, attributed *rai* to the "bad air" of mountain winds, citing as evidence the fact that the disease was common in "distant areas of mountains and valleys" where one or two people out of one hundred were infected in contrast to cities where only one or two in ten thousand fell ill.[25] Katakura Kakuryō had a different theory of what constituted "bad air," which he believed was one of several possible causes of the disease. In his usage, "bad air" referred to the tainted air that arose from low swampy areas, latrines, and the areas where rancid fats and oils were stored or discarded. According to Katakura, the symptoms of *rai* occurred when the miasmic gases associated with such places entered the body through the nose and from the nose "attacked" (*osou*) the blood, causing it to "ferment" (*jōsaku*). The involvement of the nose, as the orifice through which bad air entered the body, explained why it frequently collapsed as the disease progressed.[26]

From the second half of the eighteenth century, the theory that *rai* was the result of an exogenous cause, be it wind or miasma, began to be challenged by physicians who argued instead that it was wholly or primarily "self-produced" (*jihatsu*), a theory that would be popular well into the nineteenth century and which again linked the disease to concerns about morality. The concept of "self-production" became increasingly popular as physicians and ordinary people embraced the concept of "life cultivation" (*yōjō*). The subject of dozens of health manuals composed for both general and specific kinds of readers, life cultivation was oriented by the idea that the prevention of illness was the responsibility of each individual, who, by monitoring and regulating his or her own body, could avoid illness and achieve a long life. According to the doctrines of life cultivation, the primary causes of sickness and disease were a flawed diet, overindulgence in sex, and other kinds of immoderate behavior.

The most famous and popular of the many manuals on life cultivation was Kaibara Ekiken's *Yōjōkun* (Instructions for Life Cultivation, pub. 1715). Kaibara, who wrote many popular Confucian texts, argued that health, longevity, and a life that accorded with "the way," as the normative moral order authorized by heaven was termed, required the control of bodily desires, such as those for food, sex, rest, and activity. He was particularly concerned with diet, warning that "disease comes from the mouth," and he provided detailed instructions on the beneficial and harmful effects of specific foods, as well as advice about food preparation, proper mastication, and the like.[27] Sexual desire required a similarly self-conscious commitment to restraint, since overindulgence could lead to a depletion of the body's essential *ki*. Kaibara discussed the frequency at which intercourse should occur based upon the age of the male participant, as well as the need for men to avoid sexual exertion when the body was already taxed by extremes of weather, emotions, and other factors.[28]

While many manuals, like Kaibara's, were written for a male readership, there were also handbooks for women that offered advice on how to produce healthy offspring by adhering to principles of life cultivation. They instructed women that miscarriage, stillbirth, difficult childbirth, sickly infants, and unruly children were the result of poor "self-care" (*hoyō*) during pregnancy. Dangerous behavior included engaging in sex after conception, eating the wrong foods, and sleeping in an immodest position. Even reading romantic novels like *The Tale of Genji* might inadvertently lead to unhealthy arousal in a pregnant woman, threatening the well-being of the fetus, at birth or in later life.[29]

The intense concern within life cultivation discourse for male vitality and female fecundity reflected not only personal concerns but also the ideological order of the early modern state, which valorized patrilineal descent and made it the rule for the warrior elite. As a result of the usual pattern of the trickle down of elite values, concern for the production of descendants and the preservation and well-being of the lineage came to permeate early modern society. For example, not only samurai but also commoners began to compose ethical treatises for their descendants that offered them advice about how to manage household affairs, including familial relations, finances, and other matters, so that their lineage could continue to prosper.[30] Similarly, as we've noted in relation to medical "schools," the lineage became the means of organizing scholarly activity and cultural pursuits. As the lineage became an object of personal, political, and economic concern, the sickness, health, and reproductive potential of its members came to be imbued with moral overtones, albeit in a configuration that owes little to the concepts of karmic or heavenly retribution.

The "return" of morality is apparent in the many discussions of diet and the self-production of *rai*. While some Chinese physicians had argued that sufferers of wind diseases should avoid certain foods, the theory that specific foods caused or were a contributing factor to *rai* loomed large in many Japanese discussions of the disease.[31] Katsuki Gyūzan, as we have seen, believed that eating meat exacerbated the disease, its origins in heavenly retribution notwithstanding. The Sendai physician Minamisono Ishin, too, believed that an immoderate diet was the primary cause of *rai*. He suggested that the consumption of meat, fowl, and even "fatty" forms of seafood such as tuna and whale produced a "poisonous heat" within the body that thickened the blood and led to the symptoms of the disease.[32] Even proponents of the environmental theory of *rai* emphasized the role of diet in the progression of the disease. Tatebe Seian, for example, cautioned against more than sixty "forbidden foods," including aromatic plants such as garlic, leeks, and green onions, but like Minamisono he was particularly concerned about the consumption of animal flesh, especially that of wild game, which he described as "very harmful."[33]

The particular concern for the ill effects of eating meat is further evidence of the mediation of medical discourse by political discourse in this period. The medical debates on *rai* unfolded as meat eating was becoming an object of critique by the shogunate and others. The consumption of wild game, including boar, deer, rabbit, and dog, had been common during the medieval period, but it came under increasing criticism after 1600. Not only was it proscribed by Buddhist doctrine; it was also forbidden as "inhumane" by the "laws of compassion" issued by the shogunate in the 1690s, and it later came to be embedded in a larger discourse on "Japaneseness" that emanated from both Confucian and nativist scholars, who argued that meat consumption was characteristic of less civilized peoples.[34] This is not to say that the eating of game meats was simply abandoned. It was not and indeed there was a counterargument that meat had health benefits, but the eating of animal flesh was newly viewed by many as problematic. As a result, new euphemisms began to be used in cookbooks and advertisements for eateries. Wild boar, for example, was referred to as "peony." The complex associations of meat eating were at play when doctors writing on *rai* faulted those afflicted for their dietary choices and their failure to control their appetite for morally ambiguous foods.

The discussion of sex and sexual desire within the medical discourse on *rai* was similarly imbued with new concern for morality and social order. The notion that sexual overindulgence either rendered one susceptible to *rai* or hindered recovery was widely shared. In a work published in 1819, the Kyoto physician Arimochi Keiri argued that no recovery from *rai* was possible unless the patient was wholly abstinent; Honma Sōken (1804–1872), a famous Edo physician who had studied with both the surgeon Hanaoka Seishū and the German physician Philip Franz von Siebold, took the proscription one step further, writing that the mere stirring of sexual desire, even when not acted upon, could compromise any effort at treatment.[35] But no one expressed greater concern for sexual incontinence than the physician Murai Kinzan (1733–1805), a domainal doctor in Higo (now Kumamoto Prefecture) who served as personal physician to the Hosokawa lord.

In the 1780s, Murai compiled a compendium of medicine recipes called *Wahō ichimanpō* (Ten Thousand Japanese Formulas) that so impressed his patron that he arranged to have it presented to the shogun. As its title suggests, *Wahō ichimanpō* was primarily a formulary: that is, a collection of recipes for medicinal compounds accompanied by some exposition. *Rai* has a singular place in this work. Although an entire chapter is devoted to the disease, it contains not a single formula. This makes sense, however, in light of Murai's stated view that treatment even by "a great and famous doctor" could not cure *rai*, "the most terrible disease."[36] Rather than treatment, Murai's concern was prevention. He wanted to raise the alarm that the dreaded disease was becoming increasingly common and that it had a specific cause. In his view, sexual morality had declined to such a degree that men and women were even engaging in sexual intercourse while the woman was menstruating, an act that Murai contemplated with disgust. Describing menstrual blood as "polluted and putrefied," he argued that when a child is conceived during such an act (something that in fact is highly unlikely) this "bad blood" (*akketsu*) would be incorporated into the developing fetus and at some point later in the child's life would erupt into full-blown *rai*.[37]

Murai was not the first Japanese doctor to advance this theory of *rai*'s etiology. Writing in the seventeenth century, a physician called Kitayama Jūan had also linked a pregnancy that occurred while a woman was menstruating to the development of *rai* in her child. Kitayama, who was born in Nagasaki, was rumored to have had a heritage that reflected the cosmopolitan nature of that city in the late sixteenth and early seventeenth centuries. He is said to have been the child of either a Japanese mother and a Chinese father, or a Japanese mother and a father who was half Dutch. Whatever his ethnicity, Kitayama learned medicine in Nagasaki and some sources state that he was educated in Dutch medicine there.[38] The European connection is important since the idea that sex during menstruation could infect the fetus with leprosy had a long history in Europe. There are references in both Christian and Jewish sources from the medieval into the Renaissance period.[39] In a manuscript work called "Jishūroku" (Notes on Learning for Our Time), Kitayama suggests that when a couple has sex just before, during, or immediately after menstruation, this "foul blood" can combine with semen to produce a child who will develop *rai*. His advice was that people follow the custom of places like Ise, where menstruating women were segregated from the rest of the household to guard against this danger.[40]

It is impossible to know if Kitayama's theory derived from information he received from European texts or informants, and Murai himself makes no mention of Kitayama's work. However, Murai hailed from Kumamoto, like Nagasaki, a city on the island of Kyūshū, and it is certainly possible that Murai had access to Kitayama's work. However, two things distinguish Murai's work from that of Kitayama. For one, Murai's discussion is animated by a new tone of moral panic. Two centuries of peace, the expanding market economy, and the growing economic power of commoners prompted much hand-wringing on the part of many officials and others who feared that a life of ease was encouraging the pursuit of sexual and other pleasures by the populace. But even more important was the context of Murai's work. It was composed as discussion of "blood" was beginning to shape discussions of *rai* as never before.

Blood was, to be sure, not an entirely new concern. Ashikawa Keishu raised the issue of blood in his discussion of *rai* in his 1687 work and so, too, did Katsuki Gyūzan, writing four decades later. But in the last decades of the eighteenth century a growing chorus of voices suggested that it was blood that caused *rai*, and blood that transmitted it. Although doctors writing in this period offered different theories about the causal factors in play, they were united in their understanding of the process that produced the symptoms of the disease: whether because of wind, bad food, miasma, unrestrained sex, or some combination thereof, the blood became unnaturally and pathologically "hot." A rich and illuminating vocabulary was deployed to explain the effects of heat on blood. The hot blood "congealed," "putrefied," "fermented," or "stagnated"; it became "dirty," "poisoned," or "polluted." Needless to say, the blood of which these Japanese doctors wrote differed from the substance as it is understood in modern biomedicine. Blood was the material manifestation of *ki*, as the term "blood *ki*" (*kekki*), which was used interchangeably with "blood," suggests. In a healthy person, *ki*, blood, and blood *ki* were supposed to move spontaneously and unimpeded around the body from one vessel (as the organs were understood) to another. In contrast to this ideal of fluid motion, the hot blood that caused *rai* was imagined to be turgid and slow-moving. When blood in this state pooled near the surface of the skin, it caused the eruption of lesions, nodules, and ulcerous sores. When it accumulated in the fingers, toes, or nose, it caused these appendages to "rot."

As blood became a focus of medical discussions of *rai*, so, too, did the female body, and not only because of menstruation. As Charlotte Furth has noted, within the Chinese medical tradition, blood was specifically associated with the reproductive processes of the female body, and physicians offered various theories about how women were involved in the development of *rai*.[41] Katakura Kakuryō, who argued that *rai* had multiple causes, including "bad air," a diet heavy with fatty meats, and too much sex, also suggested that the bloody lochia that followed childbirth was to blame. Blood that was not quickly expelled would stagnate within the woman's body, where it could turn poisonous and cause the symptoms of *rai*.[42] Arimochi Keiri, too, believed that the bloody fluid associated with childbirth was particularly dangerous, but for the infant rather than the mother. He suggested that if a newborn baby was not carefully and thoroughly washed immediately after birth, the bloody "filth" of childbirth could enter its body, presumably through the pores, and poison the infant, who would then "suffer from *rai* for its entire life."[43]

The concern here and in Murai's work for the blood of female bodies may reflect long-standing notions of female pollution. As Kitayama suggested, it was common in many regions of Japan for women to be isolated during menstruation and during and after childbirth, and menstruating women were typically forbidden from entering sacred places. But more important is that the association of the female body with "bad blood" provided an answer to the problem of transmission that had troubled Katsuki Gyūzan's student and others who noted that children born to those with the disease often developed it as well, although some within the household seemed immune. While no physicians explicitly rejected the idea that transmission could take place from an infected father, they obsessed over the danger posed by the maternal body, because it was assumed that the child came into contact with the mother's blood while in the womb, during childbirth, and even after birth, since breast milk was understood to be a form of maternal blood. In fact, many physicians warned that potential wet nurses and their families should be carefully investigated for any history of *rai*, lest the nursing infant be infected.[44]

Doctors in this period did not (indeed, could not) distinguish between congenital infection and hereditary transmission, and not only *rai* but also syphilis and tuberculosis were regarded as potentially resulting from either or both. Their language reflected this. Parent-to-child transmission was described by terms such as *densen* (which now means "contagious" or "infectious") but also as *idoku* and *iden*, terms that would later be used to describe hereditary transmission. The new anxiety about transmission led to two new ways of describing *rai*. It was *idoku no yamai* (a transmitted poison disease) and *ketsumyaku no yamai* (a disease of the bloodline). Both these neologisms imply that once acquired, *rai* would be a continuing if capricious danger to a lineage, infecting some progeny but not others. Some doctors suggested that it was not unknown for the disease to be latent for one or two generations, only to reappear unexpectedly; others believed that "bad blood," once formed, actually grew stronger as it was passed from one generation to the next, so that a child's case of *rai* would be more serious than its parent's.

By the end of the eighteenth century, the idea of *rai* as a "bad blood" disease that could be transmitted within a lineage was the new orthodoxy. And physicians writing on the disease were quick to warn of the danger it posed to families. According to Katakura Kakuryō,

There is no disease as terrible as *rai*. It is for this reason that whenever someone becomes sick with it, people avoid him, running away just as if he was a murderer or a beggar. And it is not only the sick person, but also his brothers, sisters, and relations who are avoided. So when you marry, before making the betrothal, it is necessary to carefully investigate whether there is *rai* or not. . . . This is because of fear that the lineage may be infected. It is for this reason that good people must choose good families, and families that have *rai* have no option but to marry families with *rai*. In the rural areas of our country, it seems that it is taken for granted that one must investigate the family, but the samurai, merchants, and artisans of the city are unconcerned about this.[45]

Katakura's advice to carefully avoid marriage with a "leprous lineage" (*rai-kei*), even if it was otherwise advantageous, was echoed by other doctors. Honma Sōken suggested that the virulence of what he called "spoilt blood" (*haiketsu*) was such that it would inevitably overwhelm "good blood": "even if you are born into family of a good lineage, if you marry a woman from a bad lineage, then your descendants may fall ill with *rai*."[46]

One of the few who voiced skepticism about the popular concept of "bad blood" was Ui Masatatsu, who authored a work called *Iryō sadan* (Trifling Medical Discussions, pub. ca. 1830s). Ui argued that *rai* did not inevitably affect the lineage—although he acknowledged that this view was widely held—and he pointed out that even notorious "leprous lineages" also had many healthy members. Moreover, rumors of *rai* could have a devastating effect upon a family, and malicious and false accusations of the disease, spread with an intent to damage a family's reputation, were not unknown. In Ui's view it was pointless to obsess over the question of whether a lineage was tainted by *rai*. Since the disease could be self-produced one could never be completely without worry. A case could develop even within a family "pure and clean from ancient time." Given this uncertainty, the best response to the disease was early and aggressive treatment.[47]

Prognosis and Treatment

Treatment and the possibility of a cure preoccupied many of the physicians who wrote on *rai*. In fact, many of the manuscript texts devoted to the disease are entirely concerned with therapies. An example is "Raifū ryōchi hiden" (Secret Transmissions on the Treatment of *Rai*). Consisting of only twenty-two pages of text, it is simply a list of recipes for medicinal compounds.[48] For other doctors, however, the issue of treatment raised important conceptual questions. What treatments were efficacious and why? What did the different constellations of symptoms mean? Under what conditions was a cure possible? These questions were crucial since there was a general agreement that an advanced case of *rai* could not be cured. If the eyebrows, toes, fingers, or nose had been lost, if the patient was already blind or lame, if the lesions were bigger than a copper coin, the palm of the hand, or the bottom of a plate, if the disease had been present for more than two, five, or ten years, then nothing, it was said, could be done. However, if treatment took place early and aggressively, many doctors believed the progress of *rai* could be halted, sparing the patient and his family the ostracism that would otherwise result.

Within the discussions of prognosis and treatment, blood—the substance that explained the transmission of the disease—was an object of new fascination. Physicians in this period generally relied upon diagnostic techniques such as the palpitation of pulses and the belly and the visual examination of the tongue, complexion, urine, and stool to determine their course of treatment for most diseases. Now some doctors began to argue that the inspection and testing of the blood itself was the best means to evaluate the severity of a case of *rai*.

Murakami Ryōan, the author of a treatise on the treatment of *rai*, was an early advocate of such an approach. To be sure, Murakami also made use of the usual diagnostic methods. He suggested that the palpitation of the pulses could reveal the distinctive pulse pattern known as *genmyaku* (bowstring pulse), a deep, taut pulse that was long associated with blood or *ki* stagnation, and that a peculiarly flushed complexion and cloudy urine offered additional evidence that the disease was present.[49] But to evaluate whether a case of *rai* was so advanced as to be incurable, Murakami suggested another test: prick the fingertip of the patient and let the drops of blood that resulted fall into a cup of water. If the drops of blood sank, this indicated that the blood was so heavy with "poison" that no cure was possible.[50] Tatebe Seian suggested a similar approach but for him the crucial issue was not whether the drop of blood sank in the water but whether it dissolved or retained its droplet shape. The latter was an indication that the case was too advanced to be cured.[51] Writing at almost the same time as Murakami and Tatebe, Nakagami Kinkei and Katakura Kakuryō suggested a different kind of test, advocating a procedure that resonates with Timon Screech's discussion of the late Edo fascination with optical instruments and the possibility of rendering the invisible visible.[52] After placing the suspected *rai* sufferer in a darkened room, the physician should examine his body using a piece of burning camphor, which emits a particularly bright flame, as illumination. If the patient has *rai*, they asserted, black or deep purple shadows would be apparent on the body, revealing the presence and extent of the "bad blood" beneath the skin.[53]

Based upon their understanding of "bad blood," physicians advocated for a dizzying array of treatments. Writing in the early seventeenth century, Gotō Gonzan (also read as Konzan, 1659–1733) suggested that hot-spring bathing could potentially provide a cure, advising that a year or two of regular soaks in "good waters" could cause stagnant blood to start flowing again.[54] By the end of the eighteenth century most doctors disagreed. Hanaoka Seishū, Minamisono Ishin, and Honma Sōken all argued that hot-spring bathing was dangerous, because heating the blood was likely to cause the "poison" in it to grow even stronger.[55] Like Nakagami Kinkei, many believed that the "poison" that caused *rai* could be expelled from the body via vomit or feces, and so prescribed powerful emetics and purgatives to their patients. Extraordinary substances were deployed as well. Several physicians suggested placing a live viper in rice wine, waiting until its flesh disintegrated, and then consuming this substance. This remedy originated in China, where the use of toxic ingredients (including venomous snakes, spiders, and insects) to treat *rai* had a following.[56]

But for those who took a medicinal approach to treating *rai*, no substance was more important than chaulmoogra seeds. As *A New Method of Treating Rai* suggested, the beneficial effects of chaulmoogra were known by the early seventeenth century, and the seeds featured in many of the "secret" collections of formulas. Hoashi Banri (1778–1852), a scholar and physician of Dutch learning who was known for his knowledge of Western science, was of the view that *rai* was a disease of the blood, but he suggested that with the appropriate use of chaulmoogra, two or three out of ten sufferers could be cured.[57] Hanaoka Seishū was another who embraced its use; chaulmoogra figures prominently in the recipes in his "secret notes." Evidence that the market for chaulmoogra was growing comes from the trade records of Nagasaki, the officially authorized trading port where the Dutch East India Company maintained a trading post. They reveal that the quantities of chaulmoogra seeds imported to Japan grew dramatically from the mid-seventeenth century. In addition, there seems to have been a lucrative if illicit trade in chaulmoogra based in Tsushima, the island domain authorized to conduct trade with the Korean peninsula.[58]

Physicians who treated *rai* never abandoned the use of medicinal compounds, but by the end of the eighteenth century the direct removal of "bad blood" from the body by bloodletting had become the cutting-edge therapy. For physicians seeking to both cure the disease and halt its transmission, the idea of simply removing the substance that caused it must have been an appealing proposition. As we have seen, Katsuki Gyūzan was advocating the use of acupuncture needles to extract "bad blood" in the early eighteenth century. Interest in the potential therapeutic effects of removing blood may have been spurred by knowledge of the use of blood-letting in Europe. The first published treatise on bloodletting was Ogino Gengai's *Shiraku hen* (Treatise on Piercing the Vessels, 1771), which makes mention of the European practice.[59] However, as Daniel Trambaiolo notes, "Japanese doctors soon discovered parallels in their own tradition and sought to explain its mechanisms of action in relation to their own doctrines."[60] Within a decade or two of the publication of Ogino's work, physicians were abandoning the use of acupuncture needles for lancets.

Katakura Kakuryō was an early advocate of an approach to treatment that focused primarily on blood. In his *New Theory* of 1786, he advocated for a treatment that seems to have combined aspects of bloodletting, acupuncture, and cauterization. After identifying the location of the "bad blood" within the body using the illumination of burning camphor, the physician was to heat instruments called *sanryōshin* on a charcoal brazier. The *sanryōshin* was the Japanese version of a lancet, and it featured a sharp triangular head. When the instruments were red-hot, they were to be inserted one by one into the affected area to a depth of two or three centimeters. This procedure was to be repeated for at least three days, until the patient developed a high fever and the wounds began to suppurate, symptoms no doubt of an infection but interpreted by Katakura as evidence that the poison of *rai* was being secreted through sweat and pus, as well as by the excreted blood.[61]

In the 1790s, Nakagami Kinkei, too, was making use of bloodletting, although he reserved it for only the most serious cases. Nakagami suggested that when visible signs of the disease were limited to the upper part of the body, emetics should be used, while if they were limited to only the lower part of the body, laxatives would be effective. However, once the entire body was involved, only bloodletting could stop the progression of the disease. The procedure for which Nakagami advocated had multiple steps. Using camphor as illumination, the physician should first identify where the "bad blood" had pooled and mark those spots with ink on the body of the patient; then he should use the *sanryōshin* to remove the blood; after that he should apply moxa (dried mugwort) to the wound and set it alight. Finally, a salve was to be applied to the wounds that resulted. The aim of all of this was to eradicate the poison within the body and thereby stop its spread.[62]

Another advocate of bloodletting was Arimochi Keiri, who believed that infants could develop *rai* if the bloody fluids of childbirth were not quickly washed from their bodies. Arimochi suggested that the leprous blood would first appear as a purplish-black spot on the bottom of the infant's feet in the area of the "bubbling spring" (*yūsen*) acupuncture point. This point (now known as the kidney-1, or KD-1, point) is understood to be the origin point for the kidney meridian, a central channel for the movement of *ki* around the body, and a needle inserted here is believed to relieve heat. Arimochi seems to have theorized that the "bad blood" that formed at this point, unless drained, would spread and affect the entire body. This could require multiple procedures since, according to Arimochi, "if you do not remove the blood each time it appears, then the child will suffer from *rai* for its entire life."[63]

Exclusion Revisited

The "bad blood" theory of *rai* emerged at the intersection of medical and ideological discourse over the course of the eighteenth century, and although most physicians rejected the idea that divine retribution explained the development of *rai*, this new "secular" medical discourse did not lessen its stigma. Instead, the new theories of causality reinscribed the disease with new ethical anxieties, making it the somatic sign of flawed behavior and the transgression of social norms. While some physicians expressed sympathy for sufferers, in some cases explicitly castigating the ignorance of both their fellow physicians and "ordinary people" who accepted the idea of karmic retribution, many others emphasized the danger those afflicted with *rai* posed to their children and through them to their lineage. The new concern for transmission through the blood made it possible for physicians, like Katakura and Honma, to affirm the exclusion of *rai* sufferers on medical grounds. Indeed, for Katakura, the forms of exclusion of *rai* sufferers practiced in many areas of Japan made perfect sense. He wrote approvingly of the situation in places such as Nara, where, in what seems to be a reference to the communities at Kitayama and Nishiyama, those who have *rai* live in "leper villages" (*raison*) and marry only within the village.[64]

Did the idea of "bad blood" that predominated in the medical literature inform popular attitudes towards the disease? There is certainly evidence that the idea of divine retribution continued to resonate into the early nineteenth century. We find it deployed, for example, within the anti-infanticide campaigns of the early nineteenth century, which sought to boost the birth rate following two devastating periods of famine in northern Honshū. The pamphlets and other materials produced by officials and their allies frequently referenced the karmic or heavenly consequences of the "evil" acts of abortion and infanticide for those involved, one of which was *rai*. For example, in the 1830s, when a Sendai official, Arai Nobuaki, composed a series of verses on the theme of the dangers of infanticide that was subsequently printed and distributed around the domain, he included one that warned women "who fear *rai* and difficult births" to avoid any act that might endanger their fetus.[65] Similarly, in his study of the healing activities within Soto Zen temples, Duncan Williams takes note of the presence of sufferers of *rai* among those who turned to priests rather than doctors for aid.[66]

But other kinds of popular print works from the same period provide evidence that the medicalized concept of "bad blood," too, had entered into popular discourse on *rai*. We find it referenced repeatedly in efficacy broadsheets (*kōnōsho*), a form of cheaply printed advertising material that proliferated in the late Tokugawa period as prepared medicines for all manner of ailments began to be produced and marketed. While efficacy broadsheets took a variety of forms, from single-sheet prints to multipage densely printed booklets, they typically referenced the language and concepts of medical discourse, albeit sometimes in hyperbolic or distorted terms. Given its prevalence in the medical literature on *rai*, it is not surprising that "bad blood" figured explicitly in the efficacy pamphlets for mass-produced *rai* treatments.

One example is an advertisement for Purifying Blood Pills (*sei-ketsuen*), which were produced in a village near what is now the modern city of Shibukawa in Gunma Prefecture by Tachibana Shunan, probably a local doctor.[67] The production of a cure for *rai* here was probably not accidental. Travelers to Kusatsu, a hot-spring town whose waters were believed to be especially efficacious for skin diseases, including *rai*, had to pass through the village, providing a ready clientele for Tachibana's pills. According to the text of the one-page broadsheet for Purifying Blood Pills, the symptoms of the disease—red face, loss of eyebrows, collapse of the nose, and paralysis of the hands and feet—are "all the result of bad blood" that developed either "within the womb" or because of "food poison." But this "bad blood" could be cleansed through the regular use of the Purifying Blood Pills—for the hefty price of one and a half *ryō* (the cost of approximately 150 kilograms of rice in this period) for a forty-day supply. The broadsheet also promised patients that they could avoid the dangerous and painful new therapy of bloodletting, since taking the pills for a hundred days more or less would provide a cure without the need to "remove blood."

Tachibana was not the only medicine producer who deployed the idea of "bad blood" to market a cure for *rai*. Funagoshi Takasuke, a self-proclaimed "syphilis doctor" who practiced in Osaka, published a series of illustrated works, essentially lengthy advertisements for his services, with catchy titles like *Baisō gundan* (Martial Tales of Syphilis, 1838) and *Baisō sadan* (Tea Talks on Syphilis, 1843). These works also incorporated advertisements for the prepared medicines that Funagoshi manufactured and sold. As Katakura's *New Work on Syphilis and Rai* suggests, the two diseases were often paired, since both resulted in disfigurement and both were believed to involve blood and sexual incontinence. However, *rai* was considered to be the far more serious disease. In the words of a popular proverb of the time, "The leper envies the syphilitic." In *Martial Tales of Syphilis*, Funagoshi incorporated an advertisement for a product he called Purifying Body Pills (*seishingan*), which he claimed was effective for both diseases. According to the advertisement, "*Rai* is a wretched heavenly retribution disease and the dislike of people for it extends even to one's siblings and one's descendants." Fortunately, it was possible to "avoid this shame" by taking Funagoshi's pills.[68] Five years later, Funagoshi was selling a product that explicitly evoked the idea of "bad blood." The advertisement for his version of Purifying Blood Pills (*seiketsugan*) described *rai* as a terrible disease that resulted from "food poison and sexual desire" but one that could be successfully treated.[69]

The diffusion of the idea of "bad blood" sheds new light on the evolution of patterns of social exclusion in the late Tokugawa period. For one, it offers an explanation for the peculiar nature of the leper huts and leper villages in Sendai and elsewhere, where it seems, at least in some cases, no one actively suffering from the disease resided. As *rai* became a "disease of the bloodline," social identity as "a person with *rai*" no longer required the visual display of the symptoms of the disease. Instead, one's association with an infected lineage was sufficient.

The new conception of *rai* as a specifically familial disease may also explain another new development, official affirmation of the care of sufferers within the household. Although in the seventeenth century authorities in Sendai had adopted the policy of requiring those with *rai* to enter leper hostels, in 1850 the domainal government published *Sendai kōgi roku* (A Record of Filiality and Righteousness in Sendai). Like other collections of moral exemplars published in this period, it celebrated ordinary people who lived in accordance with officially authorized social values, with the aim of encouraging their emulation. The Sendai collection contains more than five hundred entries, and among their numbers are individuals who are praised for providing care for family members afflicted with *rai*. One story, for example, told of young children who spoke out against their father's decision to abandon their stricken mother, while another celebrated a newly married young woman who defied her parents and refused to divorce her ailing husband.[70] While the celebration of familial responsibility for the *rai* sufferer took the form of a discourse on morality, it also served another social function—ensuring that knowledge of the "taint" of *rai* within a family was known to the larger community.

Perhaps the best evidence of the contesting meanings attached to *rai* in the mid-nineteenth century comes from a visual source. In the early 1850s, the woodblock artist Utagawa Kuniyoshi completed a series of prints that celebrated the sixty-nine "stations," as the towns along the highways that provided lodging and other services were known, along the Kiso Highway, an important road that stretched between Edo and Kyoto. Rather than depicting contemporary sights along the roadway, in the manner of other similar series, each print portrays a historical or legendary figure associated, sometimes quite loosely, with the station in question. Important for our purposes is the print numbered fifty-seven for the town of Akasaka-juku, which evokes the famous story of Empress Kōmyō washing a *rai* sufferer (figure 2.3). Even in the medical literature of the day visual depictions of *rai* were rare, and the print eschews the medieval iconography of the disease—spots on the face and white headcloths—and depicts quite graphically the loss of hair, large nodules, and patches of depigmented skin that characterize the lepromatous form of the disease.

There are no historical, or even legendary, associations of Akasaka and Kōmyō. Instead Utagawa relied upon a bit of wordplay to arbitrarily bring the two together. As we have seen, in Kōmyō legend, the beggar was eventually revealed to be the buddha known as Ashuku Nyorai, a name that is loosely linked to the place name Akasaka-juku (*shuku*), phonetically but also because of the associations of *shuku* with outcastes. However, in Utagawa's rendering, this famous event is portrayed neither as a part of a Buddhist rite of atonement nor as a display of imperial beneficence. While the beams of light emanating from the body of the *rai* sufferer suggest the Buddhist doctrine at the heart of the original story, the empress and her maid are represented in a homely domestic setting with their kimono sleeves tied up like industrious housewives, and a humble washbasin is nearby. Utagawa's print suggests then the complicated place of the *rai*

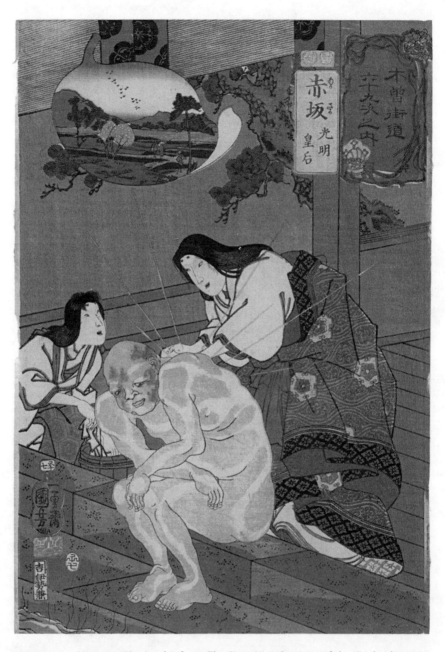

FIGURE 2.3. Utagawa Kuniyoshi, from *The Sixty-Nine Stations of the Kisokaidō*, 1852. Museum of Fine Arts, Boston.

sufferer at the end of the Tokugawa period, both in real terms and in the popular imagination. While *rai* sufferers had been associated with the liminal spaces of temple grounds, crossroads, and hostels and with marginalized people and stigmatized work, by the mid-nineteenth century they were newly understood in relation to families, lineages, and the quotidian activities of eating, having sex, and bearing children.

Over the course of the early modern period, the medicalization of *rai* did not replace the long-standing concept of karmic contribution. Instead it overlaid it with new sets of concerns—about sexual desire, diet, and place, about individual behavior and its effects on the family and social order. Doctors and the producers of prepared medicines offered the possibility, but not the promise, of a cure—for a hefty price and considerable pain and suffering. Although Minamisono had declared *rai* to be "just another disease," few of his colleagues agreed with this assessment. By the end of the eighteenth century, the leper villages could be praised on medical grounds, and people were being warned to investigate the families of potential marriage partners for the disease. The medicalized understanding of *rai* developed in this period would have a powerful and long-lasting legacy. The idea that it was a disease transmitted from parent to child would shape popular attitudes well into the twentieth century, in spite of repeated efforts by doctors and public health officials to convince the public that it was infectious. And those who were afflicted continued to hope that medicinal compounds, bloodletting, moxibustion, or hot-spring bathing might provide a cure.

Chapter 3
Rethinking Leprosy in Meiji Japan

In 1880, a man who used the name Nishiyama Kyōzan submitted a petition to the authorities of what was then Nara District in Sakai Prefecture. It stated:

> I suffer from leprosy [*repura*], that is, the heavenly punishment disease, and am a resident of Nishiyama in this village. In this province there are two such places. One is Kitayama at Tōdaiji, the other is Nishiyama at Yakushiji. From long ago, those who suffered from this disease entered these two places and spent their lives in them. . . . Based upon an edict from the time of Emperor Monmu, we began to receive blessings of rice in two seasons. That is, the rule was established that those who live at the two places Kitayama and Nishiyama twice a year could traverse the province and receive rice to save and support the sick interned within them. . . . However, after the Restoration the gathering of alms was generally forbidden and since then we have no other means of receiving support, for there is no law that saves those who are diseased, no law that offers them aid. And because each of us suffers from this serious disease, there is no occupation that we can perform daily. Even though this sickness is the result of karmic retribution, there is no method to aid those who are without support.[1]

This is but one of a series of desperate pleas that Kyōzan made to local officials in the 1870s and 1880s asking for some kind of aid on behalf of the sufferers of *rai* housed at Kōmyōin. We learn more about Kyōzan (who took the name of the temple as his surname) from a petition he submitted to the governor of Osaka Prefecture in 1881, following the incorporation of Nara District into that administrative unit. He attached a medical certificate that stated that he was forty-four years old and had suffered from *rai* for twenty years, that his arms and legs were partially paralyzed and that his speech was impaired.[2]

Carefully crafted to reference historical precedent, signs of imperial favor, traditional forms of aid, and pure human need, Kyōzan's petitions are evidence of how the 1868 revolution that ushered in the formation of the modernizing Meiji state inadvertently affected sufferers of *rai*. In 1871, the new government announced the abolition of the outcast status categories within which the *rai* huts, *rai* villages, and *monoyoshi* communities had been embedded. Although framed as an act of "emancipation" (*kaihō*) that made outcasts into commoners, in the short run the edict deprived many vulnerable people of the long-standing right to a degree of public support— albeit support acquired by begging and alms gathering—that had provided for their basic needs. In the wake of its promulgation, some communities of *rai* sufferers quickly dissolved. The *monoyoshi* village in Kyoto disbanded in 1872 after the municipal government issued an ordinance that banned begging. By 1873, all traces of the community were gone. The temple Seienji was abandoned and its land sold off.[3]

The plight of *rai* sufferers did not go unnoticed even amidst the profound social and political changes sweeping the country. This chapter explores the new visibility of the disease—on the streets of cities like Tokyo and Kyoto, but also within new forms of political, medical, and philanthropic discourse beginning in the 1870s. My aim is to excavate the tensions and contradictions that shaped responses to the disease in the last three decades of the nineteenth century, an important historical moment that has largely been overlooked in the historiography of leprosy in Japan. Significantly, in this period, the Japanese government was only occasionally and peripherally involved in the unfolding discussions about the nature of the disease, its social significance, and the issue of how to care for sufferers. Instead, it was a group of civic actors, including journalists, private physicians, and patent drug producers, who played the central role in defining the social significance of the disease for modernizing Japan while advocating for new policies for its sufferers.

Gotō Masafumi and the Origins of Modern Leprosy Relief

In 1874, a petition entitled *Thoughts on Leprosy* (*Repura-byō kō*) authored by a then obscure doctor of Sino-Japanese medicine (*kanpō*) named Gotō Masafumi (1826–1895) caught the attention of Tanaka Fujimarō, minister of education in the new government.[4] In his petition, Gotō laid out a request for public funds to establish a system of leprosy hospitals that would be under his direction and make use of a treatment regime he had developed, which he claimed could cure leprosy. The term *repura* used here, as well as in Nishiyama Kyōzan's 1880 petition, a transliteration of the term "leprosy," is evidence that the disease construct *rai* was now associated with leprosy, even though the understanding of the latter was in flux. Gerhard Armauer Hansen had identified *M. leprae* in 1873, but debate over whether it truly constituted the sole causative agent of leprosy continued for some time. In light of this new, if still tenuous, association, from this point on I will use "leprosy" to name the disease in question.

Tanaka was sufficiently intrigued by Gotō's petition to alert Ōkubo Toshimichi, then governor of Tokyo and an influential member of the new governing elite, of his proposal. A biographical sketch that appeared in the 1881 work *Meiji Success Stories* (*Meiji risshi hen*), a collection of essays on men who had risen to fame in the first decade of the new era, suggests how Gotō's initiative came to be framed.[5] It describes him as a native of Minō Province and a member of a family that had been practicing medicine for "more than ten generations." Gotō, too, trained as a doctor, but while he was still in his twenties, his career took a new turn when he decided to devote himself to discovering a cure for leprosy. This decision, according to his biographer, was motivated by compassion. Gotō pitied sufferers who were fated to become *hainin* (literally "discarded people"). It took "more than twenty years" of study and experimentation, but he finally succeeded in producing a cure.[6] According to the "success stories" account, when government officials heard of the miraculous results of his new medicine, they "ordered" Gotō to leave Minō for Tokyo and offered him a job in the clinic attached to the Higashi-kō, the government-supported medical school that would later become Tokyo University's medical school. When the clinic was closed due to lack of funds, his patients begged him not to abandon them, and so Gotō struck out on his own, founding a private clinic devoted to the treatment of leprosy in what is now Shinjuku Ward in 1872. This was the origin of Kihai Hospital (literally "Resurrection Hospital"), a leprosy clinic that in the 1880s attracted international attention.

This celebratory narrative, while it conveys Gotō's reputation in the 1880s, is not entirely reliable. Gotō himself would later write that he left Minō for Tokyo, not at the government's request, but with the aim of offering to supply the government medical school with the medicines he had developed (which he recalled took ten, not twenty, years to develop).[7] But even when detached from this hagiographic account, Gotō's petition is significant. It reveals his prescient awareness of the new politics of both poverty and health that he successfully navigated to rise to fame.

In 1870, when Gotō first arrived in Tokyo, the city was in a state of chaos. The population had fallen by perhaps 50 percent, after shogunal vassals and their retainers, family members, and servants deserted the capital for their home domains. As a result, both the consumer economy of the city and its administrative structure had collapsed. According to contemporary reports, by the spring of 1868, just months after the triumphant imperial edict that declared the emperor's return to direct rule, the city was awash in human and animal waste, and beggars, would-be prostitutes, and orphaned or abandoned children wandered its streets. Leprosy sufferers, too, seemed to have been a part of the new urban poor, "freed" like Nishiyama Kyōzan from the status system that had sustained them. Officials of the new government attempted to respond to the crisis by establishing "relief facilities" (*kyūikujo*) in several parts of the city that distributed rice from the former shogunate's granaries to the poor.[8]

Somehow Gotō found employment in one of the public relief facilities and began offering medical care to leprosy sufferers at a short-lived charity hospital. However, in 1871 the financially strapped new government abandoned its early efforts to provide for the city's poor, even though conditions had improved only marginally. It was at this moment that Gotō, newly unemployed, established his leprosy clinic in Kashiwagi Naruko Ward, near the post station known as Shinjuku. A report in one of the early newspapers provided a description of Gotō's endeavor. It relates that the twenty to thirty patients housed there cooked for themselves, with the healthier patients helping those less able. Gotō provided them with medicines, offering them without cost to some patients.[9] What caught the eye of the journalist was the newness of this effort, which made leprosy sufferers the object of a specifically medicalized charitable endeavor that focused on treatment.

The founding of Kihai Hospital coincided with a new resolve on the part of the leadership of the new government, which gradually became committed to a top-down program of social reform that aimed to transform Japan into a powerful "civilized" country. The modernization of medicine and the promotion of public health were integral parts of this plan. In 1874, the government announced its Medical Policy (Isei), an ambitious plan to transform medical practice in Japan through the establishment of new schools for doctors, midwives, and pharmacists that would train medical providers in so-called Western medicine. In addition, a system of new public hospitals was to be constructed in order to ensure that medical care was available to all.[10] The goal of what we might now call "universal access" was not to be realized until the postwar-1945 era, and in fact as medical care came to be increasingly commodified, access to trained physicians came to be out of the reach of many, but in the mid-1870s there was great enthusiasm for the idea of publicly funded medical care for the poor.

Gotō's *Thoughts on Leprosy* deftly acknowledged the goals of medical modernization and public health. But as the name of his most famous medicine—Seiketsuren (Purifying Blood Compound)—implies, Gotō's understanding of leprosy reflected the early modern medical discourse on the disease. Leprosy, he wrote, was either "self-produced" or resulted from "inherited poisons" acquired from one's parents at conception or within the womb. However, he couched the theory that leprosy was a "bad blood" disease within a new and self-consciously "scientific" vocabulary: "[Leprosy] is caused by nothing other than the weakening of both the red and white cells. . . . As their structure weakens, their mysterious activity slows, and then the normal blood becomes poisoned. [The poison] attacks the nerves and causes paralysis; it attacks the skin and causes lesions; it attacks the joints, and the patient is unable to stand."[11] While Gotō referenced European medical knowledge, citing, for example, Christoph Wilhelm Hufeland's *Enchiridion medicum*, a canonical work for the doctors of "Dutch medicine" who staffed the new Bureau of Hygiene and the new government medical school, he was aggressive in asserting his own expertise over even such a well-known Western expert. He dismissed the theory that leprosy was spread by person-to-person contact, noting that it was common knowledge that people could live intimately with an infected spouse for decades without acquiring the disease.

Gotō's treatment for leprosy also derived from early modern therapies. The formula of his Seiketsuren was a closely guarded secret, but its active ingredient was probably chaulmoogra oil, a common ingredient in early modern treatments for leprosy, as noted in the preceding chapter. Given that chaulmoogra oil would be used until the 1950s to alleviate symptoms of the disease, Gotō's claims about the efficacy of Seiketsuren likely had some validity, and he probably did engage in experimentation to produce his compound. Chaulmoogra oil has an offensive smell and taste and is also difficult to digest, with the result that when taken orally it can induce profound nausea. Gotō's compound apparently made it possible to ingest the oil by minimizing this troubling side effect. Even so, treatment with Seiketsuren was by no means quick or easy. According to Gotō, to be effective the drug had to be administered for a period of three to twelve months under the direction of a physician who would monitor the patient and alter the dosage as needed.

The aim of *Thoughts on Leprosy* was not, however, simply to promote the use of Seiketsuren. Gotō had a far more ambitious vision, and while his understanding of leprosy and the drug he developed to cure it had roots in early modern medicine, the public leprosy hospitals for which he advocated were entirely new. Citing Antonius Franciscus Bauduin, a Dutch physician who had taught at the medical school attached to the Nagasaki Naval Training Academy in the 1860s and briefly at the government medical school in the early 1870s, Gotō asserted that cases of leprosy, once common in Europe, were now exceedingly rare. How had this been achieved? Hufeland, he suggested, supplied the answer: Europeans had vanquished leprosy by establishing a system of "national leprosy hospitals" (*kokushu raibyōin*).[12]

In fact, there is no mention of "national hospitals" in Hufeland's work. This is not surprising since European lazar houses were almost entirely run by religious orders, not governments. Moreover, Gotō left unexplained how these institutions had contributed to the decline of the disease in Europe—an important issue, given his rejection of the theory that leprosy was infectious and his stance that Seiketsuren was the first-ever effective treatment. Gotō's referencing of European practice was then clearly strategic. He evoked the European model in order to assert the modern nature of his ambitious plan.

At the same time, Gotō was well aware of the economic realities of the day and hence stressed that the cost of establishing treatment centers would be minimal. His former patients, "full of joy at having cleansed their soiled name and pity for their fellow sufferers," would be willing to stay on at his hospital and care for other patients, presumably for little or no compensation. Proceeding in this way, "leprosy hospitals could be created in every province and the disease that has been regarded as incurable for a thousand years could be swept away so that it will no longer be necessary to investigate the lineage when considering a proposal of marriage."[13] Notably, even as Gotō was attempting to gain government funding, he was also moving forward with his plan to establish leprosy clinics around the country. In 1875 in response to Bureau of Hygiene survey of medical facilities in Tokyo, he submitted a report that stated that in addition to the original Kihai Hospital, he also operated a second Tokyo clinic in Honjo Ward (now Sumida Ward), and five branch hospitals, one each in Aichi, Gunma, and Okinawa, and two in Ōita.[14]

If these institutions existed, they must have been of a very small scale, given that even the original Kihai Hospital had only twenty-five patients

at the time. Even so, there is evidence that Gotō's work was already having an impact outside of Tokyo. In 1874, prefectural authorities in Miyagi
allowed a local doctor in the prefectural capital of Sendai to establish a
leprosy clinic in conjunction with the new public hospital. The announcement of its opening stated that the clinic would use the "miraculous and
unprecedented" treatment developed by Dr. Gotō of Tokyo, and it called
upon those in Miyagi who wanted to "escape the misfortune of transmitting
the poison to their descendants" to apply for treatment. The prefectural
seal of approval notwithstanding, this was apparently a for-profit venture
for the doctor involved. The basic treatment cost six yen, which did not
include room and board, a fee that likely would have limited the potential
clientele of the clinic. According to a newspaper report published eleven
years after its founding, the clinic had treated only about two hundred
patients in total.[15]

Back in Tokyo, Gotō's petition finally won him an interview in 1876
with Kusumoto Masataka, who had succeeded Ōkubo as governor of Tokyo. This sign of official interest in leprosy is striking, given that at this
time national public health policy was focused on the control of cholera
and other acute infectious diseases. The Bureau of Hygiene had been established in 1873, and it began to track the raw numbers of those infected
with cholera, smallpox, diphtheria, and dysentery in 1875. However, no
attempt was made in relation to leprosy until 1880, when it was classified
as a "regional disease" (chihōbyō), a designation applied to certain parasitic
diseases and "intermittent fevers," a reference perhaps to malaria. According to the official Report of the Bureau of Hygiene, between July 1880 and
June 1881, 288 cases of leprosy were reported, more than half in Higo (now
Kumamoto Prefecture). Many areas reported no cases at all.[16] This remarkably small number, needless to say, does not reflect the actual prevalence
of the disease; rather, it reveals a lack of interest in tracking leprosy, on the
part of both the Bureau of Hygiene and local officials.

Gotō apparently used his meeting with Kusumoto to expound upon
the remarkable properties of Seiketsuren. His pitch must have been effective, because the outcome of the meeting was a plan for an ad hoc
clinical study. It was agreed that Gotō would select three patients with
advanced cases of leprosy for treatment, monitor their progress, and report
back on the results. A year later Gotō submitted his report: one patient
had completely recovered after seven months of treatment; a second one
who suffered from both leprosy and syphilis was "on the path towards
complete recovery"; while the third, who suffered from a "weak stomach,"
had proved difficult to treat since he could not take Seiketsuren, but he,

too, was improving. The effectiveness of his treatment was clear, Gotō asserted, and so he hoped to make it widely available. To that end, he was treating five poor patients for no cost and another five for half the usual fee in his clinic, but official support was needed in order to treat the "countless impoverished leprosy sufferers."[17] Hasegawa Tai, then the director of the Tokyo Prefectural Hospital, was not impressed. He instructed a staff doctor to follow up on the three patients who were the subject of Gotō's report. Six months later this doctor offered a less-than-glowing assessment of Gotō's results. One patient, he reported, was somewhat improved, but the condition of the other two was still serious.[18] Nonetheless, in November 1877, the governor decided to give Kihai Hospital, by this time located in Sarugaku-cho in Kanda, the status of a "leprosy ward" of the public hospital, an arrangement that made it possible to provide public funding to Gotō so that he could begin treating the poor of Tokyo.

The decision of the Tokyo authorities to fund Kihai Hospital seems remarkable, given the equivocal results of the test cases and Gotō's status as doctor of *kanpō* medicine and manufacturer of proprietary medicines at a moment when such professions were already under assault by the state's plan for the modernization of medicine. The crucial factor in the success of Gotō's campaign for public funding seems to have been his new celebrity. In the early 1870s the new newspapers of the capital embraced Gotō as a popular hero, celebrating his success in treating leprosy as a worthy object of national pride. Typical of the reportage on Gotō in this period are two articles that appeared in the *Yomiuri shinbun* in July 1876. The first tells of the murder of a young female leprosy sufferer in Ehime Prefecture. Her parents, fearing "shameful rumors" if her illness became known, had employed a former samurai to murder the girl. The author of this sad tale concluded by lamenting that the victim had the misfortune to live "in such a backward place," because "here in Tokyo we have Dr. Gotō who is an expert at curing leprosy."[19] Two weeks later the newspaper followed up this article by printing what purported to be a letter to the editor. Its author related that in the aftermath of the initial report, he had a conversation with "a certain doctor," presumably a European, about the state of leprosy in Europe and North America. In these places, he reported, as in Japan, sufferers of the disease and their families were ostracized. However, according to the unnamed doctor, if only the treatments of Dr. Gotō were more widely available, the disease would surely be eliminated. From this perspective, the letter writer urged Japanese sufferers in the Tokyo area to take advantage of their good fortune and quickly seek treatment.

Taken together, these two short pieces reveal the set of intersecting themes that would shape journalistic discourse on Gotō within the newspapers of the day. Dramatic anecdotes that highlight the "backward" state of popular knowledge, as well as the desperation and despair of victims and their families, were contrasted with the hope offered by Gotō's treatment, which was celebrated as without parallel even in the West. We learn, for example, of O-Ume, the wife of a bathhouse owner, who jumped off Azuma Bridge into the Sumida River when she learned that she had leprosy, a death that could have been avoided "if only she had known of Dr. Gotō."[20] Gotō himself is depicted as a skilled physician who was also a crusader for the public good. According to an article in the Tokyo Daily News (*Tokyo nichi nichi shinbun*) from 1873, through the use of his "miraculous treatment," Gotō was able to cure even those "whose hands and feet were deformed or rotted," "whose hair had fallen out," "whose nose had collapsed"—a litany of the symptoms associated with advanced cases of leprosy. The author went on to praise Gotō's "aim of saving the poor" and concluded with the declaration, "Would it not be a great and beautiful thing if leprosy hospitals like [Kihai Hospital] were established in every region so that the citizens of the nation could be saved."[21]

In the newspapers of this era, the line between reportage and advertisement was often a thin one, and Gotō may have been instrumental in shaping the extensive coverage he received, but whatever his role, the impact of media involvement was significant. The newspapers became the discursive site where leprosy was first transformed into a social issue, where claims of its curability were celebrated, and where a chorus of voices began to call for government action to aid in the new project of leprosy relief. This new public interest in the disease, an early reflection of the new power of the press, was the context of Kusumoto's decision to provide public funds to Kihai Hospital for the treatment of the most destitute but calls for further government action continued. In January 1878, the editors of the major newspapers, including *Kanayomi*, *Yomiuri*, *Tokyo nichi nichi*, *Chōya*, and *Nichiyō*, each of which had its own distinctive readership, joined forces to undertake a public campaign to encourage donations to support Gotō's hospital.

This public campaign in support of Kihai Hospital reflected a new conception of charity as an individual imperative. Provisions of aid to the poor and sick were of course nothing new. Buddhist doctrine had long encouraged such acts by the concept of "merit," and Confucian discourse did as well by making "benevolence" the responsibility of social superiors to those beneath them. Still, in the early modern period, many provisions of aid to the sick, the dying, and the poor were compelled by official policy that required villagers and townspeople to contribute to the support of the vulnerable among them. The journalistic campaign for contributions to support Gotō's Kihai Hospital was but one example of the new celebration of individual charity. Japan's early newspapers were filled with calls to provide "relief" to specific needy individuals (an ill woman with a nursing baby, a widow with three children) as well as to a variety of groups, from veterans of the Seinan conflict, to families who had lost everything due to fire, flood, or crop failure, to communities struggling with epidemic disease and later the effects of industrial pollution.[22] Significantly, newspapers made the case that private philanthropy was the norm of modern civilized societies. It was precisely this perspective that ordered an 1878 *Yomiuri shinbun* article that described how foreign residents of Japan had gathered funds to send to China to aid famine victims, encouraging Japanese readers to do so as well.[23]

Journalistic encouragement to support Kihai Hospital was thus part of this larger phenomenon, but leprosy "philanthropy" had its own peculiar logic. The newspapers involved in the campaign printed the names of those who contributed, and the lists they compiled included the names of many patent medicine producers and journalists. Given that both professions were viewed askance by Meiji officialdom, the campaign created an ideal opportunity for those involved to demonstrate their enlightened compassion and commitment to the public good, while also drawing attention to the limits of the government's response. Meiji journalism thus made leprosy into evidence of Japan's progress towards civilized-nation status. Not only had a Japanese doctor succeeded in discovering the cure for this dreaded disease, but it was also ordinary citizens (like themselves) who had played the leading role in the campaign to aid its victims.

Within the media celebration of Gotō in these years, however, the victims of the disease were often depicted in ambivalent terms. Even as they documented the financial, familial, and other difficulties that sufferers confronted, journalists also castigated them for failing to step forward and accept treatment, portraying it as a willful refusal that only governmental intervention could counter. An article published in the *Yomiuri shinbun* during the campaign for donations stated that "to have so many lepers is a national shame," and it called for the creation of policies that could compel sufferers to avail themselves of Gotō's treatment. The author not only recommended the establishment of more leprosy hospitals but also suggested that cases of leprosy should be recorded in the household registers (*koseki*). The household registry system, established in 1872, was the government's means of compiling important demographic data. Reflecting the rise of modern patriarchy, it recorded addresses of origin, residences, births, deaths, marriages, and divorces under the name of the male family head. It also, as is well known, became an instrument for the perpetuation of old and new forms of discrimination. Members of the old outcast status groups were designated as "new commoners" (*shinheimin*), making it possible to distinguish them from other commoners, while children born to unmarried mothers were newly designated as illegitimate (*shiseiji*). In an implicit recognition of the new power of the household registry system, the *Yomiuri* author argued that inserting the disease into the household registries would make concealing the disease impossible and thus could be used to compel the sick to seek treatment.[24]

"A Race of Asian Lepers"—Entrepreneurial Doctors and the Uses of Stigma

The new concern for "national shame" and the representation within the press of recalcitrant "lepers" point to the ambiguous nature of the 1870s reportage on leprosy, ordered as it was by compassion, opportunism, and new civic pride. How this impacted sufferers of the disease is difficult to discern. Although newspapers routinely carried reports of suicides by leprosy sufferers in the first three decades of the modern era, it is unclear whether this was a new phenomenon or simply one that for the first time found its way into discourse. What is clear is that as leprosy came to be defined as simultaneously a social problem and a curable disease, Gotō and his hospital prospered. Popular philanthropy and public funding more than doubled the number of his patients, from 150 in 1878 to 387 in 1881, making Kihai Hospital a medical institution of significant scale in this period, when the Tokyo prefectural psychiatric hospital, the largest public medical institution in the country, had a capacity of only 150 patients.[25] One indication of his fame in the early 1880s, even beyond the immediate environs of Tokyo, was the response to a speech he gave in the provincial city of Kōfu in Yamanashi Prefecture in 1880. Contemporary reports estimated that as many as two thousand people gathered in the theater Mitsui-za to hear Gotō declare that leprosy was a curable disease and that victims should "come as soon as possible to Kihai Hospital where they will be examined, given medicine, eat nutritious food, recover quickly, and return to the pure and fresh appearance they once enjoyed."[26]

Gotō's success at securing public funding in Tokyo spurred similar efforts elsewhere. In 1877, Masafumi's son Masanao (1857–1908) approached the governor of Kyoto and pitched the idea of prefectural funding for a leprosy hospital, arguing that "like the support of industry, schools, hospitals, vaccination," the care and treatment of leprosy sufferers should be the responsibility of the government. After deliberating for some months, the governor agreed and authorized the establishment of a hospital in Jōdoji village, located on the northeastern outskirts of the city, in 1878.[27] In that same year, Gotō Masafumi was involved in opening a leprosy clinic in Ibaragi Prefecture. According to a newspaper article, he was to travel there twice a month to oversee treatment. In 1879, a group of physicians in Maebashi in Gunma Prefecture, apparently operating independently from Gotō, created their own charity clinic for leprosy sufferers. About the same time, a doctor in Osaka opened a clinic that the local edition of the *Asahi shinbun* celebrated as akin to the famous Kihai Hospital of Tokyo.[28] Gotō then may have felt newly confident of success when he submitted a petition in March 1880 to elder statesman Iwakura Tomomi in which he again advocated for the creation of a nationwide system of leprosy hospitals under his direction that would cure Japan's lepers, whose numbers he estimated to be at least 140,000. Evoking both a popular slogan and the pervasive anxiety about Japan's international stature, Gotō declared that not only would the cure of leprosy aid the project of "enriching the country and strengthening the military," but it would also be "a great and beautiful thing" that would bring Japan honor before all the countries of the West.[29]

Gotō's personal fame, popularity, and considerable powers of persuasion notwithstanding, it was not long before local governments began to withdraw their support. In June 1881, Hasegawa recommended ending public funding for Kihai Hospital, citing the high cost of Gotō's cure, which required patients to be hospitalized for as long as a year. A Hygiene Department memorandum cast the issue in an even more skeptical light. It, too, recommended the end of public funding, stating that "no matter what one does, leprosy is a disease that is difficult to completely cure." By this time, the Kyoto facility had already closed after being in operation for only a year. Almost as quickly as it had emerged, official interest in funding leprosy treatment began to wane. Thus, when a doctor on the staff of Kihai Hospital and the director of the public hospital in Akita city approached the prefectural government asking for money to support the creation of a leprosy clinic, arguing that the apparently small number of sufferers in Akita was deceptive and that there were in fact many "hidden" cases, officials were unreceptive. Prefectural officials replied that the shame of the disease was such that few patients would present themselves for treatment, making such an endeavor not worth the investment of public funds.[30]

While there were concerns about the effectiveness of Gotō's treatments and the size of the patient pool, the more direct cause of the withdrawal of support in Tokyo and elsewhere was national policy. In 1881, Finance Minister Matsukata Masayoshi instituted a new policy of fiscal restraint designed to control the rampant inflation then plaguing Japan. As a result, local authorities were directed to cut their budgets in order to reduce taxes and shore up waning popular support for the government, with the result that social welfare initiatives were abandoned. In this same year, Tokyo Prefectural Hospital, which had offered free care to the poor, was closed, leading to a popular outcry and the founding of a new institution, the Yūshi Community (Kyōritsu) Hospital, which relied heavily on private donations for the two years of its existence. The fate of both the prefectural hospital and public aid to Kihai Hospital reveals the experimental and ephemeral nature of many of the medical initiatives in these years, as dreams of institution building collided with hard economic realities.

The withdrawal of government support meant the end of Gotō's dream of heading a national system of leprosy clinics supported by a combination of public and philanthropic funds. With the loss of the former and new competition for the latter, Gotō abandoned the "relief" model of treatment in favor of a new approach that targeted potential consumers directly. Working with Masanao, who had studied medicine at Keiō Igakusho (later the medical school of Keiō University) and successfully passed the new licensing exam for physicians required in Tokyo beginning in 1880, Gotō senior began to advocate a new regime of "self-treatment" (*jiryō*) that called upon patients to dose themselves at home with an array of medicines they purchased from the newly established retail pharmacy of Kihai Hospital. The hospital itself continued to accept patients, but only those who were capable of paying for their own long course of treatment.

In 1882, Gotō senior and Masanao published *Self-Treatment of the Intractable Disease (Nanbyō jiryō)* to explain and promote the new protocol of self-care. It sold for seventy-five sen, a hefty amount in a time when a skilled tradesman earned about twenty-five sen per day.[31] The Gotōs addressed their readers directly, offering detailed information about self-diagnosis, the assessment of symptoms, and the progress of the disease. Typical of the tone of the work is the explanation of leprosy as a blood disease, a theory they continued to embrace. In *Self-Treatment*, the self-conscious attempt to deploy a scientific vocabulary that had figured in *Thoughts on Leprosy* was abandoned in favor of a new set of metaphors that seem to have been aimed at a popular readership: healthy blood "nourishes" the body, rendering it strong and healthy, as fertilizer enriches the soil, while the loss of eyebrows and lashes associated with the disease is described as akin to the withering of plants in poor soil.[32]

Although the Gotōs' understanding of the disease remained fundamentally unchanged, they now explicitly recognized the possibility of infection (*densen*), something Gotō Masafumi had dismissed ten years before. But the possibility of infection was simply integrated into the existing etiological paradigm that allowed for multiple causes. The Gotōs continued to assert that the disease was often transmitted from parent to child, although the term "inherited poison" (*idoku*) was replaced by the term "hereditary transmission" (*iden*), and they still identified "self-production"—the result of a flawed diet, heavy drinking, and overindulgence in sex—as its most common cause. The Gotōs' understanding of the disease at this juncture was thus a confusing mix of old and new ideas. The discussion of diet is a case in point. While early modern doctors had identified the eating of meat as the leading cause of the self-production of the disease, the Gotōs, clearly influenced by new enthusiasm for the Western-style diet, now called upon those engaged in self-treatment to eat meat often, even helpfully providing a recipe for beef soup.

The aim of *Self-Treatment* was, of course, to promote the use of the medicines sold at Kihai Hospital, and it advocated the use of eight proprietary treatments developed by the Gotōs.[33] Chief among them was still Seiketsuren, the "miraculous cure" that had figured in Gotō Masafumi's original petition. In addition, Kihai Pharmacy also sold Shichikasan, a medicine in powder form for the treatment of weeping lesions; Hijitsusen, an infusion said to prevent the inflammation of the eyes and loss of hair; and Shūigan, a pill for the treatment of anemia, jaundice, and "exhaustion." Other offerings of the pharmacy included a "release-poison strengthening bath," a powder that was to be dissolved in water to create a medicinal bath; a purgative to "cleanse the stomach"; a "skin-purifying cream" for lesions; and medicated bandages. As this array of products suggests, self-treatment was a costly and time-consuming process. The daily routine the Gotōs advocated included three doses each of Seiketsuren, Shūigan, and Shichikasan, frequent drinking of the Hijitsusen infusion, and the application of the skin cream. In addition, patients were to bathe every five days in medicated bath waters and take a dose of the purgative every seven days.[34]

It is unlikely that many leprosy sufferers would have had the resources to undertake the treatment advocated by the Gotōs. While they offered no information about prices in *Self-Treatment*, a newspaper advertisement from 1896 reveals that at that time a month's supply of just the four main drugs cost 4.25 yen, an impressive amount given that the average wages of a skilled male tradesman in 1896 were in the range of 6–9 yen per month and a farm laborer made on average less than 26 yen a year.[35] For those who wished to be treated on an inpatient basis, the cost was even higher. The cheapest room at Kihai Hospital cost about 9 yen a month, but patients also had to pay for their medicines and meals.[36] As a point of comparison, a month's stay in the Tokyo Public Asylum in this period cost the self-funded patient 1.5 yen for a second-class room and 2.24 yen for a first-class room.[37]

The Gotōs acknowledged that their treatment was expensive, time-consuming, and unpleasant, but they suggested the price of not pursuing it was even higher: "Of course it is very hard to spend money on these disagreeable substances and continue to take them for a year or more. But think about it carefully. . . . If these medicines did not exist, what would [life] be like? People would still curse you saying that you suffer from the heavenly punishment disease or the karmic retribution disease."[38] The evocation of the stigma of the disease in this way—to encourage the purchase of their products—marks an important departure from the philanthropic discourse of the 1870s. Then, ideas such as heavenly punishment and karmic retribution had been the object of derision, held up as hopelessly backward and outdated in the new era of the "cure." Now, the Gotōs themselves made much of the "shame" of the disease in order to promote the benefits of self-treatment. And "shame" was not the only emotion they tried to provoke. In the opening pages of *Self-Treatment*, readers were reminded that "the strength of the nation depends on the health of its citizens" and admonished to aggressively seek to cure themselves "to ensure the prosperity of your family and the strength of the nation," a handy phrase that linked personal concerns and national goals. And in a telling statement that reveals the influence of both early modern medical discourse and the nascent category of race, the Gotōs stated that "when families with bad blood intermarry, then the poison their descendants inherit will grow stronger and stronger, and in the end this could even produce a race of Asian lepers [tōyō raibyō jinshū]."[39]

The Gotōs' new willingness to evoke the stigma of the disease in light of new ideas of class, nation, and race was driven by the financial exigencies of maintaining their business, but their abandonment of the philanthropic rhetoric that celebrated "saving" poor sufferers was part of a new public discourse on leprosy. In the 1880s, private physicians writing on the disease began to make use of language and ideas drawn directly from the public health discourse on acute infectious diseases. The incorporation

of leprosy into the paradigm of infectious disease is most explicit in Kobayashi Hiroshi's 1884 *A New Treatment for Leprosy* (*Chirai shinron*),
the first modern work on leprosy written specifically for an audience of
physicians. Unlike Gotō Masafumi, Kobayashi was the very model of the
new physician. He was a graduate of Tokyo University's medical school,
and in the 1880s and 1890s, he authored a series of books on contemporary
Western clinical medicine, including one on tuberculosis and another on
dysentery. In *A New Treatment for Leprosy*, Kobayashi suggested that there
was a particularly pressing need for a medical discussion of leprosy since
to this point only one work on the disease was available. This he dismissed
as beneath discussion, stating that "it was not written for doctors but for
ordinary people, so it would simply be childish for a doctor to attempt a
serious refutation of this work."[40] The work in question was none other
than the Gotōs' *Self-Treatment*. This is not the only evidence that Gotō
Masafumi's fame prompted Kobayashi to take up leprosy. He also noted
that in 1881 he had accompanied Erwin Bälz, a German doctor who taught
at the medical school of Tokyo University and treated the Meiji elite, on a
visit to Kihai Hospital. They were, however, refused entry by the Gotōs,
with the result that Kobayashi stated that it was impossible for him to
evaluate their treatment.[41]

Given Kobayashi's training and his clear disdain for the Gotōs' work,
it is not surprising that *A New Treatment of Leprosy* plunges us into a
discursive world very different from that of *Self-Treatment*. Instead of
folksy metaphors and beef soup recipes, this work is littered with foreign
names and Latin and German medical terms that have been painstakingly
transcribed into the Japanese syllabary. Even more striking, however, is
Kobayashi's lack of interest in the issue of treatment, the title of his book
notwithstanding. Instead, he focused on the social implications of what is
described as the "leprosy pandemic."[42] As the use of this term, popularized
with the rise of germ theory, reveals, Kobayashi was aware of Hansen's
work and its implications. He wrote, "Following Mr. Hansen's identification of the *M. leprae* there have been several years of experimentation and
now the theory of infection is emphasized. In spite of this, there are still
many people who discuss leprosy, and their debates branch off in many
directions.[43] Kobayashi's summary of these debates is succinct and ac-
curate: they centered on the question of whether vulnerability to infection
was influenced by some other factor, such as heredity, diet, or miasma, or
whether the bacterium in question was simply weak and therefore mildly
contagious.

Kobayashi devoted considerable time to relating the history of the disease in Japan, with the aim of contributing to this discussion. According to his account, immigrants from the continent introduced leprosy to Japan in the sixth century. Even with the passage of more than a thousand years, the disease continued to be prevalent in western Japan where these immigrants settled. According to Kobayashi, many "old leprous families" (*kyūraike*) resided in Kyūshū, Shikoku, and Okinawa. In contrast, the disease is rare in northern Honshū. The source of this demographic data is unclear, given that the first national survey of leprosy did not take place until 1900, but Kobayashi used it to conclude that "leprosy is a contagious disease that has a hereditary component and therefore it takes the form of a regional disease."[44] Thus, while he explicitly abandoned the "multiple cause" paradigm of Gotō and his early modern predecessors and embraced the concept of infection, Kobayashi theorized that susceptibility to the disease must be hereditary given the pattern of its distribution.

The significance of Kobayashi's extended discussion of the history and epidemiology of the disease becomes clear only in the final chapter of *A New Treatment*. Rather than treatment, its central concern was, in fact, prevention. Japan, he declared, was already one of the "leprous countries" (*tarai kokudo*) of the world, and the available treatments could do little to halt the spread of the disease. The Japanese government must follow the example of European countries and institute new national policies. The best option would be to relocate all sufferers to an island or another isolated location, but if this proved too difficult, an alternative would be to construct "leprosy hospitals" around the country and require the removal of all infected people to them. Significantly, the term "leprosy hospital," used by Gotō Masafumi since the early 1870s, was now employed to describe a very different kind of institution. These were not to be treatment centers from which the cured would eventually emerge to fully participate in civic life but institutions of confinement meant to segregate sufferers from the rest of the population. And this was only part of Kobayashi's plan. He was also concerned about the threat posed by those who, although not yet infected, came from leprous lineages and thus were susceptible to infection. To control this danger, Kobayashi suggested making use of the household registry system. However, unlike the *Yomiuri* correspondent who wanted to use the household registries to force sufferers to seek treatment, he proposed enacting laws to prevent those from infected families, whose status would be demarcated within the registries, from intermarrying with "healthy people" (*kenjin*).[45]

Leprosy in the Medical Marketplace

The strategies Kobayashi advocated and his rhetoric, which centered on the need to "improve the race" and "strengthen the nation," reveal his engagement with social Darwinist ideas that were enjoying considerable popularity at the time. But if his aim in writing *A New Treatment* was to capture the eye of policy makers, he failed completely. His book elicited no response from officials, even though its publication coincided with the first signs of interest in leprosy at Tokyo University's medical school, following the appointment of Murata Kentarō as the first professor of dermatology and syphilology. In 1887, the newly founded *Journal of the Tokyo Medical Association* (*Tōkyō igakkai zasshi*) published a talk by Murata titled "The Treatment of Leprosy." Murata described leprosy as a treatable, if not curable, condition, and he made no mention of the "danger" of leprosy to nation and race and issued no call for government intervention.[46]

In fact, Kobayashi found his most enthusiastic reception among patent medicine producers and entrepreneurial doctors, a readership he seems unlikely to have welcomed. In the 1880s, the medicine marketplace quickly became the site where medical entrepreneurs offered up both information on leprosy and the promise of a cure. Writing in 1890, Arai Saku, who had founded his own leprosy hospital, Shūsai Hospital (literally "Public Relief Hospital"), in Sendagi in Tokyo in 1885, listed more than thirty leprosy treatments then available, although he claimed that most were ineffective—unlike, of course, the drugs that he himself was selling.[47] Some of the remedies on the market were worse than ineffective. In 1883, the Home Ministry revoked the license of the Kagoshima-based manufacturer of one leprosy "cure" after several people died from taking it.[48] While many of the remedies Arai examined were, like this one, marketed as "secret family recipes" (*hikaden*) and sold out of homes or peddled on the streets to a purely local clientele, others were part of the emerging nationwide trade in modern proprietary medicines.

Raichigan (literally "leprosy-curing pill") is an example of this new kind of drug. It was manufactured and sold by Mori Kichibei, the proprietor of Chōjudō, a pharmacy in Osaka. Born in 1854, Mori began his career at age ten as an apprentice to a wholesaler of Chinese materia medica in the Osaka neighborhood of Doshōmachi, where the trade in the raw materials for Sino-Japanese medicines was based. In the late 1870s, he was one of a number of Doshōmachi merchants who abandoned the raw medicine business to get involved directly in drug production and the lucrative retail market. Beginning in the 1880s, Mori's new pharmacy began to sell a

number of Western-style drugs, including Hebarugan, which claimed efficacy for "sensitive stomachs" and "infectious disease." The latter term
was an oblique reference to cholera, and Hebarugan was in fact a diarrhea
cure. Cholera treatments were sure sellers in this era of frequent epidemics and launched the careers of several manufacturers, most notably that
of Morita Jihei, whose drug Hōtan was perhaps the best-known patent
drug of the 1870s and 1880s. Hebarugan, too, met with some success, and
Mori soon expanded his product line, introducing two leprosy treatments,
Raichigan, a medicine in pill form, and Pattosan, a bath additive that, like
Gotō's similar concoction, claimed to make it possible to replicate the
benefits of hot-spring bathing in one's own bathtub. A two-month supply
of Raichigan cost six yen and Pattosan cost ten sen per treatment, making
Mori's treatment less expensive than Gotō's, but not by much.[49]

Important for our purposes is the understanding of leprosy that Mori
evoked to market his treatments. Like the Gotōs, he, too, produced a booklet designed to promote his product. Called *A Popular Account of Leprosy*
(*Tsuzoku raibyō monogatari*, 1887), it sold for only six sen but consisted
largely of materials lifted directly from Kobayashi's book, including the
historical discussion of the spread of leprosy, the summary of the debates
that followed Hansen's discovery of *M. leprae*, and the conclusion that
leprosy was an infectious disease with a hereditary component. Left out
of Mori's book was any part of Kobayashi's culminating chapter, with
its advocacy of a government program of confinement and surveillance.
Instead, in an extraordinary passage that frames paragraphs from *A New
Treatment* with the idea of "rights" and the Enlightenment conception of
"progress," Mori turned Kobayashi's discussion of prevention on its head,
arguing that far from being modern, confinement was actually an approach
taken in the distant past, when the rights of individuals were ignored:

> In Europe at around the end of the thirteenth century, the authorities made
> it an official policy that leprosy should be hated, and in France especially
> the sick were treated as though they were already dead. Moreover, strict
> laws were established that required sufferers to wear special clothing so
> they could be seen from afar, and those identified as lepers in this way
> were ostracized. On top of this, it was then decided that the sick must be
> separated from the healthy. As in ancient China, officials drew lines to
> designate leprosy districts and the sick were required to move there and
> were not allowed to leave. In our country, too, in Nara's leper villages
> and in Kyoto's Hiden'in, although there were some small differences, the

right of all human beings to be independent [*ningen jishu no ken*] was usurped. This is something to be pitied and deplored. But now in Meiji, the era of progress when culture advances day by day, of course it is a different world from that time. Among the many great men of this era, there are those like Professor Ogata Sessai, who has developed a miraculous medicine that cures leprosy, the disease regarded as incurable. And I have the great honor of being entrusted to sell this product to the world.[50]

This is the earliest injection of the discussion of "rights" into the discussion of leprosy that I have identified. The term *ken* that appears in this passage began to be used as a translation for "rights" in the European political sense of constitutional or natural rights only in the 1860s. As Douglas Howland has indicated, before this time its meaning was closer to "power and privilege," and it referred to the prerogatives of social elites.[51] The term *jishu no ken* (the right to independence) figured prominently in Nakamura Masanao's translation of Samuel Smiles's *Self-Help*, one of the first modern best sellers in Japan.[52] While this may have helped *ken* and *kenri* become the accepted terms for individual rights with the connotation of personal freedom, ambiguity remained. The character *ken* also figured in another neologism, *kokken*, or "state sovereignty" (literally "state's rights"). In the late 1870s and 1880s, the question of the relationship of the state's rights to the rights of individuals shaped the struggle known as the Freedom and People's Rights Movement. This popular movement for democracy and constitutional government was harshly criticized by members of the governmental elite as an illegitimate attempt to infringe upon the sovereign powers of the state—and the sovereign himself, the emperor.

To be sure, it is unlikely that Mori intended his readers to parse the meaning of *jishu no ken*, but its inclusion in this bit of marketing is suggestive of the power of commercial discourse at this time, for the marketing of both products and ideas. Mori's aim was to establish the backwardness of confinement in relation to the modernity of treatment. His pointed attribution of the development of his product to Ogata Sessai, a standard feature of his print ads, also served to make this point. The adopted son and heir of Ogata Kōan, the renowned Osaka "Dutch learning" scholar, Sessai was a prominent figure in the movement to modernize medicine in Osaka in the 1870s and 1880s. In 1869, he played an important role in the formation of the city's first hospital and its medical school, the precursor of Osaka University's medical school, and twenty years later he joined other city leaders to establish Osaka Charity Hospital to extend free medical care to the poor. Mori's evocation of Sessai's name in this way thus linked his drug directly with modern medicine, distinguishing it both from competitors and from the uncivilized practice of confinement.

Mori was not the only medical entrepreneur to make use of Kobayashi's work for his own purposes. In 1890, Arai Saku responded to *A New Treatment* in a work he called *Experiments on Leprosy Treatment* (*Chirai keikensetsu*), written to promote his Shūsai Hospital. At its peak in 1889, this institution, located in Hongō, housed almost seven hundred patients, with another three hundred receiving treatment on an outpatient basis. In contrast, by this time the popularity of Kihai Hospital, now located in Shiba, not far from Shiba Park, seems to have waned. Its total clientele had fallen to less than three hundred patients.[53] No less than Mori, Arai was overtly critical of the policy of confinement that Kobayashi advocated. Segregation, he wrote, would accomplish nothing, except "great inconvenience for those who are sick," because leprosy is not an infectious disease. Information about Arai's background before he founded his clinic is elusive. In *Experiments*, he wrote that his search for a leprosy cure stretched back to 1876, when he traveled to Germany to learn more about the disease. However, eventually recognizing that German medicine had nothing to offer in terms of leprosy research, he departed for India in 1881. There, he took up residence in an "island province" populated by leprosy sufferers and began researching treatment methods. Returning to Japan in 1882, he founded his clinic and began testing his treatments, which drew upon Western, Chinese, and Japanese medical knowledge, with the result that he eventually "completely cured" more than 150 people.[54] In fact, there is no corroborating evidence for this story, and given the considerable financial, linguistic, and bureaucratic difficulties involved in undertaking overseas study privately in the 1870s, it seems likely that Arai invented his tale of research abroad as a means to legitimate his treatment and enhance his reputation.

Kihai Hospital and Shūsai Hospital were the largest, best-known, and most successful leprosy hospitals in this period, but there were many others as well. In the period between 1880 and 1908 at least eighteen private hospitals and clinics that advertised themselves as specializing in the treatment of leprosy were in operation in various parts of Tokyo. As map 2 indicates, these institutions were scattered around Tokyo, with one, Aisei Hospital, only a short walk from the environs of the imperial place. Most were located near train and streetcar routes. One popular site was Kyōbashi Ward, one of the most densely populated areas of the city; another was the area around Ueno Station. Ueno was an important node in the transportation system, and it was also located near Tokyo University Hospital. Patients often turned to this, the premier hospital of the time, for a second opinion after a diagnosis of leprosy by a local doctor. Enterprising physicians may well have established their clinics nearby with the intent to attract those who had just received devastating confirmation of their condition. What is clear is that these institutions were by no means concealed or relegated to the periphery of the cityscape of Tokyo. Rather they were positioned with visibility and ease of access in mind.

Some of the leprosy clinics and hospitals were in business for a relatively short time (see table 1). As Wei-ti Chen has demonstrated, setting up a new practice in this period was an expensive proposition for a young

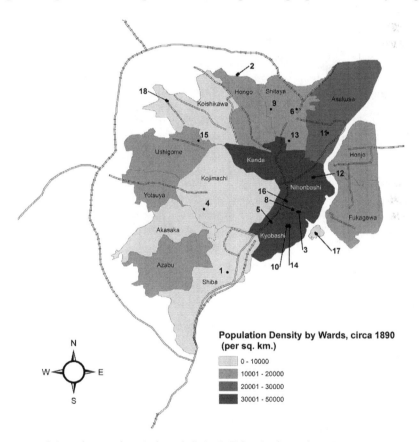

MAP 2.   Private leprosy hospitals and clinics in Tokyo in the early 1890s.

TABLE 1. Clinics and hospitals in Tokyo offering treatment for leprosy, 1883–1909.

ID	Name	Location	Years in operation	Diseases and conditions treated
1	Kihai Hospital	Shiba	1883–1905	Leprosy
2	Shusai Hospital	Hongo	1886–ca. 1905	Leprosy
3	Katō Hospital	Kyōbashi	1892–1906	Leprosy, syphilis, skin diseases
4	Aisei Hospital	Kojimachi	1890–1909	Syphilis, leprosy, skin diseases
5	Yamamoto Clinic	Kyōbashi	1890–1905	Syphilis, hemorrhoids, leprosy, uterine disease
6	Sakuragi Hospital	Shitaya	1891–1893	Leprosy, ringworm
7	Religion Hospital Kyūsekan	Ikegami village	1892	Leprosy
8	Kuyōdō Clinic	Kyōbashi	1893	Leprosy, skin diseases
9	Tokyo Geka Hifu Hospital	Sakuragi	1893–1895	Ear, nose, and throat diseases; leprosy, syphilis, skin disease
10	Marumo Hospital	Kyōbashi	1895–1909	Internal medical conditions, skin diseases, leprosy
11	Oda Clinic	Asakusa	1895–1903	Leprosy, ringworm, syphilis
12	Junseidō Clinic	Nihonbashi	1895–1905	Leprosy, syphilis, gonorrhea, diseases of the reproductive organs
13	Wada Clinic	Shitaya	1898–1899	Syphilis, leprosy, skin diseases
14	Menkandō Clinic	Honjo	1898–?	Leprosy
15	Tokyo Dermatology Specialty Clinic	Asakusa	1898	Leprosy, syphilis, gonorrhea
16	Aiseikan Clinic	Nihonbashi	1900–?	Leprosy, syphilis, tuberculosis, hemorrhoids
17	Sekizendō	Kyōbashi	1901	Leprosy, syphilis, gonorrhea
18	Gotō Leprosy Clinic	Koishikawa	1904–?	Leprosy

ID numbers in this table correlate with those used in map 2.

doctor and especially challenging in Tokyo, where graduates of the new medical schools preferred to remain, a situation that gave rise to intense competition for patients. It is likely that some doctors began to specialize in treating leprosy with the aim of carving out a place for themselves in the overcrowded medical marketplace of Tokyo.[55] From this perspective, it is not surprising that many of those who operated leprosy clinics also advertised their expertise in relation to other stigmatized diseases, especially sexually transmitted diseases such as syphilis and gonorrhea.

Commercial motives notwithstanding, unlike Gotō, with his roots in early modern medicine, and Arai, who would later be characterized as a quack, some of those involved in the new leprosy trade were well-educated modern doctors.[56] Katō Hospital, which specialized in the treatment of syphilis and leprosy, was founded by Katō Tokijirō. The son of a physician, Katō began his medical education in 1877 in the short-lived Forensic Medical School that was established by the Tokyo Police Bureau. He then entered Tokyo University's medical school but left after only one year, apparently because of financial difficulties. The rest of his medical education came via a stint in the private Saisei Academy, a cram school that prepared students for the medical licensing exam. Katō successfully passed the Tokyo licensing exam in 1882 and for a time was employed in a syphilis clinic operated by the Tokyo police and as the "ward doctor" for Kyōbashi Ward in Tokyo. In 1883, however, he married into a wealthy family of medicine wholesalers, an event that significantly improved his prospects. After successfully passing the new national licensing exam, he left for Germany, where he studied medicine from 1888 to 1890 and encountered socialism for the first time. After his return to Japan, he founded his hospital in Kyōbashi, where he was already well known. At the same time, he became active in the famed Commoners' Society, an early socialist organization. His interest in left-wing politics notwithstanding, Katō was well connected with Tokyo's medical and public health elite. He played a prominent role in an organization called the Popular Hygiene Society, led a campaign against efforts by doctors of Sino-Japanese medicine to be licensed, and later joined medical luminaries such as Kitasato Shibasaburō, Japan's celebrated bacteriologist, to create an organization to support military doctors during the Russo-Japanese War.[57] Katō's hospital, then, was no fly-by-night operation.

The credentials of Dohi Keizō, who was director of the short-lived Tokyo Dermatological Hospital, were even more impressive. Like Katō, Dohi, too, was the son of a physician, and he went on to excel at the medical school of the Imperial University, as Tokyo University was re-named in 1886. After graduating in 1891, for a time he worked as an assistant to Julius Scriba, the German doctor who taught surgery at the medical school, before moving on to Tokyo Dermatological Hospital, which was located in front of Ueno Station. Ads instructed potential patients that it was near the Panoramakan, a popular attraction that immersed visitors in panoramic landscapes and representations of historical events. Reflecting Dohi's prestigious credentials and presumably his knowledge of leprosy's infectiousness, newspaper ads for the hospital stressed that leprosy patients would be housed separately from others and that treatments were based upon "academic research." His stint as director was cut short, however, when Dohi was selected to study in Germany on a government scholarship only a few months after taking on the directorship.[58] Upon his return to Japan, Dohi joined the faculty of the university medical school as a professor of dermatology and urology.

Not every commercial leprosy hospital was medical and modern in its orientation. The most extraordinary institution of this period was the Dai Nippon Kyūsekan (literally "Great Japan Saving the World Institute"). Advertised as a "religious hospital" (shūkyō byōin), it was the brainchild of Tanaka Chigaku and Ota Kōsaku. Tanaka was an ardent proponent of Nichiren Buddhism who later became famous for his promotion of "Nichi-renism," an interpretation of Nichiren doctrine that promoted emperor-centered nationalism. The central object of worship in Nichiren Buddhism was the Lotus Sutra, and leprosy sufferers were known to gather on the grounds of Nichiren temples. In contrast, Ota was an enterprising physician who specialized in the treatment of syphilis, leprosy, and dermatological ailments. In 1888, he had published an English-language booklet advertising his skills, presumably with the intention of appealing to foreign residents and travelers.[59] By 1891, he was also the proprietor of Sakuragi Hospital, which like Dohi's Tokyo Dermatological Hospital was located near Ueno Station.

Like Gotō, Mori, and Arai, Ota, too, published a treatise on leprosy designed to promote his services. Entitled A Refutation on the Pathology of Leprosy (Raibyō byōri benmō), it reiterated the familiar theory that leprosy was a blood disease, originally self-produced, that was spread from parent to child.[60] The work also laid out familiar rules for controlling the disease, including the use of medication, a long list of forbidden foods, and the proscription of any kind of sexual stimulation. However, Ota framed his discussion of leprosy's etiology around a new claim, arguing that the rising rates of both leprosy and "lung disease" (a popular euphemism for tuberculosis) were the unintended result of the government policy of promoting smallpox vaccination. According to Ota, smallpox had in fact been "nature's good medicine," because it aided the expulsion of "fetal poison"(*taidoku*), a substance widely believed to pass from mother to child within the womb and that Ota argued caused both leprosy and lung disease. He argued that when children failed to develop smallpox and thereby expel the poison, they were fated to suffer from these more serious diseases and later to pass them on to their children. The notion that smallpox resulted from fetal poison had a long history in Sino-Japanese medicine. It had figured in pregnancy manuals for women dating back to the eighteenth century. Ota's innovation was to relate this familiar idea to popular anxieties surrounding compulsory vaccination and to concern that cases of leprosy were on the rise.

It is unclear whether Ota believed this theory or was seeking to exploit popular resistance to vaccination to advertise his clinic—although his subsequent actions in relation to the Kyūsekan support the latter conclusion. The "religious hospital" was established on the grounds of Ikegami Honmonji, a famous Nichiren temple located in a village south of Tokyo. According to an article published in *Meikyō shinshi*, a Buddhist newspaper associated with the Pure Land sect, its aim was to "use Buddhism's boundless love for the public to contribute to the mutual aid of the nation by providing comfort and treatment to leprosy sufferers who are the most unfortunate people in mankind." What was remarkable about this institution was its explicit use of the theory that leprosy resulted from karmic retribution. The author of the *Meikyō shinshi* article wrote that through sermons and teaching the hospital would offer the patients a chance to "recover from their illness by reducing their karmic burden."[61]

Ota himself actively promoted the idea that leprosy resulted from karmic retribution. In 1892, he published a booklet to advertise the services of the Kyūsekan. In this work there is no mention of smallpox. Instead, while still characterizing "bad blood" as the primary cause of the disease, Ota suggested that when a case of leprosy proved intractable, it was possible that karmic retribution was also involved. This was where Kyūsekan came in. "High-ranking priests" of the Nichiren sect would offer patients guidance in Buddhist practice, while Ota prescribed medicines, a two-pronged approach described as akin to "adding a steam engine to a sailing boat." Like his competitors, Ota was quick to frame this endeavor in nationalistic rhetoric: Kyūsekan would contribute to the advancement of hygiene in Japan while promoting what he called "Japanese religion" around the world.[62]

Unfortunately for its backers, the peculiar mixture of Buddhism, medicine, and nationalism on offer at the Kyūsekan apparently attracted few patients, and the hospital closed after only a year in operation. But Ota's efforts are revealing of the problematic nature of the "trade" in leprosy in the 1890s. Flawed though it was, the philanthropic efforts of the 1870s and early 1880s had the intention of extending treatment and the possibility of a cure to as many victims of the disease as possible. However, after the withdrawal of public funding, leprosy quickly came to be embedded in a flourishing but highly competitive medical marketplace, with the result that exaggerated claims and unsubstantiated theories came to be featured in advertisements and journalistic discourse, usually accompanied by rhetorical appeals to national pride and civic duty. Far more concerned about the impact of acute infectious diseases for its program of modernization, the Meiji government had little, if any, interest in leprosy in this moment and so it was medical entrepreneurs and their journalist allies who began to shape public perceptions. And while a few, like Mori Kichibei, deployed the new language of "rights," others like the Gotōs and Ota were willing to evoke popular prejudices, personal anxieties, and nationalist rhetoric to sell their services.

We cannot know how consumers—as leprosy sufferers were newly cast—negotiated the proliferation of newspaper articles, advertisements, pamphlets, and books, although Mori Kichibei's use of Enlightenment discourse seems to have succeeded and Ota's evocation of karma to have failed. Even more opaque is the fate of those like Nishiyama Kyōzan, who probably knew little of the costly treatments on offer in Tokyo and other cities or of the new and conflicting meanings attached to the disease that had defined his life. As late as 1886 he was still reminding local authorities that the loss of begging rights had devastated his community, and by 1896 he was dead. The last resident of Kōmyōin was a woman called Naka, described in some documents as Kyōzan's wife. The daughter of a wealthy local family, she retained possession of some assets even after she became ill and left home to join her fellow sufferers at the temple. She lived on into the 1910s, eking out a modest living by making small loans, with interest, to her neighbors.[63] By the time of her death, however, the Japanese government had begun to define a leprosy policy.

Chapter 4

Between the Global and the Local

Japan's 1907 Leprosy Law

I n 1893, Chinda Sutemi, the Japanese consul in San Francisco, was approached by a member of the board of health of that city.[1] More than ten cases of leprosy had been identified in San Francisco in that year, and their numbers included migrants from China, Finland, Singapore, and Mexico, as well as the "Bindt Brothers," as local newspapers described three young men born in Honolulu to an American mother.[2] The board of health proposed sending San Francisco's leprosy patients, who were then confined in the municipal quarantine center known as the "pesthouse," to Kihai Hospital for treatment. Chinda sent a detailed report of this proposal to the Foreign Ministry in Tokyo, noting that Gotō Masafumi, who had been approached directly by a San Francisco official, was of the belief that an affirmative response would "not only be of credit to his hospital but would also be in the national interest." Chinda disagreed. He characterized this as an attempt on the part of San Francisco authorities to use Japan as a "garbage dump" (*suteba*) for its leprosy sufferers and argued that for the "self-defense of Japan" the government needed to emulate the United States and ban entry to the country by anyone suffering from the disease.[3]

This minor incident in the global history of leprosy is a window into the new international politics of the disease in the age of high imperialism. Zachary Gussow has argued that leprosy, all but forgotten in much of the Western world by this time, was rediscovered and "re-tainted" as Europeans and Americans began to encounter its sufferers in their colonies and among migrant populations from Asia and elsewhere. They reacted with "lepraphobia," casting the disease as a threat posed by racial and ethnic others, an attitude exacerbated by Hansen's discovery of *M. leprae* and the confirmation it offered of leprosy's infectiousness. Gussow suggests that this attitude began to shape attitudes towards the disease in places where it continued to be endemic, marking it with new forms of stigma.[4]

Much of the recent work by Japanese scholars on Japan's leprosy policy parallels Gussow's discussion of the formation of lepraphobia. The Japanese state, it is argued, came to view leprosy as a national "shame" that undermined Japan's place among the advanced nations, and the government responded by quarantining its sufferers, "sacrificing" them on the altar of civilization, to paraphrase Sawano Masaki.[5] This chapter seeks to complicate this narrative by reexamining the international context in which Japanese policy took form. I argue that at a time when the coerced confinement of sufferers was endorsed by leading scientists, proposals to implement such a policy in Japan led to a prolonged and divisive debate centered on different conceptions of citizenship and the reach and responsibility of the modern Japanese state. The 1907 law that resulted from this debate was a limited one that reflected growing concern about poverty rather than infection.

Japan and International Medical Discourse

While the endemic nature of leprosy did not go unnoticed by the foreign tourists and sojourners who began to travel to East Asia in increasing numbers from the 1870s, Japan escaped the label of a "leprous" country that was widely used to characterize neighboring China. Instead, Japan quickly gained a worldwide reputation as a place where the disease could be successfully treated. The new medical internationalism of the late nineteenth century, which propelled discussion of leprosy as a public health threat, has often been understood in light of the rise of international organizations, congresses, and treaties, but a variety of private, nonstate actors were also involved in the circulation of ideas about disease, treatment, and health, among them doctors, patients, journalists, missionaries, and ordinary travelers.[6] It was via these informal patterns of movement, transfer, and exchange that Japan's private clinics and hospitals began to attract international attention.

Given his domestic fame at the time, it is not surprising that Gotō Masafumi played an important role in establishing Japan's reputation as a center of cutting-edge leprosy treatments. In 1879, an American businessman residing in Yokohama wrote to a member of the Board of Health of Hawai'i informing him of Gotō's success in treating leprosy and alerting the board that he was sending samples of Gotō's proprietary compounds to Honolulu, presumably to cultivate an overseas market.[7] The Hawaiian government had adopted the policy of confining leprosy sufferers to the remote Kalaupapa "colony" on the island of Moloka'i more than a decade before, but interest in treatment continued. The board followed up on this report, seeking further information from Duane B. Simmons, an American doctor who had set up a private practice in Yokohama. His response to the board's inquiry was not encouraging. While he acknowledged that Gotō was well known among "the natives," Simmons expressed doubt that this "man of little or no scientific attainment" could really cure leprosy.[8]

In spite of Simmons's skepticism, in 1881 when the Hawaiian king David Kalākaua traveled to Japan as a part of an official trip around the world, he visited Kihai Hospital and consulted with Gotō about his treatment methods, an event widely reported in the Japanese press. Following the king's visit, information about Kihai Hospital made its way back to Hawai'i with remarkable speed. In the early 1880s, at least three American residents of the islands, a wealthy businessman named Gilbert Waller and a woman named Frances and her teenage daughter, all came to Japan to seek treatment at Kihai Hospital, by this time in its third and final location in Shiba Ward.[9] The fate of Frances and her daughter is unclear, but Father Damien, the Belgian priest who famously contracted leprosy while at Kalaupapa, wrote to a colleague about the experience of Gilbert Waller. According to Father Damien, Waller had returned to Hawai'i after three years in Japan "with all the appearance of a cure."[10]

Prompted by reports like this, in 1885 board of health officials in Hawai'i invited the Gotōs to visit Hawai'i and treat patients there so that their methods could be evaluated. Masanao, the son, savvily responded with a request for a two-year contract.[11] The board of health agreed to his terms, and Masanao arrived in Hawai'i in 1886 with a substantial supply of the Gotōs' medicines. In addition to his official duties, Masanao also operated a private clinic, where he treated people of means who hoped to avoid forced relocation to Moloka'i. His patients in this period included Father Damien, who became an enthusiastic supporter, as did many of those he treated on Moloka'i, some of whom were released after their condition improved dramatically following treatment.[12] Damien of course was not so lucky. He died in 1889, becoming arguably leprosy's most famous victim.

By the time of Damien's death, Masanao, whose contract with the board of health had expired, had moved on to San Francisco, where he briefly enrolled at Cooper Medical College, a not unusual course of action for an ambitious young Japanese doctor at a time when overseas study was a mark of distinction, but he also seems to have used his sojourn in California to advertise the services of Kihai Hospital. In 1887, Masanao returned to Japan, but he was soon followed by two American women from San Francisco, a mother and daughter, who entered Kihai Hospital in 1888 for a course of treatment that would last two years.[13]

By the early 1890s Kihai Hospital seems to have been well known even beyond Hawai'i and the West Coast of the United States. When the German ophthalmologist Julius Hirschberg visited Japan, he toured the hospital (as well as other medical institutions in Tokyo), an event later recorded in his popular account of his world tour, which brought a distinctively medical perspective to the familiar genre of the travelogue. To Hirschberg, it was remarkable that patients entered the hospital voluntarily and were free to leave at any time—a reflection of his knowledge and acceptance of the policy of coercive confinement already in place in Hawai'i and Norway. The claim that featured in some print ads for Kihai Hospital—that it was famous "all around Japan of course, but also in England, America, France, Germany, Hawai'i, and every other foreign country"—was not entirely an exaggeration.[14] Other medical entrepreneurs, too, began to promote their treatments abroad. Arai Saku, for one, prepared a slick pamphlet in English to advertise his hospital outside Japan. It described him as the "President of the Leper Hospital of Hongo, Tokyo," and offered up a lengthy explanation of his expertise, including the claim that of the 4,875 people he had treated (including 106 foreigners from the United States, China, and India), 4,008 had been cured. Treatment "in pleasant and home-like" surroundings was offered at ten dollars a month.[15]

As Tokyo's private hospitals began to attract an international clientele, so, too, did another site, the hot-spring resort town called Kusatsu in Gunma Prefecture, about two hundred kilometers from Tokyo. As discussed in chapter 2, in the early modern period, some doctors believed hot-spring bathing could worsen the symptoms of *rai*. Many patients, it seems, disagreed, and the sulfurous waters at Kusatsu gained a reputation for efficacy for leprosy and other skin ailments. In this period, most of those who traveled to Kusatsu for treatment were apparently transient visitors. While they bathed alongside other guests, people with leprosy stayed in special inns known locally as "leper inns" (*kattaibōya*).[16] In 1871, however, a disastrous fire struck Kusatsu and destroyed much of the town. In its aftermath, the town's leaders began a publicity campaign designed to attract more visitors in order to finance rebuilding. The pamphlet they designed made much of the local water's effects on leprosy, and leprosy sufferers, newly emancipated and able to travel freely, began to arrive. Some settled there, investing in property and establishing businesses.[17]

The rising number of people with leprosy at Kusatsu, both visitors and residents, coincided with new interest on the part of foreign residents of Japan in the potentially curative properties of Kusatsu's waters. Hydrotherapy was popular among Europeans at this time, and mineral-water spas were much in vogue as an international tourist and leisure activity. Regular periods of rest and bathing at hot-spring resorts were believed to be particularly beneficial to residents in the colonies, whose health was endangered by the physical, cultural, and social hardships of life among non-Europeans.[18] Japan of course was not a colony, but this view prevailed among foreign residents nonetheless. In 1878, Erwin Bälz, the German physician on the faculty of Tokyo University's medical school, visited Kusatsu for the first time. He came away much impressed with its potential to become a modern European-style spa and played a role in promoting it among Tokyo's foreign residents.[19] Situated in a beautiful spot in the shadow of several volcanic mountains, Kusatsu soon began to attract international visitors, and it gained a place in the guidebooks and travelogues intended for Western readers.

The opportunity to view leprosy sufferers seems to have been a part of the Kusatsu tourist experience. The Irish travel writer Lewis Strange Wingfield described Kusatsu in his 1889 *Wanderings of a Globe-Trotter in the Far East*, remarking on the stark contrast between the beauty of its natural surroundings ("nature divinely fair") and the bathers one encountered there, who offered the opportunity "for studying the most fell of diseases in all its horrors."[20] The British Japanologist Basil Hall Chamberlain expressed similar sentiments in his popular guidebook, *A Handbook for Travellers in Japan*, remarking that "the horrors that walk the streets must be seen to be believed."[21] As Kusatsu gained new popularity among both foreign and domestic travelers, town leaders began to reconsider their earlier strategy of marketing the spa to leprosy sufferers. They decided that the town's tourist economy would be better served if residents with the disease, some of whom by this time operated inns, restaurants, and other businesses that served their fellow sufferers, were to relocate outside of the central part of the town. This led to the founding of a new community that became known as Yunosawa (literally "hot-spring marsh") on what had been wasteland. This did not mean that leprosy sufferers were confined to this area. Rather they continued to move freely around the town, although they now bathed in separate facilities.[22]

If some Western writers emphasized the voyeuristic appeal of Kusatsu, others took note of the therapeutic benefits of its waters. The

French journalist M. Louis Bastide described Kusatsu as equipped with special facilities for the three hundred or so leprosy sufferers in residence. A summary of this report, originally published in the popular monthly *Revue des deux mondes*, was subsequently reprinted in some of the most prominent medical journals of the day, including the *British Medical Journal*, *Journal of the American Medical Association*, and the *Medical Record*. Equally impressed by Kusatsu was W. K. Burton, a British engineer in the employ of the Japanese government. In an 1891 article first published in the *Annals of Hygiene*, Burton described the Kusatsu baths as offering a cure for leprosy—a point he emphasized through the inclusion of a rare photograph of a Japanese leprosy sufferer, freshly emerged from the hot waters.[23] It was around this time that Bälz, too, became interested in leprosy and began to publicize the curative properties of Kusatsu's waters in German medical journals.[24] By 1900, reports about Kusatsu were appearing in the American mass media. In that year, for example, the *San Francisco Chronicle* published a lengthy article celebrating "Wonderful Japanese Baths, Where the Leprous Are Made Clean."[25] Not only were the waters said to have a miraculous effect on "all skin diseases, gout, and even rheumatism," but they could also cure "leprosy in its early stages permanently" and temporarily arrest the progress of the disease in even advanced cases. The anonymous author emphasized, correctly, that the "leper village" was separate from the rest of the town and had its own facilities, but he also marveled that "strangely enough, the afflicted town was busily engaged in all sorts of business just like human beings [*sic*]."

In the 1880s, some critics of the rising tide of lepraphobia internationally began to point to Japan as an example of a reasonable and humane approach to the disease. In this period, colonial physicians and missionary doctors often positioned themselves as medical ethnographers of the countries where they worked, publishing case reports, discussions of new therapies, and translations and summaries of medical treatises for the benefit of their colleagues at home.[26] Erwin Bälz published often on Japan in German medical and scientific journals, and while much of this work was predictably tinged with the orientalism of the day, his reports on leprosy were different. They were written to criticize European attitudes towards the diseases.[27]

Bälz contributed the first of a series of essays on leprosy to Japan to a volume of essays called *Lepra Studien* (Studies of Leprosy), which was published in Hamburg in 1885.[28] His contribution was one of two ethnographic reports on the disease (the other was on Norway), in a volume otherwise devoted to histological studies. In the 1880s, the international medical community was still bitterly divided over the question of whether leprosy was truly an infectious disease, with many doctors expressing doubt that Hansen's discovery of *M. leprae* had settled the issue. Even those committed to the theory of infection were troubled by their inability to explain the path of transmission or why so many people seemed resistant to infection even in the face of prolonged exposure.[29] In his essay, Bälz deployed information from Japan in a manner that would become increasingly common in the next two decades, arguing that the country's considerable number of leprosy sufferers made it a veritable laboratory for the clinical study of the disease.[30]

Citing the depth of his experience in Japan, Bälz addressed what he recognized as the most important question of the day, the issue of leprosy's infectiousness. He agreed that it was indeed infectious, but only mildly so since "the presence and even reception of the bacilli is not sufficient. . . . The point is that the bacilli find the proper soil for their nutrition and this favorable soil is a mostly hereditary weakness of the tissues."[31] The conclusion that some kind of hereditary susceptibility must be involved was by no means unique (nor in fact was his soil metaphor), but Bälz supported his position by a lengthy discussion of evidence from Japan. He noted that while inmates in Japan's new prisons were exposed to leprosy for a prolonged period, in close contact and in poor conditions, the disease did not spread, and while the disease was rarely seen in the densely crowded slums of the cities, it was common in impoverished and insular rural areas. E. H. Ackernecht has argued that the late nineteenth–century debate on contagion versus hereditary transmission was never merely a matter of scientific inquiry: it was always implicated in the social and political issue of whether leprosy sufferers should be quarantined.[32] This was true in the case of Bälz. In his 1885 essay, he referenced his experiences in Japan to argue passionately against the ascendant view that strict segregation of sufferers was necessary, stating, "Let him who in the face of these experiences has the courage to demand the exclusion of all leprosy sufferers from human society, do so. I cannot."[33]

In 1897, Bälz returned to the issue of leprosy in a German medical journal, this time in response to the outcry that followed the discovery of a cluster of cases of leprosy in Germany near the Baltic seaport town of Memel (now the city of Klaipėda in Lithuania) in 1889. The appearance of the disease within the German Empire caused widespread consternation, particularly since it could not be traced to the kind of racial others then associated with transmission. The German bacteriologist Robert Koch investigated the "outbreak" and eventually attributed it to recent migrants from the Baltic states, evidence that there were still pockets of endemic leprosy in various parts of Europe.[34] Bälz again argued that the disease posed no great threat to the general population. As evidence, he pointed to the Tokyo Poorhouse, where nurses cared for "lepers of the worst kind, with mutilated limbs and covered with ulcerations" in very unhygienic conditions, and yet in sixteen years none of the staff had been infected.[35]

Included in this essay were the case studies of four non-Japanese leprosy sufferers (three Americans and a German, all adult men) whom Bälz treated in the 1890s, apparently as part of his private practice. Bälz wrote that these patients came to Japan from Hawai'i immediately after their diagnosis in order to avoid transfer to Moloka'i. He treated them with a combination of chaulmoogra pills, the extensive use of a salicylic acid salve, and months of bathing at Kusatsu, and concluded that this regime had produced a remarkable improvement of their symptoms, if not a complete cure. One man, he noted, was so transformed that the public health officer who had diagnosed him in Hawai'i could find no evidence of the disease upon his return from Japan. Based on this evidence, Bälz asserted again that the segregation of leprosy sufferers was unnecessary: the disease was infectious, but weakly so, and eminently treatable.[36] However, his attempt to calm fears in Germany notwithstanding, a leprosarium was created in Memel in 1899 and in 1900 a statutory requirement for confinement was established.

If evidence from Japan failed to quell the wave of lepraphobia, it was also open to alternative interpretation. The American doctor Albert Ashmead used the example of Japan to argue for, not against, segregation. A native of Philadelphia, Ashmead had arrived in Japan in 1873 and taken up a position in the government-supported charity hospital, a job offer that resulted from his successful treatment of a Japanese nobleman who fell ill while on a trip to the United States. Not long after his arrival in Tokyo, Ashmead first encountered cases of leprosy. In a report he sent to the *Philadelphia Medical Times* in 1874 Ashmead described what he called "Japanese leprosy," a term he devised to characterize "a disease found here which I have never found in any medical work or journal."[37] Later Ashmead grasped that there was nothing specifically "Japanese" about the disease he had observed, and upon his return to New York in 1876, he quickly set about establishing himself as an expert on leprosy by referencing his experiences in Japan, citing Japanese practices, folklore about the disease, and his own observations as evidence to assert that not only was leprosy infectious, but it could also be spread by intermediaries, such as mosquitoes, which could transfer the infected blood of an infected person to the healthy.[38] In other words, he believed that the disease could spread without direct person-to-person contact.

Ashmead would hold this position for the next three decades, and it made him a passionate proponent of both segregation and immigration restrictions. He supplied American newspapers and medical journals with a steady stream of warnings about the threat of leprosy until his death in 1911. Typical of these was an opinion piece published in the *New York Times* in 1901, in which Ashmead suggested that Japanese immigrants to the United States, infected with leprosy, threatened the health of residents of the Pacific Northwest who fished for salmon in the Columbia River. According to Ashmead, the Japanese were passing the disease to the fish, which in turn infected those who caught and consumed them.[39] As this baseless theory suggests, Ashmead was an old-school clinician with no understanding of modern bacteriology, and he was treated with contempt by Hansen and other scientists.[40]

Ashmead's views were also colored by his xenophobia. While he argued that "Orientals" posed the greatest threat to the health of American citizens, his animosity extended to Norwegians as well. He repeatedly charged that Norway's resolution of its leprosy problem had been accomplished by exporting its infected citizens to the American Midwest.[41] Ashmead was, however, a fan of Gotō Masafumi, with whom he was personally acquainted, and in 1894, he published an English summary of Gotō Masafumi's 1882 *Self-Treatment of the Intractable Disease* in an American medical journal. In his introduction, he describes Masafumi and his son as "the most eminent leprologists in Japan," who are "in charge of the largest Japanese leper hospital." They were friends of the late Hawaiian king, former employees of the Hawaiian government, and "as good authority as can be wished for on the subject of leprosy."[42]

Public health officials in San Francisco may have learned of Gotō's success in treating leprosy via publications such as this one or from Gotō Masanao. Although Chinda concluded that they were seeking to rid their city of leprosy at the expense of Japan, it seems there was a genuine interest in treatment. After the Gotōs bowed to the wishes of the Foreign Ministry and declined to accept the San Francisco patients, the board of health used a combination of public funds and private donations to purchase a large quantity of their proprietary medicines. Reports in the *San Francisco Chronicle* suggest that hopes were high that a cure was possible. A headline from July 4, 1896, declared, "There Is Joy at the Pesthouse: The Gato [*sic*] Remedies Arrive," while one from October of the same year stated, "Curing Lepers at the Pesthouse: The Wonderful Goto Cure."[43] Initially, as in Hawai'i,

Gōto's medicines seemed to be effective. Within a few months, the famous Bindt brothers were so recovered that they successfully absconded from the pesthouse, an event that the *Chronicle* reported was evidence that "hope has been restored to them through the medium of the Goto remedy."[44]

Rod Edmond has argued that the interest of British and American doctors in indigenous treatments for leprosy in South and East Asia reflected an imperial perspective that rendered "the natives" useful informants about local remedies.[45] The remarks of Ashmead, Bälz, Hirschberg, and others suggest that Japan had a more complicated place in international medical discourse. The Japanese lack of concern for infection prompted some to reflect upon the rising tide of lepraphobia and its human costs; others, to display their racism, cruel curiosity, and crude humor. To desperate sufferers of the disease, Japan offered hope that they might escape the stigma of the disease, elude confinement, and perhaps even be cured. Meanwhile, Japanese physicians and newspapers used their plight for advertising purposes and as fodder for a nationalistic celebration of Japan's medical achievements.

Japan and the Berlin Conference

The 1880s and 1890s were marked by the optimistic view that leprosy could be successfully treated, but that celebratory moment came to an end around the turn of the century as medical opinion began to coalesce around the conclusion that leprosy was both infectious and incurable. Chinda's recommendation in 1893 that Japan follow the United States and establish immigration restrictions to keep foreign leprosy sufferers from entering Japan was an early sign of shifting attitudes. In that same year, Gotō Masanao returned to Hawai'i, again at the invitation of the board of health, which installed him as the resident physician at the colony on Moloka'i. While he continued to be popular among patients, it soon became clear that he could only relieve the symptoms of the disease; he could not cure it—an unacceptable outcome from the perspective of the board, although patients disagreed. In 1897, he was dismissed for the second time and departed from Hawai'i, never to return.

The first International Leprosy Conference took place in this transitional moment, as ideas about causality and curability were beginning to solidify, and its final pronouncements ushered in new national policies towards leprosy around the world. The initiative for the event came originally from Albert Ashmead and Jules Goldschmidt, a French citizen who was superintendent of the leprosarium on the Portuguese island of Madeira.

Both were avid segregationists, and both believed that the movement of leprosy sufferers across national borders posed a profound international public health threat. Their ambitious, even grandiose, goal was to create an international organization made up of representatives of "civilized countries," who would forge a system of segregation and surveillance that would operate at both the national and international levels. But while Hansen and the other scientists involved in leprosy research initially expressed support for a conference, they soon began to distance themselves from its organizers, a stance that reflected their discomfort with the less than scientific views of Ashmead and Goldschmidt and tension over the funding of the conference. After the two groups parted ways, Hansen and his allies took control of the meeting and redefined it as primarily a scientific meeting. Even so, the conference had a policy aim as well. Its organizers wanted to provide guidance to countries around the world to aid them in formulating national policies to control the spread of leprosy, newly cast as an international public health threat of the highest order.[46]

When the conference opened in October 1897, its participants included 180 doctors, scientists, and public health officials from the countries of Western Europe (France, Germany, Italy, and Belgium), from North America (the United States, Mexico, and Canada), and from leprosy hot spots such as Hawai'i, Eastern Europe (Russia, Rumania, Bulgaria, and the Governorate of Livonia), and Scandinavia (Norway, Finland, Denmark, and Sweden). The Ottoman Empire was represented, as were Chile, Brazil, and Colombia.[47] There were notable absences as well. The British government declined to send an official delegate, although some of its colonies were represented. The notable exception was India, well known for its large number of cases. British policy in India held that the threat of infection was so slight that quarantine was unnecessary, and the British government was unwilling to participate in an event dominated by pro-segregation figures.[48] Nor did anyone from China attend in either an official or unofficial capacity, although like India, it, too, was known for the prevalence of leprosy. These absences meant that the Japanese attendees were in a peculiar position; they were the only official representatives of an Asian country where leprosy was endemic.

Japan was represented at the conference by two young physician-scientists, Dohi Keizō and Takaki Tomoe, and Japan's premier bacteriologist, Kitasato Shibasaburō (1853–1931). Dohi was the young dermatologist, a graduate of Tokyo University's medical school, who had briefly been director of the Tokyo Dermatological Hospital in Ueno before he left for study in Europe in 1891. Takaki, also a graduate of the medical school, was an employee of the Infectious Disease Institute, at the time still a privately funded laboratory under the direction of Kitasato. In 1894, Kitasato had achieved international fame for his identification of the microorganism that caused plague. In that same year, he also began to examine leprosy patients at his Tokyo institute, treating a total of 208 between 1894 and 1896. In 1896, he declared that he had created an antitoxin serum (tentatively named Leprine) that could be used to treat leprosy, an announcement that was greeted with hefty doses of both acclaim and skepticism.[49] According to the *Yomiuri shinbun*, it was planned that Takaki would announce at the conference that Kitasato's serum had succeeded "in curing 8 or 9 out of ten cases [of leprosy]."[50] However, after it became apparent that Leprine was a failure, the plan to celebrate Kitasato's achievement was dropped.

Takaki's announcement would have disrupted the unacknowledged but explicit division of labor that ordered the conference. Representatives from Europe and Scandinavia made presentations on "hard" scientific research, while those from the "non-West" and from the colonies provided ethnographic reports that addressed clinical issues, popular attitudes, and the facilities in place. With no grand announcement to make, Takaki and Kitasato were relegated to the role of observers, although Kitasato made a presentation on the demographics of his institute's leprosy patients. He never addressed whether his pool was representative of the general population but concluded nonetheless that "leprosy is spread almost equally across the Japanese empire, with no difference between coastal and mountainous areas."[51] The question itself seems to have been driven by the early modern medical concern for environment and the belief of many that leprosy was more common in some regions than others, further evidence of the endurance of long-standing ideas about leprosy, even in the most elite medical circles.

Dohi, on the other hand, not only played an active role in the conference; he also managed to successfully bridge its organizational divide by giving two very different presentations. One was a straightforward scientific report that summarized his histological research. In contrast, the other presentation was carefully crafted to intervene in the international politics of the disease.[52] It began by noting that "foreign physicians," including some who had spent little time in Japan, had been actively publishing reports on leprosy there, and Dohi cast his remarks as an attempt to correct the misinformation that had resulted from their efforts. The presentation was organized around four intertwined claims. First, Dohi evoked Japan's long tradition of leprosy research and treatment, pointing to examples such as Katakura Kakuryō's work in the late eighteenth century, the effectiveness of the treatments provided at Kusatsu, and the success of private leprosy hospitals. He also took pains to establish his own credentials, implicitly challenging the expertise of many of his fellow attendees. Not only had he treated more than fifty patients personally, he had also observed several hundred cases of the disease. Secondly, while Dohi admitted that the disease was still to be found in Japan, he emphasized that it was on the decline. As evidence, he pointed to the so-called leper villages, noting (as discussed in chapter 2) that in some not a single case of the disease could be found. This, he asserted, called into question the speculation of "Bälz and others" that there were ten or twenty thousand victims of the disease in Japan. Dohi suggested these estimations were wildly inaccurate and exaggerated the real extent of disease by a factor of ten.

The explanation of the declining prevalence of leprosy was Dohi's third point, and he noted with pride that it had been achieved without "coercive segregation such as was practiced in medieval Europe," a pointed criticism aimed at Western advocates of segregation. In a curious valorization of the stigma of the disease, Dohi argued that it had a certain social utility. Families who confined stricken members at home rather than risk being ostracized by their neighbors prevented the spread of the disease. Dohi was honest enough, however, to acknowledge the limits of relying on stigma as a means of disease control. Close and sustained contact within the household made family members particularly vulnerable to infection, and this pattern of transmission also contributed to the popular but mistaken belief that the disease was hereditary in nature. Moreover, because some sufferers fled their homes to save their families' reputations or were forced to leave by unsympathetic family members, there were those who survived by begging along established pilgrimage routes. These people, Dohi argued, posed the biggest risk to public health.

This discussion was a preface to Dohi's final and most important assertion. He stated that in recent years leprosy had largely been brought under control by means of an effective combination of private and public efforts. The government policy of criminalizing begging was gradually reducing the numbers of itinerant sufferers, who were newly housed in institutions that provided care and medical treatment. These included prefectural and public hospitals, private leprosy hospitals, the community at Kusatsu, and finally a new facility located in Gotemba in Shizuoka Prefecture.

Dohi used this final institution, Fukusei Hospital (literally "Resurrection Hospital") to portray the situation in Japan in the best possible light, but this required some dissembling. Fukusei Hospital had its origins in a hostel for leprosy sufferers that was established by a French Roman

Catholic priest, Father Germain Léger Testvuide, in 1886.[53] Testvuide had arrived in Japan as a missionary in 1873 and by 1880 was in charge of Catholic missionary activities in eastern Honshū, with Gotemba, a town not far from the foot of Mount Fuji, as his base. According to the story Testvuide later told (which was strikingly similar to the accounts of other missionaries who became involved in leprosy relief), he was drawn into leprosy work by his first encounter with a pitiful victim of the disease, a blind and disfigured young woman who had been abandoned by both her husband and her natal family. With the support of the Church, he eventually purchased property in Koyama, a village just outside Gotemba, where he established Fukusei Hospital. It grew rapidly, from fourteen patients in 1889 to seventy-two in 1892.

Fukusei Hospital was one of three missionary institutions for leprosy sufferers in Japan at this time. The Ihaien (literally "Comforting the Disabled Sanitarium") was established in Meguro village, not far from central Tokyo, in 1894 by Kate Youngman, an American missionary associated with the Presbyterian Church.[54] Kaishun Byōin (Rejuvenation Hospital) was founded the following year in Kumamoto by Hannah Riddell, a British missionary associated with the Church of England's Church Missionary Society.[55] Dohi had left Japan in 1891 and probably had no knowledge of these two institutions, but they were evidence of growing missionary interest in leprosy relief worldwide. For some Christians, biblical references to Jesus "cleansing lepers" made the disease a potent symbol of compassion and the possibility of salvation, and providing for the care of its victims helped missionaries to win both financial support at home and converts abroad. In 1874 Wellesley Bailey, an Irishman who had worked as a teacher in British India, organized the Mission to Lepers, which aimed to bring both Christianity and care to Indian sufferers of the disease. The organization expanded rapidly, and by 1893 it was operating ten "asylums" for sufferers on the subcontinent and providing support for ten more.[56]

In the years that followed, Hannah Riddell in particular and the other missionaries as well would become powerful and vocal advocates of quarantine, which they cast as a response that was both compassionate towards those with the disease and necessary to protect the larger public. Their stature as representatives of powerful nation-states, the association of Christianity with "civilization," and their personal ties to powerful figures in Japan all gave the missionaries' advocacy of quarantine considerable weight in the public discourse on the disease. At the same time, however, their participation in the debates over national policy irritated many. As D. George Joseph has noted, missionaries involved in leprosy relief "pursued the dual but inseparable goal of 'evangelization' and 'civilization,' advancing not only a religious program but also a political and cultural one."[57] For example, in soliciting donations from their home countries, missionaries portrayed Japanese with leprosy as pitiful victims who, rejected by their fellow countrymen and ignored by their government, survived only because of the beneficence of enlightened European, British, or American Christians.[58] If this pitch appealed to donors' sense of moral (and perhaps racial) superiority, the implication that Japan needed the charity of foreigners offended many Japanese, both within and outside government.

Dohi then had many reasons for glossing over the fact that the Gotemba hospital was founded, funded, and managed by Catholic missionaries, and in his presentation he mentioned only in passing that there was a Catholic chapel on-site. Ignoring its religious nature, he described its scale (a total of 150 beds), its charitable nature (the sick paid nothing for their care), and the availability of high-quality medical care. Characterizing both the hospital and the Kusatsu community, Dohi emphasized their progressive nature. Beginning in the mid-1890s the so-called colony model of care had begun to be discussed in Japan in relation to the care of the mentally ill, a population that many in government viewed with far more concern than leprosy sufferers. Advocates of colony care, such as Kure Shūzō, who was later to be chair of psychiatry at the Imperial University's medical school, referenced its popularity in Europe and its therapeutic potential and low cost, and Dohi cast Fukusei Hospital in similar terms.[59] Those who were physically capable engaged in productive labor, such as agriculture and handicrafts, and they also helped care for their fellow patients.

Kusatsu and Fukusei, in Dohi's account, were cast as humanistic endeavors that reflected contemporary approaches to the care of the chronically ill in Europe. His presentation thus carefully negotiated the international discourse on leprosy in order to establish that Japan was not one of the "uncivilized" countries whose leprous citizens threatened the health of the international community. Instead, it was a center of research and treatment, a country where leprosy had been brought under control through humane and progressive measures. By the end of the conference, however, it was apparent that Dohi's carefully composed argument against coercive segregation was at odds with the consensus on leprosy control that emerged under the leadership of Hansen. As chief leprosy officer of Norway, Hansen had pioneered his country's so-called mixed model, which required the confinement of poor leprosy sufferers but allowed those with means to remain at home. By the time of the Berlin conference, Hansen had changed his mind about the desirability of this approach, after a study he conducted using Norway's National Leprosy Registry revealed that the prevalence of the disease was declining only gradually, leading him to conclude that the isolation of all leprosy sufferers was necessary to rapidly eradicate the disease.[60] This was the position Hansen took in his plenary address, and it was supported by the scientists who made up the bulk of the conference attendees. The final resolution of the conference declared that the confinement of all people with leprosy was the best means available to control the disease.[61]

The Berlin conference thus sent a strong message that modern sovereign states should act to control the disease by developing strategies to quarantine its victims. In the decade that followed, the confinement of leprosy sufferers began around the world. One of the first governments to react was the British colonial government of India, which quickly reversed its earlier stance against segregation. It issued the Lepers Act of 1898, which required the isolation of all leprosy sufferers. Contemporary estimates put the number of those with the disease at 250,000, but from the outset it was clear that the British did not plan to undertake mass incarceration. Instead, they actively encouraged missionary involvement in constructing institutions of quarantine, effectively passing the cost of confinement to religious entities. Missionaries were quick to respond. By 1910, at least 10,000 Indians were being cared for in "leper asylums" funded by the Mission to Lepers.[62]

Elsewhere, other governments did become directly involved in funding new facilities of quarantine. In 1898, a new law in Iceland required the segregation of leprosy sufferers in a public asylum, and one was established at Laugarnes in Reykjavík to house the 236 leprosy sufferers who had been identified. The following year, the German government established the leprosarium at Memel. In Colombia, the state of Cundinamarca had established a lazaretto at Agua de Dios, a town about 114 kilometers from Bogotá, in 1864. In the aftermath of the conference, however, it ordered new measures to ensure the segregation of the patients. The section of the town where the lazaretto was located was cordoned off, surrounded by barbed wire, and put under police surveillance. In 1902, the US authorities in the Philippines made the island of Culion the site of a new "leper colony," and Spain created a leprosarium at Fontilles. In 1904, Finland converted an unused army barracks into a leprosy hospital, and it soon housed almost one hundred patients. In 1905, the state of Massachusetts established the Penikese Island Leper Colony; it continued to function until the establishment of the US National Leprosarium in 1921. The colony of Queensland also embraced the island model of segregation and designated Peel Island, in Moreton Bay east of Brisbane, the site of a new leper colony in 1907.[63]

Debating Leprosy Policy in Japan

The governments that acted quickly to establish institutions of segregation had, in most cases, only a small number of leprosy sufferers in their jurisdictions: the Massachusetts colony, for example, had a peak population of only seventeen, and the Memel institution initially housed only sixteen. Segregation in such circumstances was unnecessary but also relatively easy to effect. It also proved easy in places like Queensland, where confinees were initially racialized others (indigenous Australians) and recent immigrants (Chinese), and there was little public outcry over coerced isolation from the white population.

The situation in Japan was very different, with even the lowest estimates acknowledging that thousands of people—Japanese citizens—suffered from the disease. As a result, the formulation of a national policy proceeded slowly and with considerable debate. By this time, the medical entrepreneurs who had played an important role in defining popular perceptions of the disease for three decades were passing from the scene: Gotō Masafumi had died in 1895, and his son Masanao would live only until 1908; Mori Kichibei of Raichigan fame died in 1900; and by 1901 Arai Saku was either dead or no longer active in public life. In their place, a different set of actors took the lead in shaping the debate over a national leprosy policy. And while issues of national strength, international reputation, and Japan's status as a civilized country had played a role in the early Meiji discourse on leprosy, these concerns became even more overt in relation to the discussion of public health policy.

Prompted by the international conference, the Japanese government first took up the issue of leprosy in 1900, when the Home Ministry ordered a national survey to determine the prevalence of leprosy. While little information is available about the design of the survey, the collection of data was put in the hands of the police force, which was charged with the enforcement of public health policy, an arrangement that, as many have noted, gave the impression that to fall ill with an infectious disease was a criminal act. The investigation, carried out secretly at the prefectural level, sought to identify the number of "leprosy patients," "households of leprous lineages," and "members of households of leprous lineages."[64] While this first category may seem unproblematic, in fact measuring the prevalence of leprosy in a specific population is notoriously difficult.[65] The only definitive way to diagnose the disease is to examine a skin smear (a scraping of dermal tissue) in a laboratory, a costly and time-consuming procedure. Instead, the police relied on the visual identification of symptoms, an unreliable method given that symptoms such as skin lesions and depigmentation are not limited to leprosy. Complicating matters further is that *M. leprae* replicates very slowly, so that someone can be infected for many years with few noticeable symptoms. Finally, of course, because of the stigma of the disease, the afflicted and their families often sought to conceal its occurrence.

The initial survey gave the number of leprosy patients as 33,359, or 7.4 cases per 10,000 population, substantially more than the earlier estimate by Bälz that Dohi had criticized. Proponents of segregation within the Diet would later characterize this figure as a gross underestimation, with some arguing that the true number was actually double.[66] In 1907, Kubota Seitarō (1865–1946), head of the Bureau of Hygiene, acknowledged that the survey results were unreliable. He suggested that the number of patients was about 50,000, a figure he derived by applying the incidence of the disease discovered by army doctors while examining potential conscripts (1.3 per 1,000) to the total population.[67] The issue of prevalence became even murkier when a second national survey was carried out in 1906. It gave the number of patients as 23,815, a drop of more than 25 percent in just six years, a figure that was widely rejected as deceptively low, although there was no sustained discussion of how the results came to be skewed.

The pattern of the distribution of the disease, as exposed by both surveys, also raised questions. As map 3 reveals, rates of prevalence varied dramatically by region. According to the first survey, the prefectures on the island of Kyūshū had startlingly high rates of prevalence: Kumamoto, 26 per 10,000; Miyazaki, 21 per 10,000; Ōita, 16 per 10,000; and Saga, 15 per 10,000. Initially, many thought that this distinctive pattern resulted because leprosy sufferers from other areas of Japan had relocated to Kyūshū and clustered at certain religious sites that were rumored to offer the possibility of a cure to those who worshipped there. The best known of these was the temple Honmyōji in Kumamoto, where the deified spirit of the sixteenth-century warlord Katō Kiyomasa was worshipped. This was where the missionary Hannah Riddell said she first encountered leprosy sufferers, in conditions so pitiable that she was inspired to found Kaishun Hospital. Katō was rumored to have suffered from leprosy, and it was widely believed that in his deified form he had both the ability and the inclination to cure the disease. But another theory for Kyūshū's high rates of the disease also gained currency in this period, one that had been first advanced by Kobayashi Hiroshi in *A New Treatment for Leprosy*. Leprosy, it was said, was an "alien" disease introduced to Kyūshū, the point of contact with the continent in ancient times, from Korea and China.[68] Ignored when Kobayashi first advanced it, this theory now gained a following, reflecting both the emergent ethnic politics of the Japanese Empire and the increasingly racialized international discourse of leprosy.

In contrast to the discussion evoked by the rates, prevalence, and patterns of distribution exposed by the survey, the number of "households of leprous lineages" (199,075) and of "members of households of leprous lineages" (999,300) went almost unscrutinized, although these figures pose an interpretive conundrum on several counts. Why include "lineage" within

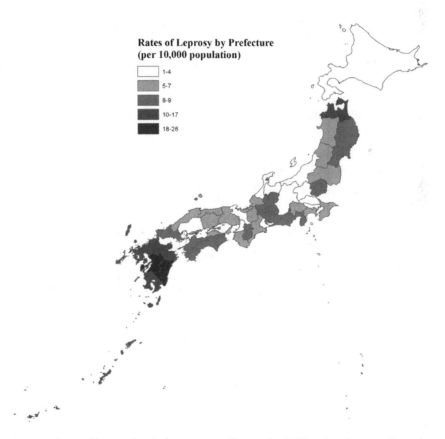

MAP 3.   Rates of leprosy by prefecture according to the 1900 national survey. Note the high rates of the disease in Kyūshū.

the survey given the official acknowledgment that leprosy was an infectious disease? It is unclear whether the concern for lineage reflected the still current belief that leprosy was a heredity disease, a new awareness of the pattern of intrafamilial infection, or the durability of the notion that a disease can have multiple causes. If the rationale for including this category is unclear, so, too, was the method for deriving the number of households within a lineage. According to the survey, Wakayama, for example, had 388 identified patients, but 7,452 households of leprous lineages, while Shimane was said to have 390 identified patients but only 1,755 households of leprous lineages. Given that family size and structure did not vary significantly from one prefecture to another, it seems likely that in some areas local police included all the households connected to a lineage where a case of leprosy was rumored to have occurred, even if there were no actual cases at the time, while elsewhere they adopted a more rigorous standard.

Although the figure of 999,300 conflated real and potential cases of the disease, it proved immensely attractive to the proponents of segregation—and to the newspapers, which were quick to exploit it. In the reportage and political debates that followed, it was this number, rounded up to the rhetorically useful "one million," that appeared most often. And as the inflated figure gained credence, the journalistic celebration of Japan's international success in treating leprosy quickly gave way to articles that asked whether high rates of leprosy did not call into question Japan's place among the "civilized" countries of the world. A case in point is one from the *Tokyo Daily News* (*Tōkyō nichi nichi shinbun*) that stated, "In the number of leprosy sufferers, our country is second only to India, and if one considers the ratio of that number to the general population then this is indeed the most leprous country in the world."[69]

Japanese newspapers also used the figure of "one million" to emphasize the threat leprosy posed to individual health and well-being. A 1902 *Yomiuri* article opened with the headline "One Million Leprosy Patients." While the text of the article went on to explain that this was the number not of sufferers of the disease, but of those who had a relative who was infected, it was the threat posed by the latter that was emphasized: "People from such lineages work in businesses that sell food and drink and in this way the poison of this sickness is spread."[70] Perhaps as a response to this kind of rhetoric, officials within the Home Ministry dropped the category of "leprosy lineage" from the 1906 survey. Instead, this second survey tracked the number of households with one or more actual patients and the number of those living within such a household. According to the 1906 survey, there were 22,887 "leprous households," which collectively included

102,585 people. While ostensibly a more reasonable way of estimating "potential patients," given that it was recognized that transmission occurred most often with sustained and intimate contact, it still implied, implausibly, that a 100 percent rate of infection was possible. Although still inflated, this new number was a tenth of the celebrated figure of "one million," but it was largely ignored by the mass media.

The Berlin conference, the confirmation of leprosy's infectious nature, the new international enthusiasm for institutions of confinement, and the national surveys all contributed to what can, without much exaggeration, be termed a "paradigm shift" in conceptions of leprosy—at least for some members of Japan's political and medical elite. In the midst of calls for the systematic isolation of leprosy sufferers, there was new interest in the premodern forms of exclusion examined earlier. In 1902, Mitsuda Kensuke, whose name was soon to become synonymous with the forced confinement of leprosy sufferers, published an essay called "On the Need to Establish Isolation Centers for Leprosy," one of the first calls for a policy of total quarantine.[71]

Mitsuda's rapid rise to prominence as Japan's premier leprologist belied his humble origins. The expected path to an elite medical career required a university medical education and study abroad with government sponsorship, most often in Germany. In contrast, Mitsuda gained his medical credentials by attending a medical cram school, working as an "assistant" (shosei, a live-in student) in the household of a wealthy doctor, and taking the licensing exam, an educational background that typically led to a career in private practice. He veered from this path when he took a job in the Tokyo Poorhouse (Yōikuin) in 1896. Founded in 1874 to house the indigent of the city, this institution was under the direction of Shibusawa Eiichi (1840–1931), a Japanese industrialist who was well known for his interest in education and social welfare. Not surprisingly, Mitsuda discovered leprosy sufferers among the residents of the Poorhouse, and like Albert Ashmead and Erwin Bälz before him, he, too, capitalized on his experience to establish himself as a leprologist and a public figure in this period of growing concern for the disease.

In his 1902 essay, Mitsuda made much of the danger posed by those deemed "vagrant lepers" (furō raisha), the indigent sufferers who survived by begging at temples, shrines, and markets, charging them with "spreading poison" wherever they went. But even more dangerous, he argued, were those who lived "normal lives," that is, "the person who is not a beggar, but works on a ship, or preparing food and drink, or something else, or the barber whose parents are lepers and the woman whose husband is a leper who works serving food and drink."[72] He contrasted this state of affairs with the situation in Germany and elsewhere, where quarantine laws had been recently established. But the segregation of leprosy sufferers, Mitsuda asserted, was not a custom foreign to Japan. He wrote, "In our country too, before the Restoration, as a principle of social order those of leprosy lineages were excluded by the public, and so they naturally came together to form villages and in this way the spread of the disease was forestalled, but after the Restoration, as all the old ways were destroyed, the leper villages to came to be forgotten."[73]

Unlike figures such as Dohi and Mori Kichibei, who had favorably compared Japan's lack of exclusionary laws with the coercive policies of medieval Europe, Mitsuda made Japan's premodern practices a blueprint for future action. He was not alone in attempting to map modern institutions of confinement onto premodern forms of exclusion. In 1902, the *Kyoto Journal of Medicine and Public Health* (*Kyoto iji eisei shi*), then an important journal of medicine and public health, published a series of articles on premodern "institutions" for the sufferers of leprosy. Writing on the history of the Kitayama shelter in Nara, Sawa Riichirō framed his work around the now commonplace assertion that Japan's "one million lepers" made the country "the most leprous country in the world."[74] He stated that his aim in examining the history of the Nara shelter, which he described as "something to be proud of before the rest of the world," was "to arouse the determination of the Japanese people to create new leprosy hospitals."[75] A few months later, the journal began to serialize a long article on the history of leprosy in Kyoto. Like Mitsuda and Sawa, its author, Takahashi Seii, lamented the fact that the premodern tradition of exclusion had been forgotten.[76]

Of course, neither the leprosy shelters of the medieval period nor the "villages" of the early modern period bore any resemblance to the "isolation centers" and "hospitals" for which these authors were advocating. Ignoring their embeddedness in Buddhist conceptions of karma and merit and disestablished forms of status, Mitsuda, Sawa, and Takahashi advocated for the creation of modern institutions of medical quarantine by appealing to an indigenous Japanese "tradition" of confining leprosy sufferers. In 1902, the claim that quarantine was a Japanese tradition was front and center in the "Proposal for the Control of Leprosy Sufferers" submitted by Diet member Saitō Hisao to his colleagues. The proposal began with a description of the Kitayama hostel, a "leprosy hospital" that Saitō stated was established 1,450 years [*sic*] earlier, evidence of a long-standing tradition of segregating leprosy sufferers that had unfortunately been allowed to lapse.[77]

Saitō was a physician who had earlier been involved in public health legislation, but he also hailed from Gunma Prefecture, where Kusatsu was located, and so perhaps had reason to be particularly interested in leprosy policy. While he misdated the founding of the Kitayama shelter by almost a millennium, he was acutely aware of the contemporary international politics of leprosy. In his proposal, he drew attention to the policies of "civilized countries," citing the laws of countries and colonies around the world that required the confinement of leprosy sufferers and describing Japan's inaction on this issue as "a great failure." Within weeks of the submission of his proposal, Saitō convened a special Diet committee on the leprosy issue. When members of the committee met with Hasegawa Tai, the official involved in the decision to fund Gotō Masafumi's Kihai Hospital in the 1880s and the head of the Bureau of Hygiene since 1898, they pressed for government action, citing again the "national shame" of failing to enact a leprosy policy. Hasegawa disagreed: it was both logistically and financially impossible to house a population of 30,000 or more for years or even decades. He argued, instead, that private philanthropic efforts should be encouraged, in order to "confine those who should be confined, and treat those who should be treated." In support of this position, Hasegawa had his own international precedents to cite, pointing to private, charitable involvement in public health initiatives in Britain and Germany.[78]

Hasegawa's stance was consistent with policies enacted in relation to other chronic diseases in this period. In 1900, the Diet had passed the Law for the Protection of the Mentally Ill (Seishinbyōsha Kangohō), legalizing what was known as "confinement within private residences" (*shitaku kanchi*), the forcible confinement within the home and by their families of those deemed mentally incompetent, a measure that reserved the few public asylum beds for the poor and the criminally insane. While the law was harshly criticized by members of Japan's new psychiatric profession, it relieved the government of the burden of establishing public institutions to house those judged to be mentally ill. In the same year, the government passed Rules for the Regulation of Prostitutes and Entertainers (Shogi Torishimari Kisoku) in response to growing concern about the spread of syphilis. It required brothel owners to cover the cost of regular examinations of prostitutes in their employ as a condition of their licenses to operate and to pay for the treatment of those discovered to be infected, a policy that left their male customers free to spread the disease.[79]

The issue of the government's role in the prevention of tuberculosis provoked far greater debate. In 1899, the first national survey of tuberculosis identified the number of sufferers as 66,480, almost double the number of those with leprosy identified in 1900.[80] In response to reports of high rates of the disease among factory workers, some social reformers called for new laws to improve working conditions and thus protect workers' health. Others argued for a government-sponsored educational campaign that would educate housewives and local doctors about the disease and involve them in prevention. Kitasato Shibasaburō echoed Hasegawa's stance by calling for private philanthropic efforts to provide care for impoverished TB sufferers. In the end, the Tuberculosis Prevention Ordinance, established in 1904, took a different approach. In the words of William Johnston, its "central assumption was that the state, through legal measures, could force changes in behavior that would control tuberculosis." The behavior that aroused the most concern was spitting in public places. Fines were now attached to spitting anywhere but in a spittoon, and spittoons were required to be available in public places, including schools, hospitals, train stations, theaters, and hotels and inns.[81]

Underlying all three laws was the assumption that responsibility for the chronically ill lay with civil society, a stance that reflected less a well-defined ideological position than the economic realities of the time. The 1895 Sino-Japanese War and the 1897 adoption of the gold standard had left Japan heavily in debt, and war on the Korean peninsula was looming, leaving little money available for public health. The concern over finances explains the reaction of the Tokyo Prefectural Assembly when Mitsuda and Shibusawa approached them with a plan to create a public leprosy sanitarium for the city. In 1903 Mitsuda, alarmed at the growing number of leprosy sufferers housed in the Tokyo Poorhouse, had successfully lobbied Shibusawa to create a new leprosy ward in order to separate them from the larger population. When the number of leprosy patients outpaced the capacity of the ward, Mitsuda and Shibusawa petitioned the assembly to create a new institution for them. The contemporary clamor about leprosy in official circles notwithstanding, the assembly rejected this request on fiscal grounds.

In the aftermath of this decision, Shibusawa was instrumental in crafting the kind of public-private partnership for which Hasegawa had advocated. He approached the Ihaien, the Protestant missionary sanitarium in Meguro, which at the time was financed almost entirely by donations from abroad. Under the agreement Shibusawa negotiated, patients from the Poorhouse were housed within the Ihaien at the discounted rate of twenty sen per day. While this arrangement saved public funds, it put leprosy sufferers under the authority of the Christian missionaries and converts who ran the Ihaien, and they compelled those transferred from the Poorhouse, like all Ihaien residents, to attend prayer services morning and evening and church on Sunday, rules established to encourage conversion.[82]

The decision to turn the Poorhouse residents, doubly marked by their poverty and their disease, over to a missionary establishment points to the question that haunted the Diet discussions in the years that followed. What was the place of leprosy sufferers within the Japanese nation-state? Were they vulnerable citizens in need of care, a financial liability to the public coffers, a national shame, a threat to individual and national well-being? To be sure, this ambivalence was not entirely new. As we noted in chapter 3, even in the midst of the optimism of the 1880s, there had been calls for the use of household registries to compel leprosy sufferers to treatment or to police their intimate lives. But as the debate over leprosy policy progressed, this ambivalence became more pronounced and gave rise to increasingly divisive positions.

The central proponent of segregation within the Diet was Yamane Masatsugu (1857–1925). Yamane was one of the first generation of modern physicians trained at Tokyo University's medical school. After graduating in 1882, he became an instructor in the Nagasaki Medical School. A port city in an era when the unequal treaties made it impossible to inspect incoming ships for disease, Nagasaki was ground zero for several devastating epidemics. When cholera broke out in 1886, sparking an epidemic that would kill at least one hundred thousand people, Yamane became deeply involved in attempts to control the spread of the disease through quarantine and other measures. His efforts not only made him a lifelong advocate of interventionist public health measures, but they also brought him to the attention of the Ministry of Justice, which dispatched him to Germany and Austria for four years to study forensic medicine and public health policy. After his return to Japan in 1891, Yamane became medical director of the National Police Agency and later chief quarantine officer within the Home Ministry. In 1902, he left the bureaucracy for politics and was elected to the Diet for the first of six terms.[83]

Beginning in 1903, Yamane's self-appointed mission became the expansion of Japan's public health system. In a speech to the Diet in that year, Yamane declared, "What are the misfortunes of our country? The greatest is that our people are unhealthy. . . . Each unhealthy person becomes an unproductive person."[84] Yamane argued that the 1897 Law for the Prevention of Infectious Diseases, which defined a lengthy list of measures designed to control acute infectious diseases (including requirements for quarantine, disinfection, the immediate cremation of corpses of those who died of infection, and restrictions on travel and commerce in times of epidemic disease) should be expanded to address the threat posed by diseases such as tuberculosis, syphilis, trachoma, but most pressingly leprosy, because this disease in particular was evoking international criticism. In remarks that suggest his reading of the international reportage on leprosy in Japan must have been highly selective, Yamane claimed that foreign newspapers "laugh at how we deal with [leprosy sufferers], leaving them to beg in places that make them a danger [to others] and discarding them so that they can roam about."[85] Two years later, Yamane submitted a proposal to revise the Law for the Prevention of Infectious Diseases to include leprosy with a specific provision for the quarantine of its sufferers.

Yamane's proposal evoked a lengthy series of debates that culminated with its rejection by the Diet in 1905. Representing the government's position was Kubota Seitarō, who served as the director of the Bureau of Hygiene from 1903 to 1910. Unlike his predecessors in this position, Kubota was not a doctor. He was a graduate of the law faculty of Tokyo University and was appointed to the Bureau of Hygiene after joining the Home Ministry. Kubota had been involved in the formulation of the Law for the Prevention of Infectious Diseases under Gotō Shimpei, then the head of the bureau, and he was also a member of the Council on Leprosy Prevention (Tai Yobō ni Kansuru Kyōgikai). This latter organization was founded by Shibusawa, and its members included politicians, bureaucrats, and physicians.[86]

In his remarks to Diet members in February 1905, Kubota steadfastly rejected Yamane's proposal to incorporate leprosy into the infectious disease law. He argued that not only were diseases like tuberculosis and syphilis a greater public health threat than leprosy but also that any attempt to quarantine thousands of people would serve only to cripple the country financially and at a time when military spending was a priority. While Kubota acknowledged the global wave of regulation that had followed the Berlin conference, he argued that public health priorities must reflect domestic needs, noting that "our Japan is a country with many infectious diseases, and in this way we are very different from the countries of Europe." As for international precedents, Kubota suggested that the country would do better to emulate France's policy of supporting scientific research and establish a national research facility like the Pasteur Institute. Rather than quarantine, he argued, research to cure or control disease was the best means to improve the health of the Japanese people.[87]

Kubota's remarks sharply countered the arguments of Yamane and his allies, but he did not reject the idea of a national leprosy policy out of hand. According to Kubota, while victims of leprosy could be found among the wealthy no less than the poor, it was the plight of indigent sufferers, particularly those who survived by begging in public spaces, that should be addressed. An effective policy, he suggested, would "protect" (*hogo*) and "manage" (*kantoku*) this specific population. Twenty-eight years later, Kubota wrote a brief essay reflecting on the role he played in the formulation of leprosy policy at this moment that allows some insight into his views.[88] In it, he noted that there were two types of leprosaria, those that were established to aid people with the disease and those that sought to protect the larger public from infection. According to Kubota, the leprosy law he championed in 1904–1907 aimed to create institutions of the former type because "no one was in more urgent need of relief [*kyūsai*] than leprosy sufferers." Moreover, he did not believe leprosy posed a risk to the general public: "I thought that while leprosy was an infectious disease to be sure, whether one came to be infected or not depended upon one's physical makeup."[89]

Kubota's remarks reveal that the debates over leprosy policy were implicated in a new political cleavage over the issue of state responsibility for the welfare of vulnerable citizens. Although many within the government, like Hasegawa Tai, continued to view charity as the most expedient way to fund social welfare initiatives, by the turn of the century others had begun to argue that "relief" was a state responsibility that could not simply be left to private philanthropists. Kubota was an advocate of the latter position. Beginning in the 1890s he published a series of articles on poverty in journals like *Society* (*Shakai*) and *Philanthropy* (*Jizen*), and in 1899, he joined with others interested in social reform to found the Poverty Study Association, a group that David Ambaras has described as combining "academic exchanges with ground-level surveys of Tokyo slums."[90] In his writings on poverty, Kubota asserted that its cause could not be reduced to simply the moral failures of the poor. In formulating policy, it was necessary to distinguish between the poor who were incapable of supporting themselves (the young and the old, but also those who were sick, infirm, or disabled) and those who had the ability to perform useful labor but lacked education, skills, or discipline. Support for the former, Kubota argued, was a legitimate responsibility of modern ethical government. The "able poor," too, required government action but of a different sort. Direct aid risked turning this group into perpetual dependents, and so the state should develop policies that would transform them into productive citizens by providing opportunities for education and work.[91]

It was this analysis of poverty, which made it a state responsibility to support the biologically vulnerable, that framed Kubota's approach to leprosy, but it was countered by powerful figures within the Diet. Yamane was the author and sponsor of a draft leprosy prevention bill that would have given the state unprecedented authority over leprosy sufferers. In addition to requiring each prefecture to create a sanitarium, it made doctors responsible for reporting any case of leprosy to public health authorities within three days of a diagnosis, so that local officials could record it in the household registry. The bill also required anyone suspected of the disease to submit to a medical examination and to open their homes to physicians or officials for purposes of disinfection; those with a confirmed diagnosis were required to get official permission to travel by steamship and were forbidden from selling food, drink, and children's toys, and they were banned from employment in schools, factories, public baths, and barbershops. In addition, prefectures and local governments were made responsible for the costs associated with enforcing these provisions, and the bill laid out a system of heavy fines for noncompliance by physicians, the sick, and public officials.[92]

As discussion of the draft bill unfolded, Yamane and his supporters reiterated now familiar arguments, referencing the Berlin conference's recommendation, the international embrace of quarantine, and the threat the disease posed to public health and national prestige, as well as the "shame" of leaving Japanese sufferers in the care of foreign missionaries, but the draconian provisions of the bill provoked dismay on the part of many within the government. Okano Keijirō, the chief secretary in the Ministry of Law, was one critic. A former professor of law at Tokyo University, he noted that the bill's provisions infringed on the civil rights of Japanese citizens and that any attempt to impose them was likely to evoke unrest.[93] He also had more mundane objections, expressing concern that local authorities would be overburdened by the web of regulations created by the law and the potential cost of their enforcement.

Kubota and his counterpart in the Bureau of Local Affairs countered the segregationist politicians with their own version of a leprosy law. It retained some of the policing measures of Yamane's draft, including the requirements for reporting and disinfection and the provision for the compulsory examination of suspected cases. However, most of the articles addressed the indigent and itinerant population of sufferers that concerned so many. The 1906 survey had numbered this population at 1,182, a fraction of even the most conservative estimate of the prevalence of the disease.

The government's draft allowed local authorities to forcibly return those "unable to care for themselves and without someone to help them" to their families if they could be identified but authorized their transfer to public or private sanitaria if no family support was available. Under an unprecedented plan, the public sanitaria were to be created jointly by two or more prefectures as directed by the Home Ministry, with the national government providing one-sixth of the costs and the prefectures involved jointly sharing responsibility for the remainder.[94]

It was this bill, virtually unrevised, that became Japan's first leprosy law. In essence, it made indigent leprosy sufferers a special kind of vagrant, a designation that reflected Kubota's theory of poverty and state responsibility but which also anticipated the Police Ordinance for Criminal Offenses (Keisatsu Hanshobatsu Rei) that was issued by the Home Ministry the following year. Vagrancy laws had existed at the local level for decades, but the Police Ordinance made "the offense of vagrancy" part of a new category of misdemeanor crimes, in relation to which the police were authorized to impose fines and jail offenders without going through the criminal courts. Under the ordinance, "the offence of vagrancy" was punishable by a jail sentence of no more than thirty days. In contrast, the leprosy law called for ongoing confinement, which was envisioned as "protection" rather than punishment.

This new conception of confinement as a form of "protection" for those who were vulnerable and indigent elicited intense debate, particularly among the members of the House of Peers committee, perhaps because they tended to be better educated and more cosmopolitan than many rank-and-file members of the lower house. Miyake Hiizu, a physician trained at Tokyo University, expressed bewilderment at the bill, asking why leprosy prevention was suddenly being treated as a matter of great urgency. In his words, it was as if the familiar disease "had suddenly turned infectious just now." He pointed out that the law was likely to stigmatize anyone suspected of leprosy, even those who suffered from more minor dermatological ailments.[95] Several members of the upper house committee directly questioned both the motives and the impact of the law. Hirozawa Kinjirō asked what provisions for treatment would be made available within the new institutions and declared that unless treatment was available, "what you are calling 'sanitaria' would be nothing more than slaughterhouses for human beings."[96] Takagi Kanehiro (1849–1920), a physician who had studied at St. Thomas's Hospital Medical School in London, questioned whether confinement would not be "spiritually" (seishinteki) difficult for the patients, and both he and Miyake argued that the new sanitaria should be established adjacent to the religious sites where leprosy sufferers gathered in hope of a cure in order to respect their "freedom of belief."[97] Takagi also questioned how children would be accommodated within the new sanitaria: what provisions would be made for their education?[98] Ishiguro Tadanori (1845–1941), who had had a long and illustrious career in military medicine, asked—discretely—how the sexuality of those confined would be managed within the sanitaria, perceptively raising an issue that would trouble administrators of leprosaria around the world. Would couples be allowed to live together? What would happen in the case of pregnancy?[99]

Kubota and his colleague Noda Tadahiro, a physician by training, struggled to answer these questions, which required them to imagine a new kind of public institution. While they assured the members of the upper house committee that the sanitaria would be staffed by medical professionals with expertise in leprosy, they were vague about how many aspects of institutional life would be handled. According to Kubota, the location of the sanitaria was a matter for prefectural authorities to decide, and educational policy fell under the jurisdiction of the Ministry of Education. He also sidestepped a discussion of how sexuality and reproduction would be dealt with within the new institutions, stating only that a child born in a sanitarium could not be allowed to remain for long because of the risk of infection.[100]

In contrast to the generally circumspect responses he put forth in the committee discussions, Kubota's 1933 essay suggests that he was deeply concerned about the issues raised by Miyake, Takagi, and the others. Kubota recollected that while many at the time called for the sanitaria to be located on "distant islands," he himself thought this would be a "blow to the spirits of the patients" and advocated for the establishment of the institutions in relatively central locations. He was also concerned about the design of the new facilities. In his view, it was essential that they not resemble prisons, because those they housed would be patients, not prisoners. Kubota also discussed the issue of sexuality at some length, writing that he had weighed different approaches to this "difficult problem." One option was to house men and women separately and to prevent any interaction. However, according to Kubota, this would have "made the men extremely aggressive and may well have led to violence." On the other hand, if relations between men and women were allowed to become "dissolute," "children would be born one after another," a result described as "unpleasant." At stake was the protection of female patients, whom Kubota speculated would be vulnerable to unwanted sexual advances by the stronger, more numerous men. While suggesting that there was no easy solution, Kubota stated that he had favored a "generous approach" that did not insist upon absolute separation of men and women but instead called upon patients to police one another.[101]

This chapter began by exploring the place of Japan in the new global politics of leprosy that emerged in the late nineteenth century. I argued that Japan initially had an ambivalent place in the international public health discourse on the disease. Unlike China, India, and other places where the disease was endemic, Japan was not cast as a "backward" country whose "leprous" inhabitants threatened the health and well-being of the civilized world. Instead, in both the medical press and the popular media, it was celebrated for the medical achievements of its doctors and for providing a chance for effective treatment and even a cure. But as a new consensus emerged that leprosy was both incurable and infectious, things began to change. In the aftermath of the Berlin conference's endorsement of quarantine, as a growing number of countries began to establish institutions of confinement, advocates of quarantine in the Diet pressed the government to act, deploying political rhetoric that cast people with leprosy as both dangerous and shameful.

What is important in this context is that the government ultimately resisted calls to emulate the quarantine policies that were enacted elsewhere. Rather than treating leprosy sufferers as a danger to the health of the nation, Kubota and his allies successfully argued that their care was an issue of social welfare and that a modern state had a responsibility to support its vulnerable citizens. However, as Kubota's equivocal responses to the issues raised by the members of the upper house revealed, the 1907 law left fundamental questions unaddressed. How far did state responsibility extend? Did it need to provide treatment and an education to those in its care or simply a minimal level of support? And what were the rights of those deigned in need of care? Could they marry and have families? Could they refuse the "protection" of the state rather than accept the "management" it entailed? Kubota himself was honest enough to admit that the five public leprosaria established under the 1907 law did not fulfill his vision of institutions that would become "the seed of the happiness and consolation of the patients."[102] The next chapter explores the struggles that accompanied efforts to create these unprecedented institutions and the tensions between competing visions of citizenship that shaped them.

Chapter 5

Not Quite Total Institutions

The Public Sanitaria and Patient Life

In October 1912, *Without the Camp*, the quarterly journal of the Mission to Lepers (MTL), described an incident at Fukusei Hospital that had taken place a few months before. In an organized protest of conditions at the hospital, "practically the whole of the lepers made their escape but were re-captured by police and sent back. Subsequently, however, they ran away by ones and twos, alleging misgovernment and inhuman treatment." The author of this piece offered little information on the patients' grievances and instead used the "strike," as it was termed, to make a sectarian jab at the Catholics' treatment of patients and to contrast it with the "truly Christian treatment" that prevailed in the Protestant-affiliated institutions supported by the MTL.[1] We learn more from a patient's account composed a decade later. He recounted that he and his compatriots grew disgruntled with conditions at Fukusei Hospital as rumors reached them about the public sanitaria that had opened three years earlier. After hearing that those in the public institutions received better medical care and higher pay for fewer hours of work and were allowed to pursue sexual relationships, they decided to leave the missionary facility and make their way to one of the public institutions.[2] After they were forcibly returned to the hospital, patients sent a petition to the governor of Shizuoka in which they demanded better food, medical care, hygiene, and wages.[3]

That some leprosy sufferers had actively pursued confinement in a public sanitarium seems unimaginable in light of much recent scholarship on these institutions, with some authors describing them as akin to the Nazi concentration camps, in a reckless bit of hyperbole.[4] This chapter explores the establishment of the first public sanitaria, Japan's first effort at building social welfare institutions on a national scale. I argue that they took form as

132

a prolonged experiment in long-term quarantine shaped by the conceptual ambiguity between "protection" and "management," financial constraints, tensions with local communities, and the need to negotiate with patients who were never passive in the face of institutional power. What emerged from this process were not "total institutions," to borrow Erving Goffman's famous term, but complex communities that defy easy characterization as prison, hospital, village, colony, or sanctuary.[5]

The Politics of Place

In the aftermath of the passage of the 1907 leprosy law, Bureau of Hygiene officials divided the country into five zones that overlapped roughly with established conceptions of region (see map 4), and committees made up of local officials and representatives of the bureau and the national police began to consider where the regional sanitaria for which they would have joint responsibility should be located. Home Minister Hara Takashi ignored demands of segregationists in the Diet that the sanitaria be located on isolated islands, following the much-discussed example of Kalaupapa on Moloka'i, and provided explicit instruction on site selection that reflected the view that the sanitaria were to be institutions of relief established by the benevolent state. Those to be confined were Japanese citizens and thus deserving of empathy, and the sanitaria should be located in places that would allow them to live as comfortably as possible. An appropriate location would be near a major city or town with good transportation facilities, and it would have clean air, fresh water, and a pleasant natural setting, allowing "patients"—as those to be confined were now termed in Bureau of Hygiene documents—to take walks, raise vegetables, and engage in other kinds of healthy activities.[6]

These careful instructions notwithstanding, the sanitaria came to be located in sites that had little in common with the Home Ministry's vision of a setting that would be both centrally located and pleasantly bucolic. In some places, the change of plans was pragmatic, with local officials privileging the acquisition of state-owned lands over the ministry's requirements; elsewhere, social relations at the local level forced officials to abandon their first choice of location in favor of a less desirable one. A case in point is the controversy that surrounded the founding of the zone one institution. Zone one included twelve prefectures and the city of Tokyo, making it the most densely populated of the five zones. Zensei Hospital, as the zone one institution came to be known, was eventually established in Higashimurayama village, about forty kilometers from central Tokyo

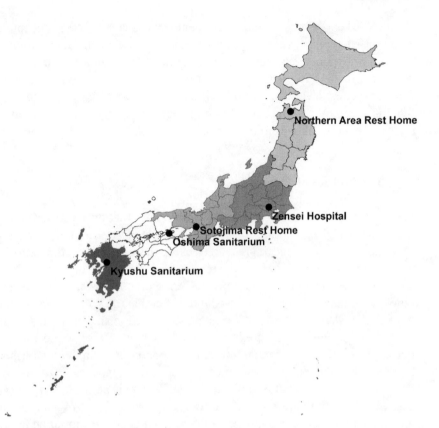

MAP 4. The regional zones created by the 1907 law and the location of the public sanitaria within them.

near the border with Saitama Prefecture. It was as far from the city as one can get and still remain within Tokyo Prefecture, and at the time, rail connections with the capital were poor. Mitsuda Kensuke, who became Zensei Hospital's first medical director, tellingly described Higashimurayama as "a cold village in an isolated area that was the Hokkaidō of Tokyo Prefecture."[7]

Higashimurayama was not the first or even the second choice of those charged with selecting a site for the zone one sanitarium. In the summer of 1908, six places were under consideration: Kusatsu in Gunma, Ikegami in the southern part of Tokyo, Narita and Nakayama in Chiba Prefecture, Tatsu no Kuchi in Kanagawa, and Minobu in Yamanashi.[8] This short list reflected concern for the comfort of those to be confined. These places would have been familiar to many, and all but one reflected the still potent religious resonances of the disease. The exception was Kusatsu, which was clearly considered because of its well-known community of leprosy sufferers and the popularity of its thermal baths. All the other sites were associated with popular Buddhist temples. Sites associated with Nichiren temples predominated because the Lotus Sutra, famous for its reference to *rai* as karmic punishment, was a principal object of worship for many sufferers. Ikegami is the site of Honmonji, the Nichiren temple where the short-lived Religious Hospital had been established in the 1890s. Nakayama was home to the famous Nichiren temple Hokekyōji, and Tatsu no Kuchi, of Ryukoji, another Nichiren temple. Minobu, too, had a famous Nichiren temple, Kuonji, but it was significant for another reason as well. It was the location of the only modern Buddhist-run shelter for leprosy sufferers. Known as Jinkyōen, this institution was established in 1906 by Tsunawaki Ryūmyō (1876–1970), a Nichiren priest who was inspired by Christian involvement in leprosy relief. Although it initially had only ten patients, Jinkyōen attracted considerable attention after Tsunawaki began canvassing nationwide for contributions.[9]

Absent from this list, though, was the site that was initially selected for the zone one facility. In late August, a notice in *Kanpō* (Official News) announced that the zone one sanitarium would be built in Meguro, the village where Ihaien, the Protestant leprosy facility, was located.[10] (See map 5.) Although the reasons for its selection were not specified, Meguro had a number of attractive features. It was near Tokyo, the largest population center in zone one, and the closest rail station, Meguro Station, had recently been incorporated into the expanding national railway system.[11] Meguro was easily accessible to physicians studying leprosy at the country's premier institutions of medicine and science. Researchers at Kitasato's Infectious Disease Institute had been examining Ihaien patients for almost a decade.[12] It was also home to a popular temple, known as Meguro Fudōson. According to the notice in *Kanpō*, the governor of Tokyo planned to expropriate lands adjacent to the temple to establish the new sanitarium.

The announcement in *Kanpō* suggests that officials did not anticipate opposition from Meguro residents. After all, the housing of leprosy sufferers at Ihaien had taken place without incident, and even the far larger commercial establishments of the 1890s, located in densely populated urban residential and commercial neighborhoods, had aroused no alarm. However, protests broke out in Meguro almost immediately. Beginning in early September, residents organized not only to protest the planned sanitarium but also to call for the relocation of Ihaien from the village. The

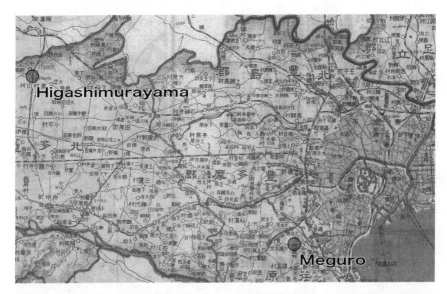

MAP 5.   Proposed and final location of the zone one sanitarium. Detail from *Tōkyō-fu Zenzu*, 1920. Map collection of the International Research Center for Japanese Studies.

Asahi shinbun reported on October 20 that 150 people had staged an angry demonstration against the planned sanitarium that ended only when the police intervened; eight days later the paper described how angry villagers armed with hoes and rakes jeered at a contingent of Bureau of Hygiene officials who had arrived to inspect the site and threatened to pelt them with human excrement.[13]

The reaction of Meguro residents has been interpreted as evidence that the 1907 law prompted a deepening of the stigma of the disease and new discriminatory attitudes towards its sufferers. While in the past people avoided marriage with those in "leprosy lineages," now it seemed they wanted to avoid all contact with sufferers. But a closer look at the protests suggests that a more complicated mix of motives was involved. Meguro, like other villages adjacent to the city, was undergoing a process of rapid urbanization at the time. Over the course of two decades, the village landscape of paddies and dry fields interspersed with woodlands had come to be dotted with new industries, including a beer brewery and a gunpowder factory. Both were established in 1887 and expanded rapidly. The size of the brewery quadrupled in just fifteen years until it occupied more than fifteen acres (six hectares) of former agricultural lands, and its workforce grew from several dozen people to almost five hundred in the same period.[14]

The gunpowder factory underwent a similar expansion, spurred by demand created by the two wars of the Meiji era. In 1907, urbanization got another boost when the Meguro Horse-Racing Track, Tokyo's first, was opened in Meguro not far from Ihaien.[15] New residents flooded into Meguro, increasing the population by more than 80 percent between 1898 and 1908.[16] The result was a community in flux. Land prices were rising and construction was booming, and there was increased competition for labor, developments that benefited some and dislocated others.

Contemporary newspaper reports suggest that the protests were driven less by anxieties about the disease than by competing economic interests. The *Asahi shinbun* reported in early September that tenant farmers were participating in the protests at the order of their landlords, whose land was under threat of expropriation.[17] Two months later, the newspaper described the protesters as a mix of farmers and artisans, with the latter comprised of those who worked in the construction trades and commercial landscape nurseries. When questioned by the *Asahi* journalist, some protesters denied that they were concerned about the threat of infection from leprosy, insisting instead that the village's "reputation" (*meiyo*) was at stake, a reference to its popularity among the new middle class.[18]

But if the protests primarily reflected tensions surrounding the boom economy, it is also true that some Meguro residents did not hesitate to evoke the stigma of leprosy. When interviewed, two of the village leaders pointed out that Meguro's horse races were popular among Tokyo's foreign residents and tourists and declared that the sanitarium would "advertise to the world that Japan was a leprous country."[19] Others suggested that "filthy" sufferers would befoul the temple grounds and wondered whether the waste from the proposed institution would not pollute the Meguro River.[20] Three months after the protests began and with organizers vowing to take the battle to court, the Home Ministry abandoned Meguro as a potential site. Protests in the village, however, continued with a new target, the attempted expropriation of land for a new elementary school, further evidence that opposition to the sanitarium had more to do with economic and social tensions than with leprosy.[21]

In the aftermath of the riots that had followed the end of the Russo-Japanese War, Tokyo officials were increasingly wary of public protests, and ignoring the Home Ministry's requirements, they abandoned the idea of a location close to the city and began to look farther afield, specifically to the still-rural area known as Tama in the western part of Tokyo Prefecture. There was for a time considerable interest in Tanashi, a former post station along the Ōmi Highway, an important route into Tokyo. However, when village leaders proved uncooperative, officials quickly moved on to another candidate, Higashimurayama, a struggling agricultural village.[22] This time the negotiations with the mayor, a man named Tatekawa Ibei, took place in secret, and with his help those in charge of zone one succeeded in purchasing twenty-four and a half acres (ten hectares) of land from a local man at a cost of fifty-four thousand yen, more than three times the usual price of such a plot in this area.[23] On February 21, 1909, the *Asahi shinbun* announced the future site with the jaunty headline "The Sanitarium Is Welcomed!" It described the benefits of the site in terms that had little to do with the Home Ministry's original directives. The purchased land was on the border with Saitama, far from any residences. It consisted of "mountains and forests," and the stream that ran through it was not used as a source of drinking water.[24]

Unbeknownst to officials in the city, who were no doubt relieved to have finally settled this troublesome issue, all was not well in Higashimurayama. When members of the planning committee, guided by the mayor, arrived at the site on the morning of February 27, they were set upon by an angry mob, and two people were seriously injured. Fifty-four residents of Higashimurayama and neighboring villages were soon arrested and charged with various crimes, including assault. When they went on trial, jointly, in June in front of a packed courtroom, testimony revealed that villagers had heard rumors that the "poison" of leprosy threatened their health and could taint the soil of their fields. Regional and class tensions were at play as well: one defendant testified that he was angry that an institution rejected by villagers in wealthy Meguro was to be foisted upon Higashimurayama.

But most of the testimony focused not on the disease, but on village politics and the resentment some villagers felt upon learning the details of the secret land sale and the high purchase price. The defendants argued that the matter should have come before the village council, that Tatekawa must have been bribed with a cut of the proceeds, and that the land's owner had failed to honor his obligation to provide his displaced tenants with some compensation from his windfall.[25] Tatekawa apparently had some knowledge of his constituents' grievances, since he later donated five thousand yen to the village coffers, but this generosity seems to have only fueled suspicion of malfeasance.[26] In the end the court showed considerable leniency to the defendants. While all but eight were found guilty, only the twelve men judged to be leaders received prison sentences, with the longest set at twenty months. All the rest received probation.[27]

Site selection in zone five, comprised of the prefectures on the island of Kyūshū that had the highest rates of leprosy in the country, proved almost as controversial. As in Tokyo, officials initially favored a place already associated with the care of leprosy sufferers. They wanted to locate the sanitarium in Hanazono village, just outside of Kumamoto city, the capital of the prefecture with the highest rate of leprosy in the country. This was the location not only of the temple Honmyōji, where a "hamlet" (*buraku*) of leprosy sufferers housed in ramshackle dwellings had taken form, but also of a small missionary-run leprosy hospital, Tairōin, which had been founded in 1898 by a French Franciscan priest, Jean Marie Corre.[28] However, when the mayor of Hanazono expressed his village's reluctance to allow the purchase of agricultural lands, officials quickly moved on and eventually decided to locate the sanitarium on state-owned property in Kikuchi county, about ten kilometers outside Kumamoto.[29]

In contrast to the uproar that accompanied site selection in Tokyo and Kumamoto, the process in zones two, three, and four went relatively smoothly, largely because the planning committees in these areas ignored the Home Ministry's requirements from the outset. In zone three, it was decided to locate the sanitarium in Osaka Prefecture, apparently because Shintennōji, a temple where leprosy sufferers were known to gather, was located in Osaka city and because the city was a departure point for the famous Kumano pilgrimage route in neighboring Wakayama. The site chosen was a small peninsula of reclaimed land that jutted out into Osaka Bay near the mouth of the Shinyodo River. It was low-lying, sparsely populated, and a considerable distance from the main part of the city, and consequently there was no local opposition to its selection.[30] Twenty-five years later the expedient choice of location would prove to be disastrous. In 1934 a typhoon struck Osaka, causing a tidal surge. The sanitarium was flooded and 187 people, staff and patients, died.

In zone four, officials decided to locate the sanitarium on Ōshima, a small island in the Seto Inland Sea off the coast of Shikoku. Shikoku was the site of the most famous pilgrimage route of all, and it was a favored destination for many sufferers who sought divine aid. Ōshima was apparently chosen not only because of its proximity to Shikoku, but also because it had only a few residents and was made up primarily of state-owned lands.[31] Although the acquisition displaced no one, there were some protests from local officials in Takamatsu, the port closest to Ōshima, who argued that a large number of leprosy sufferers passing through their town would pose a danger to residents, and from fishermen, who charged that waste from the institution would pollute their fishing waters, but these began and ended with angry words. In contrast, in zone two, which encompassed the Tōhoku region, an area with a long-standing reputation for poverty, village leaders in Aomori, the prefecture chosen as the location for the sanitarium, actively vied to house the institution, presumably because of the jobs it would bring.[32]

The public sanitaria thus came to be located in places both more remote and less developed than the Home Ministry had directed. There were financial consequences to this change in plan. Scarce building funds had to be diverted to site preparation, including land clearing and the building of access roads. The less than ideal sites impacted the early institutions in other ways as well. Both Zensei Hospital and Ōshima Sanitarium (Ōshima Ryōyōjo), as the zone four institution came to be known, were plagued by a shortage of water in the early years. At Zensei, it took several years and considerable expense to build wells deep enough to provide a steady supply of water.[33]

If the compromises over site selection shaped the early sanitaria, so, too, did differing visions of what the institutions were to be. This was reflected in the names chosen for the new institutions. The Home Ministry instructed local committees that they were free to name their facilities as they wished, with the provision that the inclusion of the word "leprosy" should be avoided so as not to provoke local opposition.[34] Only the Tokyo institution was identified as a "hospital," and the term *zensei* (full life) was presumably meant to be uplifting, reflecting the custom of aspirational names that had prevailed during the era of the private hospitals and among the missionary institutions. In contrast, elsewhere the names chosen simply referenced location and eschewed "hospital" in favor of *hoyōjo* (rest home) or *ryōyōjo* (sanitarium), which left the question of whether they were to be medical institutions ambiguous. Names could of course be misleading, and although Zensei alone took the name of "hospital," it was one of only two sanitaria that were initially headed by members of the police force; the other was the zone three institution in Osaka. In contrast, doctors served as the directors of the sanitaria in Aomori, Kumamoto, and Ōshima.

These issues were not insignificant. At the time, there were few domestic models for medical institutions designed for long-term confinement. The only public psychiatric facility was the Tokyo prefectural psychiatric hospital; a public tuberculosis sanitarium was not established until 1917. We can recollect Kubota Seitarō's stance that the sanitaria were not to be modeled upon prisons. He may well have had in mind Sugamo Prison on the outskirts of Tokyo. Completed in 1895 under the direction of the Home Ministry, it was, in the words of Daniel Botsman, a "monument to Meiji Japan's attainment of modernity and civilization."[35] Surrounded by a massive five-meter-high brick wall, the prison's design reflected Jeremy Bentham's famous plan for a "panopticon." It consisted of two tall watchtowers from which radiated five large cell blocks.

The original plans drawn up for the public sanitaria are extant, and they reveal that while the new institutions had a number of features in common, they were neither monumental nor particularly modern in their design.[36] Unlike Sugamo Prison, the sanitaria, with the exception of the naturally isolated facility on Ōshima, made use of ditches, hedges, and gates to demarcate the institutional space. Demarcation, however, did not necessarily imply an intent to forcibly confine. Rather, the plans suggest that the sanitaria were originally porous by design.

Figure 5.1 is the original diagram for the planned Northern Area Rest Home, as the zone two institution in Aomori was named. It reveals that there were seven points of entrance and exit in the low earthen wall that surrounded the institution, and while a guard station was positioned near the main entrance, there is no evidence of an intent to exercise surveillance over other points of access. The situation was the same for the other three sanitaria on the main islands. The wall around Kyūshū Sanitarium had two entrances, and Zensei Hospital and Sotojima Rest Home both had four. It

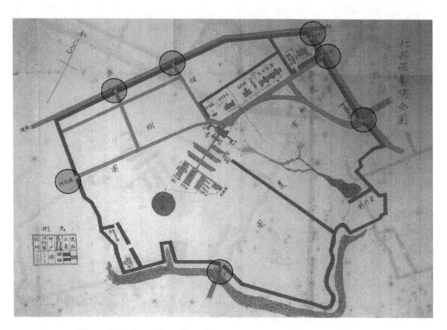

FIGURE 5.1.   Plan of Northern Area Rest Home, circa 1909. The circles have been inserted to indicate points of entry and exit. Aomori Kenshi Hensan Group.

seems, then, that planners were not concerned with designing institutions that would contain people against their will, because they did not anticipate that patients would want to flee.

The plans suggest that it was not surveillance but the distinction between staff and patients, the healthy and the sick, that informed the layout of the sanitaria. The layout of Zensei Hospital (figure 5.2) is revealing of this spatial logic. It shows that administrative buildings and staff residences were separated from the residents' living area, with the medical facilities situated between them as a kind of buffer. Early photographs suggest that architectural style visually reinforced the spatial divides. Administrative buildings reflected the Western-influenced style favored for public buildings, while the patient dormitories were traditional row houses (*nagaya*).[37] The latter were wooden structures with tiled roofs (originally thatched in the case of the Ōshima and Kyūshū facilities) that were divided into rooms of about twenty square meters each. Each of these rooms, fitted with twelve and a half tatami mats, housed eight people, a tight fit even by the standards of the day, when one tatami mat was regarded as sufficient sleeping space for a single person. At first, sanitary facilities consisted of outdoor wells from which water had to be hauled, latrines, and a communal bathhouse.

According to Mitsuda Kensuke, the Tokyo prefectural psychiatric hospital provided a model for those involved in planning the zone one sanitarium. He may have been referring to the asylum when it was still located in Ueno, when it did indeed consist of a series of *nagaya*-type wards arranged around the grounds, although after its relocation to Sugamo in 1886, the hospital was rebuilt as a single structure with connected wings.[38] This institution may have seemed a reasonable choice at the time, given the dearth of other available models, but Mitsuda complained of the inappropriateness of this design. Leprosy patients, many of whom were blind or had limited mobility, had difficulty moving between buildings separated by unpaved paths, and the tatami flooring in the dormitories was easily soiled by those with oozing lesions. Its name notwithstanding, Mitsuda found the medical facilities at the new "hospital" to be completely inadequate. There were no provisions for surgical procedures and no separate building to quarantine those who suffered from acute infectious disease.[39]

If those charged with the design of the sanitaria were ill informed about many aspects of patient life, they were acutely concerned with one issue. In each of the institutions, planning committees sought to inscribe the division of the sexes into the built environment. As the plan in figure 5.2 reveals, at Zensei Hospital shared facilities for leisure and religious activities were situated between the male and female dormitories to form a

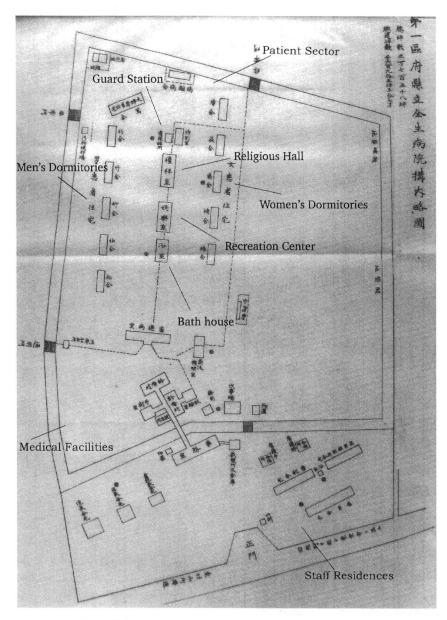

Guard Station

Patient Sector

Religious Hall

Men's Dormitories

Women's Dormitories

Recreation Center

Bath house

Medical Facilities

Staff Residences

FIGURE 5.2. Plan of Zensei Hospital, circa 1909. National Hansen's Disease Museum of Japan.

barrier, and there was a guard station as well. Similarly, the zone three institution, known as the Sotojima Rest Home, established the sexual divide by placing two large ponds and a hall for religious observances in between the male and female dormitories. The Kyūshū Sanitarium took the most direct approach; it placed a guard station in the area between the male and female dormitories, one of two on the grounds of the sanitarium. The second stood between the medical facilities and the staff residences.

Transforming the Sanitaria

The public sanitaria opened on April 1, 1909, with the exception of Zensei Hospital, where the delay caused by site selection meant that its construction required an additional six months. Over the course of the next weeks and months, leprosy sufferers began to arrive at the new institutions. It was the job of the police to identify those who fell under the authority of the 1907 law, but they were required to fully investigate whether there was an alternative to the transfer to a sanitarium. Specifically, were there family members who had the means to provide support? Any information the police obtained was forwarded to the Bureau of Local Affairs within the Home Ministry, which made the final determination on whether the person in question should be entrusted to a family member or placed within a sanitarium.[40] During this period, authorities at the local level (village, town, or city) were required to house and otherwise care for potential patients. In Tokyo, Ihaien served in this capacity; elsewhere, prefectural hospitals and even cheap inns were used. This burdensome procedure, which often took several months, reflected the ethos of poverty relief that was at the heart of the 1907 law. That is, it sought to provide care for the truly indigent but strived as much as possible to shift the responsibility to families.

Patient recollections of how they came to enter the sanitarium in these years reveal that there were both differing interpretations and unintended consequences of this procedure. Some sufferers, exhausted from life on the road, were anxious to enter a sanitarium.[41] One man later related that he took to loitering near a Tokyo police station in hopes of being picked up. When that failed, he made his own way to Higashimurayama and presented himself directly to Zensei Hospital, only to be told that admission required police involvement.[42] In some cases, patients who were not indigent came to the attention of the local police when a doctor they had consulted reported the diagnosis, as required by the 1907 law. Some families, whose poverty, profession, or crowded living conditions prompted police to press for confinement of an afflicted member, refused until the requirements for home confinement imposed by the local authorities proved too burdensome, both financially and socially.[43] In other cases, the patient and his family, anxious to hide the diagnosis, actively sought transfer to a sanitarium but were denied based upon their financial resources. It was only after the disease had progressed over years and their resources had been exhausted by long stints at Kusatsu or other attempts at treatment that such patients were deemed qualified for admission.[44] Some patients would later charge that they agreed to be confined only because local police had assured them that a cure was possible in the sanitarium, with more than one noting that he fell into despair when he realized that no one recovered.[45]

The capacity of the five regional facilities was based upon the 1906 survey, which identified the geographic distribution of indigent leprosy sufferers. Zensei Hospital and Sotojima Rest Home were the largest, designed to house 350 and 300, respectively; the Northern Area Rest Home and Ōshima Sanitarium were designed for 100 patients each; and Kyūshū Sanitarium, for 180. However, six months after their opening, the Northern Area Rest Home housed only 15 people, and Kyūshū Sanitarium only 16.[46] In contrast, Sotojima and Zensei soon reached capacity, and by 1915 both housed more patients than was officially allowed.[47]

It soon became clear that delivering patients to a sanitarium was easier than keeping them there. Many quickly took advantage of the permeable borders of the institutions to run away. In his memoir of his time as medical director at Zensei Hospital, Mitsuda noted ruefully that "in the first year after the opening the number of those who ran away increased conspicuously. Even the blind were running away."[48] A report from Ikeuchi Saijirō, the director of Zensei and a former police official, to the governor of Tokyo suggests the extent of the problem. It describes how 60 patients (of 280 total) were discovered attempting to escape en masse at eight thirty on the evening of July 7, 1911, after breaking down a closed gate.[49]

The desire of patients to flee the sanitaria baffled administrators, who seem to have been confident that indigent sufferers would embrace the aid they were offered. Mitsuda would later explain the high number of runaways by pointing to the moral turpitude of those who fled. Many, he wrote, were addicted to morphine and found his attempts to wean them from the drug intolerable, while others simply disliked the constraints and boredom of institutional life, since they were accustomed to spending their time gambling, drinking, and engaging in casual sex, all activities forbidden within the sanitarium. Such remarks were colored by contemporary stereotypes of vagrants, but Mitsuda also acknowledged that despair born of their illness may have prompted some to seek relief in alcohol or opiates.[50]

A memorandum submitted by the director of the Kyūshū Sanitarium to the governor of Kumamoto in 1909, within months of the sanitarium's opening, provides a different perspective. It describes the motives of six patients who attempted on multiple occasions to escape: some were unhappy with the food and housing they were provided, while others missed their former freedom; some ran away because they were concerned about family, friends, or companions. Alarmingly, the only woman in this group stated that she ran away out of fear of what the report described as "bad elements who tried to force their animalistic desires upon her."[51] The early sanitaria were dreary and even dangerous places, and the uncertainties of life on the road may well have been seen as the better option by some patients.

The problem of runaways was particularly acute at Zensei Hospital and Sotojima Rest Home. At Sotojima, of 889 patients admitted between 1911 and 1915, 342 absconded; at Zensei, of 792 patients admitted in the same period, 232 absconded.[52] Their proximity to major cities, which offered anonymity, amusements, and opportunities for begging, may have been one reason for the high numbers. In addition, the organization of the institutions aided those who wanted to escape, since the demarcation between the patients' residential area, medical facilities, and staff housing allowed patients a good deal of autonomy in their day-to-day lives, as did the sparse staffing. At Zensei Hospital, through the 1920s, only five staff members managed the daily life of several hundred patients.[53]

Sakurazawa Fusayoshi (1899–1990), who entered Zensei in 1919 and spent the rest of his life there, wrote an illuminating memoir that offers a patient-centric perspective of life within the sanitarium. He recalled that at the time of his arrival, his fellow residents remarked nostalgically on the ease with which they had moved in and out of the institution in the first years of its existence. Some had even raised chickens in chicken coops they built adjacent to their dormitories and journeyed as far as Tokorozawa in Saitama to sell their eggs.[54]

As administrators and staff confronted the issue of runaways, they began to alter the original porous design of the institutions and to develop new policies designed to limit patients' freedom of movement. In 1911, the director of the Kyūshū Sanitarium ordered the construction of a wide "moat" (*hori*) around the patients' residential area in order to hinder attempts to leave.[55] Later, all the sanitaria began to issue patients institutional clothing in the form of kimonos with a distinctive striped pattern with the aim of making escapees easily identifiable to local police.[56] At Zensei Hospital, a new policy required patients to turn over any cash they held to staff members, who also began to open and inspect incoming mail to head off attempts at escape. The practice of allowing the patients to go outside the sanitarium to make small purchases was also curtailed, and instead local tradesmen were invited to come into the sanitarium, and sanitarium shops were established. In addition, staff began to patrol the patients' residential area at regular intervals day and night to guard against attempts at escape.[57]

Significantly, these new efforts at surveillance, policing, and control originated not from the Home Ministry but from the directors and staff of the individual sanitaria, as a set of local efforts aimed at bringing order to the institutions under their control. These measures were accompanied by efforts to improve the unfamiliar spaces and to create a sense of community among the patients. This involved both appropriating aspects of traditional community life and introducing new modern amusements not yet widely available and certainly not in isolated rural villages. At every sanitarium efforts were made to soften the harsh institutional landscapes. Flowering trees were planted, including the cherry trees necessary for the spring festivity of "flower viewing," as were maples and gingko trees, which provided displays of fall foliage. The original stockade-like facilities were gradually improved. At Zensei Hospital, for example, roofed walkways were constructed to connect patient dormitories to the bathhouse and other facilities.[58] Other construction projects followed, including the installation of a Shinto shrine and a baseball field. Electrification came in 1916, replacing the oil lamps and candles that patients and staff had relied on to this time.[59]

Religious observances became an important aspect of sanitarium life. At the Kyūshū Sanitarium, where many of the early residents had been removed from the grounds of Honmyōji temple, priests of the temple and sanitarium staff joined forces to have an image of Katō Kiyomasa, the deity worshipped at the temple, moved to the sanitarium's religious hall. The ritual transfer, held only a month after the sanitarium's opening, was a grand event attended by seven priests, three temple musicians, and dignitaries from Hanazono village, as well as by the staff and patients of the sanitarium.[60] At Zensei Hospital, Protestant religious services began within the first year of its operation, after Ōtsuka Seishin, a Japanese Christian associated with Ihaien, approached Ikeuchi, Zensei's director. Ikeuchi agreed to allow services with the stipulation that there be no attempt to undermine government policies and no criticism of other religions.[61] Buddhist services, too, took place regularly, with priests from well-known Tokyo temples journeying to Higashimurayama.[62]

Cultural activities were gradually organized, including a variety of "circles" for devotees of poetry composition, calligraphy, and board games such as *go* and *shogi*. Educated patients organized lessons for their fellow patients, especially for the children among their numbers. When a member of the Nakamura-za, one of Tokyo's kabuki theaters, entered Zensei Hospital in the early 1910s, he was prevailed upon by his fellow patients to teach them some kabuki-style dances. This eventually led to the establishment of an amateur kabuki troupe that took the name Zensei-za (Zensei theater). Within a few years, the practice began of inviting local villagers to attend its performances, which helped to improve relations between the institution and its neighbors.[63]

While many activities were modeled on long-standing seasonal practices, the sanitarium administrators also sponsored the introduction of exotic cultural activities that had not yet reached the villages of Japan. Soon after its establishment, the Kyūshū Sanitarium purchased a phonograph, which was used to hold "concerts" for the patients. In 1911 patients were also introduced to the new media of the cinema, through the charitable efforts of the recently established Kumamoto Electric Company. Zensei Hospital, too, offered film screenings, which were accompanied by live narration. There were also new kinds of events that reflected the unique aspects of sanitarium life, and through repetition these, too, became "traditions." One of the most important gatherings at Zensei Hospital was the Ireisai (Comforting the Spirits Rite), an institutionally sponsored service held each May and October to memorialize those who had died in recent months. It reflected the sad fact that the death of one's companions was an all-too-common feature of life within the sanitarium. This event was presided over by a high-ranking priest, but Zensei's director also gave a speech in which he offered a eulogy of sorts for those who had died.[64]

Patient Work and the Sanitarium Economy

As these initiatives suggest, the sanitaria were gradually transformed into places of leisure, cultural activities, and religion that created new ties between patients and with the institution. At the same time, they were also becoming sites of labor and production. The idea that work should be a part of sanitarium life was, to be sure, not new. We can recollect that in his presentation at the Berlin conference, Dohi had highlighted this as a desirable aspect of patient life at Fukusei Hospital. Evoking the image of the therapeutic colony, he described residents who nursed their less-able neighbors, farmed, and produced handicrafts. Similarly, in his writings on poverty Kubota Seitarō, author of the 1907 law, had argued that "relief" should not take the form of handouts but must require the poor to engage in productive labor.

Nonetheless, patient labor does not seem to have been part of the initial design of the institutions. *The Fifty-Year History of the Kyūshū Sanitarium* relates that patient work got under way in its second year of operation, when relatively healthy patients began to care for the more disabled, grow vegetables, and do laundry. However, according to this official history, "rather than work, this was an important source of consolation for the patients."[65] In his memoir, Mitsuda discussed at length how labor became a central aspect of patient life at Zensei Hospital but in terms that suggest that it initially had little to do with either the concept of the therapeutic colony or "consolation" for the patients, and everything to do with strained institutional finances.

The funding of the public sanitaria was complex, with the prefectures in each zone allowed to work out their own scheme. This meant that some institutions had fewer resources than others. Zensei Hospital was one of the more poorly funded institutions and was at full capacity or beyond within just a few years.[66] According to Mitsuda, in its early years, the hospital received only about sixteen sen per day per patient to cover food and medical expenses, of which about twelve sen went to the cost of meals. As a point of comparison, in this period the inns at Kusatsu that housed leprosy sufferers charged forty-five sen per day, for food, board, and the hot-spring treatment.[67] Mitsuda found it impossible to purchase the necessary medical supplies with the four sen per patient that remained. Out of desperation, he began to have patients "recycle" used bandages by washing them in disinfectant, a job that could be performed even by the blind and those with mobility impairment. The use of patients as nursing staff began out of necessity as well, since the number of those in need of care overwhelmed the skeleton professional medical staff. By the early 1920s each medical ward of twenty patients was staffed by five patients who worked as "attendants" (*tsukisoe*). Visually impaired residents, too, were assigned an "attendant," who aided them with bathing, meals, and other aspects of daily life.[68]

Unlike the use of patient labor to supplement the limited medical budget, Mitsuda suggests that farming was regarded as an amusement (*shumi*) for patients, perhaps because the allotted funds for provisions were relatively generous, at least in comparison to the paltry sum available for medical supplies. He relates that farming began at Zensei Hospital when an older woman who came from a farming family began to grow vegetables in the soil placed on top of the large trenches where waste from the institution's latrines was buried, a method of waste management to which the institution resorted out of concern that the raw sewage might carry *M. leprae*. When her efforts proved successful, the staff began to encourage patients to become involved in farming by providing tools, seeds, and advice. Eventually a wide range of crops came under cultivation including a variety of vegetables, grapes, persimmons, melons, and even tea.[69] All of these products gradually improved the monotonous institutional diet, which relied heavily on imported *indica* rice, which many patients found unpalatable. When Sakurazawa entered Zensei Hospital in 1919 he found that patients were already involved in raising livestock, including pigs and chickens for food, and rabbits and guinea pigs as laboratory animals. In addition, patients who came to the sanitarium with specific skills were encouraged to use them: patients made bamboo utensils and tofu, repaired tatami, and worked as hairdressers and barbers.[70]

Sakurazawa's memoir reveals that patients referred to the tasks they performed within the sanitarium as "work" (*sagyō*), eschewing the language of "therapy," "consolation," and "amusement" favored by administrators. From the outset, they were paid for their efforts, albeit eventually in the sanitarium's script, another innovation designed to control runaways. In 1912, the daily rate for patient labor was three and a half sen, seven times the amount paid at Fukusei Hospital at the same time, a disparity that provoked the patient strike at the private institution.[71] By 1919–1920, the initial wage was four sen per day, and patients who remained in a position were promised a raise each year. This amount was about 15 to 20 percent of what a live-in domestic servant would have earned for a day's labor at the time.[72] The low wages reflected the administrators' view of the purpose of patient wages. In an environment in which basic needs were met, wages were intended to provide modest pocket money for patients, not to allow them to live independently, provide for their families, or accumulate savings.

Wages within the sanitarium economy were, however, subject to supply and demand. In the winter months, for example, few patients were willing to wash bandages in freezing water, and a premium had to be paid to get this work accomplished. As this suggests, sanitarium labor does not seem to have been coerced. Sakurazawa reports that in the mid-1920s a large number of comparatively healthy patients opted out of work. The practice of distributing "consolation money" to patients had begun, using funds donated by the imperial family and other benefactors, and apparently some patients found this sufficient for their needs.[73] Others, like Sakurazawa himself, moved from one position to another every couple of years in search of more interesting or better-paid work. At times Sakurazawa even held multiple jobs.

The Limits of Citizenship

As the ability of patients to forgo work or to bargain for better pay reveals, patients were able to negotiate some of the institutional norms and constraints that gradually shaped life within the sanitaria. Even so, Sakurazawa's memoir suggests that he and his fellow patients were acutely aware of the staff's power over their daily lives and that they resented any behavior that explicitly expressed the unevenness of this relationship. He recalled, with considerable anger more than half a century later, that in the early years the staff "looked at us as though we were something quite peculiar and when they spoke to us they did not attach *san* to our names."[74] Ikeuchi, Zensei Hospital's first director, struggled to define his relationship with patients. According to Mitsuda, Ikeuchi worried about which second-person pronoun was appropriate when speaking to patients, rejecting *kimi* and *omae* as too familiar but unsure whether *kisama* or *sochira* struck the right combination of distance and superiority.[75] Mitsuda himself would later note that while the low staff-to-patient ratio resulted from budgetary constraints, it actually aided in the smooth running of the institution, since "as the number of staff increased, it became difficult to control the patients."[76] At Zensei Hospital and Sotojima Rest Home, limited forms of self-governance were permitted. Dormitory heads, who were elected by residents of each dormitory, came together to form a council that managed day-to-day issues in the residential area and negotiated with the staff over matters of policy, addressing issues such as dormitory overcrowding, the lack of variety in meals, and improvements to the facilities, with varying degrees of success.[77]

A conflict at Zensei Hospital in 1913 reveals both the methods that patients could deploy to contest sanitarium policies and their sense that the institution had specific obligations towards them. The dispute involved the quality of medical care provided to patients. The most effective treatment for leprosy continued to be chaulmoogra oil, although many patients could not tolerate the side effects of its oral use. As a result, Mitsuda Kensuke began to experiment with subcutaneous injections, something that doctors in the Philippines and the United States were also attempting. He eventually concluded that the best course of treatment was the injection three times a week of two to five grams of chaulmoogra oil.[78] However, Ikeuchi, who as director of Zensei had control of the budget, refused to authorize the purchase of sufficient quantities of chaulmoogra oil, and patients received only one injection of two grams each week. Whether his intention was to pit the patients against Ikeuchi is unclear, but Mitsuda apparently complained to them about his inability to acquire enough chaulmoogra oil, blaming bureaucratic penny-pinching for the shortfall.

Angered at being denied optimal treatment, the patients put together a written petition addressed to Ikeuchi requesting more frequent injections at the higher dosage. When he failed to respond, they requested a meeting where they again made their case, stating that the regimen of three injections per week was being followed at other sanitaria, information they could have obtained from Mitsuda or from someone who had relocated from one of these institutions to Zensei Hospital. When Ikeuchi rebuffed their efforts, in terms that some patients interpreted to mean that they were unworthy of expensive medical treatment, a group of patients decided that they would escape and make their way to Tokyo in order to confront the prefectural governor. As this plan suggests, like the patients at Fukusei Hospital, those at Zensei, too, believed they had the right to demand a certain level of care, and they were also well aware of the larger political structure within which the sanitarium figured. Significantly, their protest was effective. The group made it only as far as Tanashi, a distance of about eight kilometers from Higashimurayama, before they were overtaken by Mitsuda, who had pursued them on his bicycle. He convinced them to return, promising them that he would ensure that they received appropriate treatment. When Ikeuchi resigned not long afterward and Mitsuda became director, some patients interpreted this as the result of their protest.[79]

Events such as this reveal that just as the relationship between citizens and the state was under negotiation outside the sanitaria, so, too, was it within them. And as the appeals to figures such as prefectural governors and later Home Ministry officials suggest, patients recognized that decisions on the part of the sanitarium directors and staff did not necessarily reflect government policy. However, successful protests such as this one notwithstanding, the most direct means of resistance continued to be simply to run away, and it was only in the 1920s that the number of those who escaped began to drop.

The inability to control patients gradually led to new policies that strengthened the authority of the directors. In 1916 in response to the large number of runaways and other infractions of sanitaria rules, the Diet amended the 1907 law to give the directors of the public sanitaria the authority to punish noncompliant patients. When Nakagawa Nozomu of the Home Ministry presented the amendment to members of the lower house, he initially characterized it as a "simple matter." However, in discussing problem patients, he acknowledged the tensions of institutional life: "Patients . . . are separated from the rest of society and they have few consolations. Since they are idle, there are not a few instances where they do bad things." Nakagawa related that he had consulted with his counterpart in the Ministry of Justice, evidently because he was concerned about the legality of giving disciplinary power to sanitarium administrators. The Ministry of Justice had declined to become involved, on the grounds that the breaking of the sanitarium rules did not rise to the level of crime, and in any case the country's prisons were not equipped to house leprosy patients.[80]

In contrast to the intense debates that led to the 1907 law, Nakagawa's proposed amendment elicited little commentary, although Yamane Masatsugu, champion of a statist approach to public health, took a hard line, suggesting that jails should be established on sanitarium grounds.[81] In the end, the directors were authorized to use verbal reprimands, loss of privileges, reduction of meals to half rations for up to seven days, and solitary confinement for up to thirty days to punish patients. By this time, it seems no one shared Kubota's concern that the sanitaria avoid any resemblance to a prison. Ironically, however, the severest punishment of all was expulsion from the sanitarium, further evidence of the ambiguity that continued to surround these institutions and their mission.

Sexuality and Reproduction in the Sanitaria

No sanitarium policy proved more contentious than that of sexual segregation, which had been central to the original design of the institutions. Mitsuda, who was to play a leading role in formulating policy towards patient sexuality and reproduction, provides an unintentionally comic picture in his memoir of the battle that ensued between patients and staff over attempts to maintain sexual segregation at Zensei Hospital. When a three-meter-high fence was installed between the male and female dormitories, patients tore it down in a single night; after a sturdier partition was constructed, patients successfully tunneled under it. On another occasion when staff made an unannounced check of the women's dormitories, surprised male patients fled "one after another" in the dark. In the mayhem one patient fell off a veranda, injuring himself. One of the more successful efforts at policing involved placing a flock of geese near a dormitory that housed adolescent girls—the birds honked noisily whenever someone approached, frightening off intruders and awakening the staff.[82]

The information that reached Fukusei Hospital in 1912 about the accommodation of sexual relationships was correct. In the face of persistent patient resistance, the staff of the sanitaria abandoned their attempts to control patient sexuality. Mitsuda later defended this decision, arguing that the expectation of abstinence was unreasonable and unnatural, particularly for men, for whom the suppression of sexual desire often led to violence, an observation that reflected the prevailing view of male sexuality. Moreover, he argued that leprosy sufferers, who were denied many of the comforts of an ordinary life, should at least be allowed to enjoy the consolation of (heterosexual) sex, albeit ideally within stable conjugal relationships.[83] As the rules were relaxed, the sanitaria were soon confronted with pregnant patients, a not surprising development given the demographics of the patient population in these early years. Most were between the ages of fifteen and forty and had never been married.[84] According to Mitsuda, more than ten children were born each year in Zensei Hospital in the early 1910s, and within a few years, there were thirty infants being raised in the female dormitories.[85]

This unanticipated and unwelcomed baby boom provided the medical staff of the early sanitaria with their first real research opportunity, with the result that research became yet another role of the sanitaria. By the turn of the century, Japanese doctors had already begun to document that pregnancy had an adverse effect on women with leprosy, observations borne out by more recent clinical studies.[86] Not only did some women first develop symptoms while pregnant, but the condition of many worsened during pregnancy and following childbirth. As infants began to be born, sanitarium doctors defined new questions that were both pressing and newly amenable to investigation. Could infants born to a mother with leprosy be infected in utero or during delivery, or did infection occur after birth in infancy?

The physicians who were most actively engaged in research on mother-to-child transmission were Nakajō Suketoshi, director of the Northern Area Rest Home, and Sugai Takekichi, medical director of Sotojima Rest Home. Neither had particularly strong training in laboratory research. Like Mitsuda, they had not attended a university medical school and had instead obtained their qualifications by examination. However, as babies began to be born at their sanitaria, both took up the question of mother-to-child transmission. In research published in 1914–1915, Nakajō reported that he had examined the placentas of five patients who had given birth but found no sign of *M. leprae* in the tissue. However, he noted that one infant whose placenta had been examined subsequently showed signs of leprosy at three months of age, leading him to believe that this was a case of in utero infection. Nakajō concluded that the examination of tissue from a stillborn or miscarried fetus might offer more information.[87]

At about the same time, Sugai Takekichi was also researching mother-to-child transmission. In the early 1910s, he examined blood drawn from infants born at Sotojima as well as the amniotic fluid and breast milk of their mothers, looking for the elusive *M. leprae*. Like Nakajō, he, too, believed that fetal tissue might be the key, and since skin tissue was known to be a favorite environment of the mycobacterium, he began to examine samples of fetal skin tissue obtained from both still and live births. According to an article published in 1921, over the course of ten years with help from his colleagues at the other sanitaria, Sugai had managed to obtain ninety-seven samples, twenty-seven of which were from live births. He reported that five of the twenty-seven infants later developed lesions, although these appeared to spontaneously heal, something that recent medical research has confirmed to be a characteristic of what is now classified as "indeterminate" leprosy, that is, a form of the disease that sometimes resolves spontaneously.[88]

Research on the question of mother-to-child transmission would continue into the 1950s, and decades later more than a hundred preserved fetuses were recovered from various sanitaria. To the lawyers who authored the 2005 *Final Report of the Verification Committee on the Hansen's Disease Problem*, this was evidence that the "sense of medical ethics" of sanitarium doctors "had become paralyzed."[89] However, while the use of human biological material for research purposes continues to be controversial, the practice was, at the time, both legal and commonplace not only in Japan but around the world. It was only in 1964 that the World Medical Association issued the Declaration of Helsinki, a set of ethical guidelines for medical research, and national legislation in Japan, the United States, the United Kingdom, and elsewhere took decades to formulate due to intense resistance from researchers.[90] The use of biospecimens in sanitarium laboratories, without donor consent, raises important questions about medical authority, but it does not mean that the sanitarium doctors regarded leprosy patients as "less than human" as the authors of *The Final Report* and others have charged. Moreover, the questions that oriented the work of Sugai, Nakajō, and their colleagues were valid. Scientists have continued to probe the route of infant and early childhood infection up to the present, with one recent study noting that even in the age of effective multidrug therapy 20 percent of children born to mothers with leprosy will develop the disease.[91]

Sanitarium doctors were legitimately concerned about the medical and epidemiological consequences of reproduction among their patients, but they regarded pregnancy and birth as problematic for other reasons as well. The public sanitaria were ill prepared to cope with infants and young children, given the crowded communal living arrangements, the pressing needs of the many disabled patients, and the limited budgets. In response to concerns about both infection and order, staff tried to remove children from their mothers as soon as possible. In the case of Zensei Hospital, Mitsuda first tried placing infants in the Tokyo Poorhouse, his former employer, which was charged with the care of orphans and abandoned children, but he was dismayed when two babies he placed there died within a month. Upon investigating, he concluded that Poorhouse staff had systematically neglected them. Unwilling to entrust infants to such "care," Mitsuda then attempted to place them with local families, but while he succeeded in identifying potential foster parents, he could not come up with funds to pay them, the customary practice in fostering arrangements.[92]

It was in light of this set of issues that Mitsuda came to advocate for what he believed to be the solution to the intertwined issues of sexuality and reproduction within the sanitaria—the sterilization of male patients through the use of vasectomy. Developed originally as a means to address prostate problems, vasectomy began to be promoted as a method of sterilization in the United States as interest in eugenics was growing in the late nineteenth century. In 1897, A. J. Oschner, a Chicago surgeon, published a paper entitled "Surgical Treatment of Habitual Criminals" in which he argued that the procedure offered, in the words of historian Philip R. Reilly, "a socially acceptable method of doing away with hereditary criminals from 'the father's side.'"[93] The surgery seems to have been all but unknown in Japan at the time, but Mitsuda would later write that he had learned of it from a pamphlet authored by Ujihara Sukezo, a bureaucrat within the Bureau of Hygiene.[94]

The work in question has been identified as *National Hygiene* (*Minzoku eiseigaku*), an eighty-page booklet that Ujihara published privately in 1914.[95] Sheldon Garon has described Ujihara as "the Home Ministry's leading spokesman on prostitution in the 1920s," a role that led him to stoutly defend the licensed prostitution system on public health grounds, but in this work he was explicitly critical of the Japanese government's approach to biopolitics, which relied primarily on the criminalization of abortion and limiting access to contraception as the means to promote population growth.[96] Ujihara cited at considerable length contemporary German and American works on eugenics to bemoan the fact that in Japan it was the worst elements of society who were having the most children. He advocated for a lengthy list of progressive measures designed to encourage women to have both more and healthier children, including the promotion of family planning and economic support for pregnant women, nursing mothers, single mothers, and large families.

The flip side of his plan, however, included efforts to "remove social poisons." Ujihara called for new laws that would ban alcohol consumption, control the spread of diseases such as tuberculosis and syphilis, and limit the reproduction of undesirables through the use of birth control and sterilization. (Notably, leprosy is not on the list of "social poisons.") Vasectomy was described as the ideal approach to sterilization: "a very easy and minor surgical procedure," it was without the dangers or unwelcome side effects of castration and female sterilization.

In his memoir, Mitsuda wrote that he was intrigued by the potential of this method of sterilization to resolve the problems resulting from patient pregnancies at Zensei Hospital. He experimented with the procedure on animals for some time until he was convinced that he could perform it safely. Meanwhile he also sought advice about the legality of its use on human subjects. He consulted Hanai Takuzō, a liberal lawyer who had recently and unsuccessfully defended Kōtoku Shūsui and several other socialists accused of plotting to assassinate the emperor, and Makino Eiichi, a former prosecutor who had joined the law faculty of Tokyo University in 1913. Both men, although they occupied very different positions within Japan's legal culture, advised him that a prosecutor would have to find a basis to make a charge given that the procedure itself was not explicitly defined as a crime. Even so, according to Mitsuda's memoir, he was determined to implement sterilization "as lawfully as possible" and to that end sought out patient volunteers. He gathered Zensei's residents together, explained his concerns regarding the transmission of the disease to children they might have, and told them that vasectomy would allow them to "have a married life without worry." He then asked for volunteers and chose one from the several men who stepped forward. According to Mitsuda, when the success of the operation became clear, other men volunteered.[97] By 1919, Mitsuda had performed 160 vasectomies, including 10 on male residents of Kusatsu, who had sought him out after learning of the procedure.[98]

Evaluating the 1907 Law

As Mitsuda's experimentation with vasectomy suggests, at the end of the first decade of the operation of the public sanitaria, patient sexuality and reproduction had become crucial issues for those involved in formulating and implementing leprosy policy. It dominated the discussions that unfolded at an unusual two-day conference convened by the Bureau of Hygiene in October 1919 that brought together Bureau of Hygiene officials, the directors of the five public sanitaria, and representatives of four missionary endeavors, Fukusei Hospital, Ihaien, Kaishun Hospital, and St. Barnabas Mission. St. Barnabas had been founded in 1916 by Mary Cornwallis-Legh, a British Anglican missionary, in Yunosawa, the area of Kusatsu given over to leprosy sufferers. The stated aim of the Bureau of Hygiene officials in calling this meeting was to gather "opinions on the fundamental aims of the Leprosy Prevention Law," "the real conditions of each sanitarium," and "the hopes of the directors," but the comments offered by two of the non-Japanese participants, Hannah Riddell of Kaishun Hospital and Father Drouart de Lézey of Fukusei, brought the issue of sexuality front and center. Both seized the opportunity to lecture the Japanese participants on appropriate national policy.

Hannah Riddell, whose many influential patrons had made her a public figure at the turn of the century, was invited to speak first. Her written statement, which was read aloud by a Bureau of Hygiene staffer, opened with the declaration that "in eradicating leprosy, the most important requirement is to diligently segregate the sexes."[99] Riddell reiterated a plan she had already put forth in 1914 in a letter she had written to one of her major donors, Ōkuma Shigenobu, who had just become prime minister for the second time. Her solution for leprosy control called for requiring all people with the disease to take up residence in special villages newly created for them. These were to be self-governing, working communities where medical care would be in the hands of physicians in the employ of the state, while commerce, agriculture, and all administrative and social matters would be left in the hands of residents. While Riddell left unclear where such villages would be established and how they would be financed, she was adamant about one thing. There were to be separate villages for men and women in each prefecture and they should be "as far apart as possible."[100]

Riddell's plan reflected the policy of Kaishun Hospital, where abstinence was required, and her outrage at the failure of the public institutions to enforce it. In her remarks at the 1919 conference, she described sexual activity in the public sanitaria in terms that reflected her personal prudishness, her belief that chastity was a Christian virtue, and her orientalist tendency to infantilize the Japanese she was aiding. (She was delighted when Kaishun residents called her "mother.") At Kaishun Hospital, men and women were housed in separate wards, but according to Riddell, Christian morality prevailed and patients lived chastely. In contrast, at the public sanitaria, she charged, sex primarily took the form of predatory male advances on "pitiful women," who were "unable to defend themselves against the violence of male patients." The pregnancies that resulted were "a terrible evil that cannot be allowed from the perspective of morality." Riddell concluded that the only way to curtail the spread of leprosy, described as "increasing year by year," was to confine all sufferers separately to prevent sex and reproduction.[101]

Lézey agreed with Riddell's sentiments but not her plan for single-sex communities. Although the most recent survey of leprosy's prevalence, completed just the year before, had given the number of sufferers as 16,200, a drop of a third since the 1906 survey, Lézey suggested the number was far larger, "at least 150,000 or 200,000," a figure that tripled, even quadrupled the estimates made in the aftermath of the first national surveys. According to Lézey, the growing number of leprosy sufferers "threatened the nation" but attempting to confine them would be a mistake because it "exceeded the strength of the Japanese government." Characterizing the 1907 law as "utterly defective," he called for a stiff new law that would ban anyone with leprosy from marrying and for the establishment of special jails for those who did not comply.[102]

Lézey did not explain how a marriage ban would be an effective preventive measure, and it is unclear whether he was concerned about intrafamilial infection, hereditary transmission, or just sex itself. Whatever the case, Ōtsuka Seishin, the Japanese Christian who headed Ihaien, offered his support for this proposal. The police, he suggested, should carry out a door-to-door search for leprosy sufferers to conclusively determine the prevalence of the disease and to put together a registry that could be used to enforce a marriage ban. Meanwhile, individuals should make use of private detective agencies to determine whether there were cases of disease in the family of prospective marriage partners. As for patients within the public sanitaria, those who wished to be sexually active should be required to enter into legal marriages and to accept sterilization.[103]

The missionaries did not participate in the second day of discussion, and in their absence, the sanitarium directors and public health officials showed little interest in implementing a regime of leprosy control based on door-to-door surveillance and intervention in the sexual lives of the Japanese citizenry. They also dismissed the alarmist claims of Lézey and Riddell that leprosy was on the rise.[104] But sanitarium directors were in agreement that the institutions were confronting a growing number of problems, including runaways, unwanted births, and unruly patients. There was little consensus, however, about how to move forward.

Mitsuda championed the American approach in the Philippines and Hawai'i, holding up the Culion colony in particular as an example of an island "paradise" (*rakutenchi*) created for leprosy sufferers. Culion had four thousand residents by 1919, and in the words of Warwick Anderson, its American administrators "had structured the leper colony as a laboratory of therapeutics and citizenship, a place where needy patients were resocialized, where they performed somatic recovery alongside domestic hygiene and civic pride." At Culion, families lived in small houses, voted in local elections, played baseball, served in brass bands and volunteer fire brigades, and manufactured cheap goods—and until 1927 married couples raised their children there.[105] This seemingly humane policy had a tragic outcome in many cases. According to one study, close to 50 percent of children who remained in the care of their parents at Culion for more than six months developed leprous lesions by the age of five.[106]

Like Culion, Mitsuda's imagined colony, too, was to be a model of modernity in design, "a splendid new village." It would feature running water, electricity, and opportunities for work, recreation, and self-improvement. There would be no sexual segregation. Indeed, Mitsuda suggested that monogamous heterosexual relationships, in which "men and women would depend on each other," would be an essential feature of the new community. But if there was to be no sexual segregation, there were to be no children either. Sterilization was to be the rule in Mitsuda's new village.[107]

Imada Torajirō, the former police official who headed Sotojima Rest Home, supported the island colony approach, noting that although he had tried to resolve the runaway issue by establishing self-governance within the residential area, even empowering a patient council to tackle the thorny issue of punishments, it had not brought about a significant decline in the number of escapes.[108] Sugai, Sotojima's medical director, also endorsed the island option, but reluctantly, stating that doing so required him to "suppress my tears." He explained his decision by referencing his research on mother-to-child transmission. In his view, the pattern of intrafamilial infection so common in Japan required that sufferers be separated from their uninfected family members, although Sugai acknowledged that this put the national interest above that of individual patients.[109]

Not everyone embraced this solution. Kobayashi Kazusaburō, director of the Ōshima Sanitarium, noted that the isolated location of his sanitarium had proven to be difficult for both staff and patients to tolerate. In times of bad weather, the island often had no deliveries of news and supplies for days at a time, and morale and quality of life suffered. He suggested that the problem of runaways could be mitigated by providing aid to the families of those confined, since many who escaped did so out of concern for their dependents.[110] Nakajō Suketoshi questioned whether isolation, especially coerced isolation, could be achieved as easily as Mitsuda suggested. After all, the 1907 law had targeted indigent wanderers who presumably had weak ties with their families and yet they had shown considerable resistance. Could those with property, homes, and families really be expected to abandon their lives and move to an isolated island? Nakajō suggested it was necessary to proceed cautiously. Those willing to start new lives in an island colony could be relocated, while those with the means to pay should be allowed to enter the public sanitaria, although these would have to be improved. Chillingly, Nakajō suggested that the stigma of the disease could be used to loosen familial ties and encourage acceptance of confinement: "What if we were to use the method of letting the public know 'this family is a leprous family'? . . . The family on its own initiative would then be inspired to separate themselves from the leper."[111]

The Voices of the Confined

In the midst of their assessment of the public sanitaria, officials in the Board of Hygiene undertook a new endeavor that was extraordinary in terms of both the global history of leprosy and the making of Japanese domestic policy. They decided to solicit the views of patients in the public sanitaria. Takano Rokurō, a physician trained at Keiō University and an official in the Bureau of Hygiene, was put in charge of this project, which got under way in the late 1910s. He asked the patients in the public sanitaria not only to describe the course of their lives and the effect of the disease upon it but also to comment on life within a public sanitarium and to offer suggestions on how the institutions might be improved.[112] In total, the statements of 104 patients (81 men, 15 women, 8 unspecified), slightly less than 10 percent of the total population, were published. The youngest was eleven, the oldest sixty-six, but the vast majority of statements (50 percent of the total) came from men aged thirty to fifty years in age. Whether by chance or by design, the results provided a fairly representative sampling of the patient population.

The stated aim of publishing the statements, in 1923 with the title *Confessions of Leprosy Patients* (*Raikanja no kokuhaku*), was to raise public awareness of the plight of leprosy sufferers.[113] The preface indicates that only minor revisions, such as the correction of miswritten characters and the addition of punctuation, were made to the patients' statements, but this likely minimized the editor's role, since several respondents were blind and others had limited use of their hands and thus would have required assistance. That said, the statements are distinctive in length, style, content, and tone, and patients offered a range of views. Read in its entirety, the work offers a devastating picture of what a diagnosis of leprosy meant in the early twentieth century, when fear of infection, hereditary transmission, and the still potent idea of karmic retribution had become intertwined in the minds of many in Japan. In account after account, lives unraveled after the diagnosis forced patients to take to the road in search of a cure and to spare their families.

Although patients were explicitly asked to comment upon the sanitaria, many simply ended their stories at the point of their admission. A few offered unqualified praise of the institution. One forty-four-year-old woman wrote that she had contemplated suicide upon learning she was to be sent to the sanitarium, but after settling in, she was able to "begin to live again" in what she described as "this different society that is a small paradise."[114] Others simply commented that they had no complaints. Not everyone was so sanguine. Thirty-two patients explicitly called for changes, large and small. One man asked that *japonica* rice replace the imported rice that was served at all the sanitaria as a cost-saving measure, and several protested the high prices in the sanitarium shops. But the most frequent requests were for more fundamental kinds of reforms, including improved medical care, better treatment by staff, more opportunities for work and better pay, and occasional furloughs.

Surprisingly, a significant number of patients called for the confinement of all leprosy sufferers, some because they were satisfied with sanitarium life, others because they resented what they viewed as the class bias of the 1907 law, which confined only the poor. According to a forty-year-old man who had been diagnosed in 1905, "The world tells us that we are being punished by heaven and coldly rejects us." He asked for a new policy "that would not make a distinction between the rich and poor but would gather us all together and confine us to an ideal place. . . . Choose a method that allows us to continue to live freely."[115] A thirty-four-year-old man confined at Sotojima wrote, "I have no hope that hospital life here or the treatment of the doctors can be improved. We are like prisoners who are allowed no freedom. . . . Start again with a spirit of freedom and choose some place that is appropriate for all of us with this disease and confine us all to that place. Let us make a world of our own. More than medical care I hope that you will allow us some spiritual comfort."[116]

By the early 1920s, then, both the directors of the sanitaria and some of their patients were beginning to imagine the possibility of fully segregated communities that would separate all leprosy sufferers from the larger population. But different concerns led them to this shared position. Mitsuda and his fellow directors wanted more authority over their patients. In contrast, patients who advocated for a Culion-like settlement spoke of emancipation and freedom, from the sanitarium and from the stigma of the disease.

The Leprosy Sanitaria in Comparative Perspective
The growing concern over the leprosy sanitaria notwithstanding, the Japanese government's efforts to confine those with chronic diseases expanded in this period. In 1914, the Diet passed the Law for the Establishment of Tuberculosis Sanitaria with the Support of National Funds. Formulated in response to rising numbers of tuberculosis deaths (more than 110,000 in 1913), the new law required cities with a population of 300,000 or more to establish institutions to house tuberculosis sufferers "who lack the means to convalesce," a phrase that according to Sugiyama Shigorō, then head of the Bureau of Hygiene, referred to those "who were [financially] unable to seek care from a doctor." Thus, like the 1907 leprosy law, this one, too, targeted poor sufferers of the disease. There were, however, some important differences between the two laws. For one, there was to be no need-based test for admission to the tuberculosis sanitaria. In the Diet hearings on the bill, Sugiyama explained, "even if there is someone who has the duty of support, in those cases where they cannot support the tuberculosis patient . . . then that person can be treated as someone 'who lacks the means to convalesce.'" Secondly, the bill did not specifically authorize the coercive confinement of indigent tuberculosis patients. Under questioning by a Diet member, who noted that indigent leprosy sufferers resisted removal to a sanitarium, Sugiyama explained that "using the power of the police," it would be possible to persuade impoverished tuberculosis patients to enter a hospital with the promise of treatment.[117]

The import of these aspects of the 1914 law soon became clear as the public tuberculosis sanitaria opened their doors. The Osaka Municipal Toneyama Hospital was established in 1917, followed by institutions in Kobe, Kyoto, Tokyo, Yokohama, and Nagoya. Unlike the leprosy sanitaria that came to house complex communities that lived and worked together for years, the new institutions for tuberculosis sufferers functioned very differently. In practice, "those who lacked the means to convalesce" came to mean impoverished people who were in the final stages of the disease. As a result, death rates within the early tuberculosis sanitaria were staggering. According to one source, at Toneyama Hospital in the 1920s, 60 percent of patients died within three months of admission. The situation at the Tokyo Municipal Sanitarium was similar. In 1921, 75 percent of patients died within the year.[118] For administrators, at least, the grim death toll had a bright side: few patients lived long enough to challenge their authority.

In 1919, the same year the Bureau of Hygiene convened the conference on leprosy policy, the Diet passed two new laws, the Tuberculosis Prevention Law and the Psychiatric Hospital Law, both of which authorized the establishment of new institutions of confinement. The former extended the requirement that urban areas have a tuberculosis sanitarium to cities with a population of fifty thousand or more and established new restrictions on the employment of infected people. In addition, in an implicit acknowledgment that police "encouragement" did not always work, the government now authorized local officials to force tuberculosis sufferers into a sanitarium if they posed a danger of transmission. By 1930, ten more sanitaria had been constructed.[119]

In contrast, the Psychiatric Hospital Law was far less successful in propelling the establishment of new institutions of confinement. The law was a response to growing, if divergent, concern about what police estimated to be Japan's fifty thousand mentally ill people, a number that had more than doubled since 1909.[120] At the time, the Tokyo prefectural psychiatric hospital was the only public hospital for the mentally ill in the country, and although private psychiatric hospitals had been established in the major cities, they were prohibitively expensive for all but the wealthy. As a result, far more people (more than four thousand in 1918) were privately confined by their families under the provisions of the 1900 law than were hospitalized. Japanese psychiatrists, led by Kure Shūzo of Tokyo Imperial University, deplored this situation, arguing that many of those in private confinement were often denied even basic medical care and suffered greatly because of substandard housing, food, and hygiene. They called for the creation of psychiatric hospitals to remedy this situation.[121] In contrast, Hara Takashi, then prime minister, other politicians, and police officials pushed for a new law based on concerns about public order, arguing that with few institutions to house them, tens of thousands of mentally ill people roamed the streets of Japan unrestrained and free to commit all manner of crimes.[122]

In the end, the Psychiatric Hospital Law did little to appease either group. Its intent was to encourage prefectural and local governments to establish psychiatric facilities, and to that end it required the central government to cover half of construction costs and part of the annual operating costs of new institutions. But even the offer of ongoing support was not enough of an incentive for cash-strapped local governments. Fifteen years after the passage of the law, Japan had only six public psychiatric hospitals with a total of 2,140 beds.[123] Instead of establishing dedicated psychiatric hospitals, prefectures and local governments relied upon another article of the Psychiatric Hospital Law, one that had been intended as a stopgap measure. It allowed private and public hospitals to be designated as "substitute psychiatric hospitals," an arrangement that did not require these institutions to have a trained psychiatrist on staff or other provisions for the care of the mentally ill. In addition, like the Tuberculosis Prevention Law, the Psychiatric Hospital Law, too, allowed officials to order the confinement of someone deemed mentally ill, poor, and dangerous, at public expense.[124] As a result, mentally ill people who committed even petty crimes came to be confined indefinitely in institutions that offered little in the way of treatment and no clear path to release.

It is clear then that the confinement of indigent leprosy sufferers was part of a larger policy towards the impoverished sufferers of problematic chronic diseases, one that developed piecemeal over a decade and a half, and one that privileged the national interest over that of individuals. But the institutions that were established to house these different groups differed in fundamental ways. For all their problems, the public leprosy sanitaria were neither charnel houses for the nearly dead nor warehouses for those deemed dangerous. The comparative good health (both physical and mental) of the leprosy sanitaria patients and the development of communal ties between them meant that they had far greater ability to negotiate with sanitarium administrators, by asserting their rights as citizens, than those confined in either psychiatric wards or TB sanitaria.

In this chapter, I've argued that the leprosy sanitaria were shaped by the ambivalence between "protection" and "management" that was at the heart of the 1907 law. From the time site selection began and throughout the first decade and half of their existence, the tensions between care and surveillance, compassion and control, led to a series of compromises that fundamentally altered the plan of Kubota and others within the Bureau of Hygiene. While the sanitaria had been envisioned as idyllic sanctuaries where Japan's most vulnerable citizens would spend their lives in quiet seclusion, by 1919 they had become something quite different: sites of research, treatment, work, and leisure, something like a village but not entirely unlike a prison.

In the face of growing concern about their effectiveness and viability, Board of Hygiene officials had organized the 1919 conference with the aim of assessing Japan's leprosy policy, but they came away with a confusing array of opinions. Rates of the disease were rising, or they were falling but not fast enough. Sexual segregation was the solution, or it was part of the problem. The public sanitaria were not working, but there was no clear consensus on an alternative. Confronted by patients who sought to control and craft their own lives even against considerable odds, attitudes had begun to harden among Japan's leprosy "experts," although, tellingly, they rejected the authoritarian approach advocated by the missionaries, who called for a ban on marriage and sexual relations, the creation of a national registration system, and forced relocation that would have separated husbands and wives, parents and children.

Chapter 6
The National Culture of Leprosy Prevention

On June 25, 1933, two thousand people gathered in To-kyo's Hibiya Public Hall to celebrate Leprosy Prevention Day (Rai Yobō Dei), a national event inaugurated only the year before. A radio broadcast by Home Minister Yamamoto Tatsuo got the festivities under way. This was followed by a series of speakers, including former prime minister Kiyomura Keigo and Mitsuda Kensuke. Attendees then viewed two new films on leprosy prevention that had been commissioned by the Home Ministry.[1] Events took place outside the hall as well. According to an account of Leprosy Prevention Day in Tokyo from 1933, "Every street was dotted with tens of thousands of posters advertising leprosy prevention, and on every street corner someone was making an impassioned speech to the passing crowds. . . . This shrill noise was accompanied by the sound of a plane overhead making circles while dropping blue leaflets. Standing face-to-face in a crowd, we heard someone say excitedly, 'Ladies and gentleman! Leprosy is not a disease for which you need feel shame. It is not hereditary. It is within our power to eradicate the leprosy we fear so much. The only way to do this is by strict isolation.'"[2]

Leprosy Prevention Day was but one indication of the transformation of leprosy into an important element of national culture in the 1930s. To this point, the disease had only sporadically and locally concerned those outside of public health and social welfare circles; now there was an explosion of public discourse as Japanese citizens were called upon to help eradicate leprosy and support its victims. Propelling this transformation was the revision of Japan's leprosy law in 1931. The new law ended the income restrictions on sanitaria admission, leading to the rapid expansion of the patient population. At the end of the 1920s, the five public sanitaria housed fewer than two thousand people. By 1935, there were four more sanitaria, and the number of patients confined within them had nearly tripled.

Against earlier scholarship that has argued that the 1931 law sought to exclude leprosy sufferers from national life, in this chapter I demonstrate that even as patients moved in growing numbers to the sanitaria, they became increasingly important within political discourse, deployed as symbols of national unity and the inclusiveness of an imperial culture that extended even to the sick and stigmatized. But the use of the disease as a trope for the nation did not exhaust its signifying potential. Others, too, began to make use of leprosy, transforming the disease into a powerful, pervasive, but also multivalent metaphor that some used to cast critical light on Japan's modernity and political culture.

Kusatsu Revisited: Imagining "Free Convalescent Zones"

The 1931 Leprosy Prevention Law is now notorious, with critics charging that it put in place a policy of "absolute isolation" that would endure for six decades. In actuality, the law was as much an end point as a beginning, coming after almost two decades of debate about the failures and unintended consequences of the 1907 law it replaced. In the aftermath of the 1919 conference examined in chapter 5, the Home Ministry issued a report entitled *Fundamental Guidelines for Leprosy Prevention Policy* that clarified some policies and proposed others.[3] In relation to patient sexuality, this document explicitly affirmed the use of sterilization if patients agreed, paving the way for its wider adoption. To preserve sanitarium order, it called for the creation of a National Sanitarium to which those deemed "delinquent" (*furyō*) by directors of the public sanitaria could be transferred. But the Home Ministry did more than attempt to resolve issues internal to the sanitaria in the new guidelines. It also addressed the situation of those with leprosy who remained outside the institutions.

For one, there was an acknowledgment that the process used to determine if an indigent sufferer should be transferred to a sanitarium often led to new problems. The intrusive police investigation of family circumstances alerted local communities to a case of the disease in their midst. According to one Diet member, in the wake of the police investigation, families had to "endure a life so constrained they might as well be in prison."[4] There was also a new understanding that many of those deemed "vagrant lepers" had fallen into poverty only as the disease progressed, after the loss of employment, the breakdown of their families, and the futile but often expensive search for a cure. Statistical data compiled by the Bureau of Hygiene on the patient population revealed that only about 7 percent of those confined in public sanitaria between 1909 and 1915 were perennially unemployed before their diagnosis.[5] To aid those described as "patients in the home" (*zaitaku kanja*), the *Fundamental Guidelines* called for public aid to families with an infected member, expanding the sanitaria to allow for paying patients, and the establishment of what were termed "free convalescent zones" (*jiyū ryōyōchi*).[6]

Of these proposals, the concept of free convalescent zones initially attracted the most attention from politicians. At the center of the debates surrounding such "zones" was Yunosawa in Kusatsu. Three decades after leprosy sufferers were relocated there in 1887, Yunosawa had become a thriving community with a permanent population of perhaps five hundred.[7] Residents—leprosy sufferers and their family members, some of whom were not infected—owned inns, eateries, pharmacies, and other businesses that served the sojourners who came in search of treatment and who often stayed for many months. Rumors circulated in Kusatsu about the fabulous wealth of some Yunosawa residents: according to one, a wealthy innkeeper had paid the family of a beautiful "healthy" woman the amazing sum of one thousand yen to acquire her as his wife.[8]

The community also had its critics. Mitsuda Kensuke made repeated visits to Yunosawa beginning around the turn of the century and found the fluid movement between Yunosawa and the rest of the town alarming. In 1906 he wrote that the forcible relocation of the Yunosawa community away from Kusatsu to a more isolated site should be a "national pursuit."[9] Whether Mitsuda played a role in what followed is unclear, but in 1909, the town leaders of Kusatsu petitioned the prefectural government for aid in relocating the Yunosawa community outside the town, arguing that this was necessary to stop "the spread of the poison of disease," safeguard the health of other visitors to the spa, and preserve the town's prosperity.[10] The residents of Yunosawa responded by submitting their own letter of protest directly to Hirata Tōsuke, the home minister.[11] They charged that the plan to relocate Yunosawa was nothing more than an attempted land grab and called upon the ministry to intercede. It did. Unlike "vagrant lepers," who could summarily be confined, property-holding proprietors of small businesses, their disease notwithstanding, were another matter. The ministry refused to bow to local pressure and responded by ordering the town to respect the rights of Yunosawa residents. This crisis resolved, Yunosawa continued to thrive, but opinions on the community continued to be mixed, even among leprosy sufferers themselves. Some described Yunosawa as a "paradise of freedom" where the afflicted could live normal lives among their compatriots, free from the stigma they confronted elsewhere. Others portrayed it in darker terms, claiming that those who came in search of a cure were ruthlessly exploited by innkeepers and the proprietors of other businesses, who abandoned them when their money ran out.[12]

The divide between the haves and have-nots of Yunosawa was mitigated in the 1920s when the St. Barnabas Mission began to provide a safety net of sorts for those who flocked there. In 1916, Anglican missionary Mary Cornwallis-Legh drew upon her considerable personal wealth to purchase a large parcel of land situated between Yunosawa and the "Upper Village," as the original town had come to be known. In addition to a chapel, she quickly commissioned the construction of a number of "homes," for women, children, and men, respectively. Like other missionary-run institutions, this one, too, had the aim of conversion. Those who resided in the homes were expected to remain celibate, to convert to Christianity, and to devote much time to religious observances. Indeed Cornwallis-Legh herself proudly described the mission as "like the semi-monastic leper hospitals of mediaevil times."[13]

From the perspective of many in the government, the creation of free convalescent zones on the model of Kusatsu—independent communities based on the valorized political principles of private property, commerce, self-governance, and economic self-sufficiency—seemed the answer to multiple problems, providing a civil society solution to a social welfare issue, the approach favored by the state for at least three decades, and one that made the biologically vulnerable into model citizens. Not only would such sites presumably reduce the risk of infection by removing sufferers from the larger population, they would allow patients the autonomy so many desired, while protecting them from discrimination within the larger society. All this without the financial and administrative burdens involved in establishing and operating a public sanitarium. As one proponent put it, "I can imagine no better policy than this to allow patients to serenely enjoy what remains of their lives comforted by those with the same disease in an atmosphere of warmth."[14]

This view of Yunosawa led the Japanese government to forge a collaborative relationship with Cornwallis-Legh, a new development in the often strained relationship between the government and missionaries involved in leprosy work. Beginning in the early 1920s the Home Ministry began to prop up the St. Barnabas Mission with financial support from government coffers, thus contributing to the expansion of the mission and its gradual transformation into an integral part of Yunosawa.[15] Over the years the contributions of the Home Ministry grew. In 1932, the ministry contributed 20 percent of the operating cost of the mission; in 1940, 37 percent. The American Episcopal Church and the American Mission to Lepers also made sizeable donations. But the most celebrated patron of St. Barnabas was the former Taishō empress, who made "leprosy relief" her personal cause. Her contributions covered as much as 9 percent of the operating budget of St. Barnabas in the 1930s.[16] Over the course of the 1920s and 1930s, members of the imperial family became increasingly involved in providing support for the sanitaria as well, making large donations that were celebrated in the press and within the sanitaria as evidence of imperial benevolence and beneficence.

Hirokawa Waka has documented the many proposals for free convalescent zones that were taken up within the Diet between 1919 and 1937, evidence of not only intense interest in the concept of free zones but also very different ideas about how they should be organized, funded, and administered.[17] Notably, while some proponents made mention of Culion and Moloka'i as inspiration for the "zones," evoking international precedents, others recalled the "leper villages" of the early modern period, suggesting that this arrangement represented an organic solution sanctioned by Japan's own history. One such plan called for identifying the villages that already had a high number of leprosy sufferers and designating them as free convalescent zones. The sick and the healthy could be separated within the villages, with the government taking responsibility for providing medical care and other necessary support to those in the afflicted section.[18] A preliminary survey of fifteen prefectures undertaken in the aftermath of the 1919 conference revealed the fanciful nature of this scheme. Although it identified 116 "leprosy hamlets," the working definition of such communities seems to have been remarkably broad. According to the survey, Kagawa Prefecture had one such hamlet with a total of three "leprosy households" (*raike*), while Toyama Prefecture supposedly had eighteen hamlets, which together had only twenty households with a grand total of twenty-one leprosy sufferers among them.[19] Clearly, the dense clusters of people with leprosy in specific villages that some imagined did not exist.

Moreover, in actuality the hybrid solution that had emerged at Yunosawa of paid accommodation for those with means and missionary aid for the destitute was fraught with problems. According to an otherwise glowing report on St. Barnabas published in the *Spirit of Missions*, a publication of the Board of Missions of the Episcopal Church, provisions for medical care were primitive at best: the mission had only "a rude little dispensary, no white tiles or cases of gleaming instruments, no proper sinks or sterilizers in the surgery."[20] Correspondence between John McKim, bishop of the

Episcopal Church in Japan, and R. B. Teusler, a physician on the staff of St. Luke's Hospital, a missionary-run hospital in Tokyo, confirmed this report. Teusler wrote that two American doctors who had visited St. Barnabas were "horrified" by the unhygienic conditions they observed and "considered writing an article condemning the medical side of the work."[21] The problem of course was money. The chronic and progressive nature of the disease meant that over time the number of those seeking aid from the mission grew and the cost of their care quickly outstripped available resources. According to Hirokawa, by the late 1920s, about a third of Yunosawa residents were dependent upon the aid of St. Barnabas.[22] Even with the large donations she received, Cornwallis-Legh had no option but to draw upon her dwindling personal wealth to keep St. Barnabas afloat.

The New International Politics of Leprosy Control

As the debate over free convalescent zones was unfolding, the man who was poised to become the most significant figure in shaping Japan's leprosy policy for the next three decades was on his way to Europe, a journey that would profoundly influence his thinking about the disease. In 1923 Mitsuda Kensuke was dispatched by the Home Ministry to Strasbourg in France to attend the third international conference on leprosy, evidence of his increasingly influential role as Japan's premier leprologist. Unlike the two earlier meetings, held in Berlin in 1897 and Bergen in 1909, both of which had been dominated by German-trained bacteriologists, the Strasbourg conference was organized by a group of French physicians of colonial medicine. The head of the organizing committee was Edouard Jeanselme, a French syphilologist. Like many of his colleagues, Jeanselme's own medical research was ordered by ideas about race and civilization. He argued, for example, that syphilis took different forms. The "natives" of France's North African colonies, whose brains "were not developed by mental work," suffered from a form of syphilis marked primarily by dermatological symptoms, while Europeans (and Europeanized "natives") were said to be prone to neurological syphilis, the "evolved" form of the disease.[23]

In the 1920s, leprosy, too, began to be reconceived through the lens of "the colonial." Doomsday-like predictions by Albert Ashmead and others notwithstanding, there had been no leprosy epidemic in Europe or North America, and the peculiar nature of *M. leprae*—that is, that it is a weak and remarkably slow-to-reproduce organism—was becoming clear. Reflecting the waning of the intense lepraphobia of the turn of the century, the majority of the international attendees now came from areas where leprosy was endemic. There were no attendees from Germany, a country still mired in postwar depression, and the United States was represented only by a public health officer who was attached to the consulate in Belgium.[24] His presence reflected convenience, not urgency.

For the members of the organizing committee, most of whom had experience as colonial administrators, the overriding issue of the conference was the management of leprosy in European colonies. The French representatives included Jeanselme, officials from the French Ministry of the Colonies' Board of Health, several officers of the Colonial Troops (as the French colonial forces were known), and a specialist of tropical medicine from the Pasteur Institute. The non-French participants included the Belgian physician Emile Van Campenhout, who was involved in leprosy policy in the Congo, Leonard Rogers, a retired member of the Indian Medical Service, and John Hutson, the first public health inspector of Barbados.[25] In their discussions, these men consistently referenced "the natives" and "the colonies" as the object of policy.

The emerging consensus that leprosy was less a threat to the health of Europeans and North Americans than an issue of colonial governance framed the final resolution of the conference. The two previous international conferences had ended with a ringing endorsement of the confinement of all sufferers as the best means of preventing the spread of the disease.[26] In contrast, the resolution of the Strasbourg conference stated that quarantine was required only in areas where the disease was endemic, resulting in a large number of cases; elsewhere, home confinement would suffice. In either case, children should be separated as soon as possible from their infected parents as a preventive measure, since they were recognized to be particularly vulnerable to infection. It was further recommended that the form of quarantine be "humanitarian" and adapted to "the case and the country," with the hospital, sanitarium, and agricultural colony all possible solutions. Ideally, "patients should be allowed to remain near their families if compatible with treatment."[27]

In this conference shaped by ideas about race and the divide of colonizer/colonized, Mitsuda occupied an uncomfortable position. On the one hand, he was ostensibly treated as an "authority." He presented on his own research, chaired a panel, and was placed front and center just behind Jeanselme in the official conference photograph. But his interactions with his colleagues did not go smoothly. Thirty years later, Mitsuda would vividly recall his awkward participation in the discussion that followed the presentation of the French dermatologist Ferdinand-Jean Darier, part of a

session on the "comparative pathology of leprosy." Darier, who was affili-
ated with Hôpital Saint-Louis, a public hospital that treated many migrants
from the French colonies, described symptoms he had encountered among
soldiers from the French colonies, specifically hypopigmented anesthetic
lesions in which few, if any, *M. leprae* could be found. Darius concluded
that such lesions represented an "attenuated response of tissues" peculiar to
some bodies.[28] In the discussion that followed, Brazil's representative, Edu-
ardo Rabello, made the racial dimensions of this discussion explicit, com-
menting that he had seen such tuberculoid lesions "only on the negroes,"
and they seemed to be a feature of the disease "in colored individuals."
Mitsuda objected and advised his colleagues (correctly) that such lesions
were in fact an early symptom of leprosy. He later wrote that his interjec-
tion was ignored and "all of the Western scholars agreed with Darier."[29]

Mitsuda's discussion of "Prophylaxis in Japan" was presented as part
of the panel he chaired on preventive methods around the world. No doubt
to his dismay, most of the other reports focused on colonial sites, including Indochina, Trinidad and Tobago, the Belgian Congo, the Guianas, and
various British possessions. To his international audience, Mitsuda offered
a glowing account of Japan's success at leprosy control. In his description,
the public sanitaria offered a daily routine of medical treatment and light
work, with rich and varied cultural and religious events on offer. There
was no mention of delinquent or runaway patients, or of the new policy
allowing sanitarium directors to punish the recalcitrant. In contrast to his
silence on these aspects of sanitarium life, Mitsuda discussed openly what
he called "the delicate issue" of patient sexuality at some length. In his
view, attempts to impose abstinence by physically separating patients by
sex were "counter to the laws of nature," but "allowing patients freedom
with no control" would lead inevitably to the birth of "children condemned
in advance to a miserable fate." The solution, of course, was vasectomy,
which Mitsuda recommended without reservation. He concluded by suggesting that Japan was poised to enter a new phase of leprosy prevention.
"Wealthy philanthropists" were already working with the government to
create "a kind of autonomous city that would be self-governing and self-
sufficient," with the aim of eventually isolating all patients.[30]

This was obviously a creative mixture of fact and aspirational fiction
designed to showcase the success of Japan's leprosy policy and conceal its
problems. In reality, talk of free convalescent zones notwithstanding, there
was no "autonomous city" in the works and no wealthy philanthropists
ready to step in and fund it. But Mitsuda's desire to publicize the success of Japanese policy is revealing nonetheless. In contrast to the many

discussions of unruly colonial bodies that defied both standard nosological paradigms and well-intentioned polices, he suggested that Japan had crafted a thoroughly successful approach to the disease, one that was modern, compassionate, and fully respectful of the rights and dignity of its citizens.

On his way back to Japan, Mitsuda visited a series of leprosy facilities that apparently confirmed his confidence that Japan had little to learn from other countries. He was unimpressed by the Norwegian sanitarium he visited and later wrote, "I thought that in terms of facilities and other factors . . . Japan was more advanced." In India, he visited institutions in Madras, Bombay (now Mumbai), and Calcutta (now Kolkata) but found them dark and dreary. His final stop was Culion, the largest institution of quarantine in the world, and one that Mitsuda had been holding up as a model for some years. Mitsuda found its facilities "surprisingly unimpressive," although he praised the small cottages that housed the majority of residents as "simple but clean" and expressed admiration for its well-equipped research center.[31]

Aiseien: Colony and "Ideal Separate World"

Mitsuda returned home with a clearer vision of what Japan needed: a "large-scale sanitarium like that on Culion" but one that would be "an ideal separate world" for leprosy sufferers and a testament to Japan's progressive approach. The implementation of this plan, however, had to wait. While he was in Europe, a massive earthquake had destroyed much of Tokyo and the surrounding areas. Reconstruction was the new priority of the government, and planning for the national sanitarium got under way only in 1927. In that year, the Home Ministry purchased sixty-five acres (26.3 hectares) of land along the coast of the central part of Nagashima, an island in the Seto Inland Sea just off the coast of Okayama, and designated Mitsuda as the future director of the planned institution.

Nagashima was not Mitsuda's choice of locale. In 1917, the Bureau of Hygiene, already contemplating the possibility of a national sanitarium, had dispatched Mitsuda to investigate possible locations, presumably because of his outspoken advocacy for the establishment of an island colony. Concealing his real purpose to avoid the kind of public outcry that had accompanied the establishment of the regional sanitaria, Mitsuda traveled to Iriomotejima in the Ryukyus and Kakuijima and Nagashima in the Seto Inland Sea. Mitsuda favored Iriomotejima, an island closer to Taiwan than the Japanese main islands, but Nakagawa Nozomu, the director of the Bureau of Hygiene at the time, rejected this option. Iriomotejima was not only a difficult journey from every major port, it was also covered with dense jungle and malaria was endemic among its few thousand inhabitants. Mitsuda would later recollect that Nakagawa pointedly asked him, "What would you say if I ordered you to live there?"[32] Although Mitsuda enthusiastically replied that he would be happy to go, the Home Ministry never considered Iriomotejima seriously. In the end, it settled upon Nagashima, which Mitsuda had rejected as insufficiently isolated. It is located only thirty meters off the coast of Okayama Prefecture and is clearly visible from the shore.[33]

As this incident suggests, Mitsuda's views on quarantine were often more radical than those of Bureau of Hygiene officials. One thing they did agree on was that the planned national institution should differ in both scale and grandeur from the humble, poorly funded public sanitaria, and Home Ministry officials carefully designed the layout of the colony. Figure 6.1 shows the plan of the new sanitarium at the time of its opening. Administrators and staff were housed a significant distance from the main part of the new "colony," which was established along the southern coast of the island.

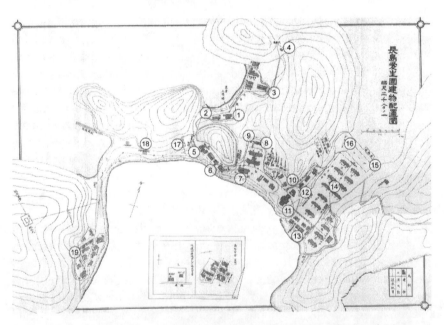

FIGURE 6.1.   Aiseien, circa 1933: (1) admission facility, (2) pottery works, (3) jail, (4) crematorium, (5) main administrative buildings, (6) medical facilities, (7) guard post, (8) critical care facility, (9) isolation center, (10) canteen, (11) worship hall, (12) sewing workshop, (13) carpentry workshop, (14) patient living quarters, (15) swimming pool, (16) sports grounds, (17) guard post, (18) childcare facility for uninfected children, (19) staff living quarters. Image adapted from *Nagashima Aiseien nenpō* 1933, front matter.

Although the topography of the island worked to demarcate this division, a guard station was established to prevent movement between the two areas. A dormitory for the uninfected children of patients occupied the middle ground between the staff and patient sections of the island—evidence of their ambiguous standing in the gray area between health and sickness.

On the northern side of the narrow island was the harbor where new patients arrived and the "reception center" where they were housed for an initial period of medical screening. Patients were then moved to the main part of the colony on the opposite side of the island. Hugging the southern coast were the main administrative buildings, the research and treatment facilities, the "worship hall," and the sanitarium store. The main patient area was a cluster of eleven dormitories, some of which were designated for cohabitating couples. It was placed adjacent to recreational facilities, which included a swimming pool and a sports field. Vulnerable patients, including children and teens, mothers and babies, and the disabled, were housed closer to the medical facilities. A third residential area, this one for paying patients, was established on the northern side of the island in 1932. Finally, unlike the early public sanitaria, sites for productive labor were demarcated in the original plan. Agricultural lands and facilities such as a poultry farm and ceramic works were situated outside the colony's center.

A generous budget of eleven million yen allowed the construction of more than a hundred buildings within just a couple of years. At the time of its opening, Aiseien was fully electrified, with its own gasoline-powered generator, and the main buildings were equipped with running water, steam heating, and telephone lines. It even had its own radio station, and the worship hall, where religious services, public assemblies, and performances would be held, had a piano and a sound system. The kitchen featured a steam-powered rice cooker that could cook 330 pounds of rice at a time.[34] The medical facilities were equally impressive. There was a research lab, a morgue where autopsies could be performed, a hospital ward for the severely ill, and another for those with acute infectious diseases. While most of the structures, including patient and staff residences, were one story and built of wood, the sites most closely associated with institutional power were built in an impressively monumental style. The main administrative buildings, the medical and pharmacy centers, the jail for delinquent patients, and the reception center were two-story buildings constructed of reinforced concrete, with high ceilings, large windows, and elaborate entranceways.

On November 18, 1930, two days before the official opening of Aiseien, Home Minister Adachi Kenzō toured the new facility and reportedly exclaimed, "Oh, it's a paradise, a paradise."[35] The Home Ministry was so proud of the new facility that it made it available for public tours, and over the next months and years, hundreds of groups from schools and civic organizations, as well as international visitors and even patient-delegates from other sanitaria, came to the island to inspect the buildings and grounds and to admire the fine facilities. Even Mitsuda would later acknowledge the wisdom of this choice of locale, noting that its accessibility made it easy for visitors to learn of the benefits of sanitarium life: "Nagashima was not a poor village or an isolated island. It was a grand new landmark (*meisho*)."[36]

The new sanitarium, however, still lacked patients. The first group of eighty-five (including sixteen women) arrived four months after the opening ceremony, having traveled from Tokyo to Osaka by train and from Osaka to Nagashima by boat. All but four members of this group came from Zensei Hospital and were handpicked by Mitsuda from his former charges. Although the national institution had originally been intended to house delinquent patients, Mitsuda was adamant that there must be a core group of model residents in place to aid in socializing difficult patients into institutional life. He asked for volunteers from Zensei Hospital and selected those he judged suitable from the more than three hundred candidates who stepped forward. In a neat inversion of the colonial discourse on leprosy that then prevailed internationally, Mitsuda dubbed this first group of patients "the colonizers" (*kaitakusha*), a term that in the age of the expanding Japanese Empire was fraught with significance, suggesting both patriotism and noble sacrifice. Of course, it also challenged the international image of leprosy sufferers as "the colonized." One of the doctors on the staff of the sanitarium, Hayashi Fumio, even composed an anthem for the new patients called "The Colonizers' Song" and taught it to them on the long journey towards Nagashima:

> Splitting open a great mass of raw metal
> We make flames emerge from the depths of the earth.
> Splitting open our sad hearts
> We alight the flames of sacrifice.
> Leaving behind our worries and sorrows
> We step ashore, ashore, ashore
> And look at the brilliant morning light
> That shines upon Aiseien.[37]

Patients thus were encouraged to think of their transfer to Nagashima not as exile but as their contribution to Japan's imperial mission. And perhaps they did. According to physician Miyagawa Hakaru, who accompanied the patients on the journey to Nagashima, they burst into cheers as they first set foot upon the island.[38]

Revising the Leprosy Law

Less than a year after the founding of this first national sanitarium in 1930, the new leprosy law was passed. Drafted by bureaucrats in the Home Ministry and passed intact by both houses of the Diet, the 1931 law fundamentally altered Japan's leprosy policy by defining the purpose of the sanitaria as disease prevention rather than poverty relief. Article 3 legalized coercive confinement in some instances, stating, "When the governmental authorities deem it necessary for purposes of leprosy prevention, ... a leprosy sufferer who is likely to propagate the disease can be made to enter a national sanitarium." But the law did more than simply redefine the purpose of confinement. It put forth a comprehensive policy for all of Japan's leprosy sufferers. Article 6 specified that the care of those who were a threat to public health would be at public expense, making the sanitarium available to those who were not destitute. Another article expanded the list of professions from which infected people were banned. In acknowledgment of the economic impact of these restrictions, the law authorized the creation of a new system of public aid for those impacted and their families. Another important initiative was prompted by concern for the stigma of the disease. It established harsh penalties for doctors and civil servants who disclosed personal information about a leprosy sufferer.[39]

While the 1931 law has been the subject of vitriolic criticism, nowhere in its twelve articles is there a specific requirement for the compulsory quarantine of all sufferers, nor is there a single reference to "absolute isolation." Fujino Yutaka has argued that the phrase "when the governmental authorities deem it necessary" provided legal justification for the mass confinement of all leprosy sufferers and that this was the ultimate intent of the law.[40] Hirokawa Waka disagrees, noting that the employment restrictions and the provisions for aid would have been unnecessary if all sufferers were to be confined. She concludes that the aim of the law was twofold, to confine in a sanitarium those who posed a public health threat and to provide public aid to those who did not. But she notes as well that because the law did not specify how the determination that someone posed a danger of transmission was to be made, it implicitly burdened those who wanted to avoid quarantine with the new responsibility to prove that they were not a threat to others. And with the legal standards for forcible confinement left undefined, overzealous local and prefectural authorities were effectively given license to coerce reluctant people to accept quarantine.[41]

Neither position, however, acknowledges the considerable confusion that surrounded the law from the outset, even among the politicians who voted for it. During the two-month period between the initial submission of the draft law and its final passage, representatives of the Bureau of Hygiene and Diet members met on multiple occasions to discuss its terms, intent, and likely effects. In this period, public health officials often complained about the public's failure to grasp that leprosy was infectious, but it is evident that some members of the political elite were equally ill informed. When Akagi Tomoharu, director of the Bureau of Hygiene, met with members of the House of Peers, Diet member Kii Toshihide stated outright, "We keep talking about infection or heredity, but it is an established fact that the disease is hereditary and that is what I believe."[42] Confronted with statements like this, Akagi was compelled to repeatedly explain the state of medical research on leprosy and to clarify that the intent of confinement was to control an infectious disease.

Still, Akagi may have preferred questions such as Kii's to those that came from better-informed Diet members. For example, he met with considerable opposition during a meeting with members of the lower house committee charged with public health matters. Akagi prefaced his introduction to the draft law by asserting that an expanded policy of leprosy prevention was necessary not only "to protect the health of the nation" but also on "humanitarian grounds" (*jindō no ue*).[43] Nakashima Takayuki, a physician educated in the medical faculty of what was now Tokyo Imperial University, challenged him on both counts. He asked Akagi why the requirements of leprosy prevention differed so radically from those for tuberculosis, given that it was more infectious than leprosy. In response, Akagi suggested that leprosy posed problems that tuberculosis did not. Not only was it incurable, but it also "troubled not only the person who was sick but also those around him and creates a tragic situation." Confinement was intended to protect patients from the public and the public from patients. Nakashima was not convinced. He argued that "underlying this law is the idea that leprosy is a disease that should be abhorred," and he predicted that the law would reinforce the stigma of the disease and make the situation of sufferers even more difficult. To this, Akagi acknowledged that popular attitudes were a problem, but he protested that statutes were not a means to educate the public. They need only to be humane.[44]

Chūma Okimaru, the chairman of the committee, was like Nakashima a graduate of the medical school of Tokyo Imperial University and a practicing physician, but his concerns and his understanding of what constituted a "humane" law were very different. Why, Chūma asked, did the law not address the reproductive potential of those who would remain in their homes? Since parent-to-child transmission was a recognized problem, shouldn't a policy of sterilization be enforced? Akagi acknowledged the use of vasectomy within the sanitaria but asserted that the state lacked the legal power to enforce such a policy on the general population, pointing out that the government had no overall policy on what he euphemistically termed "family planning." Chūma was undeterred. Ignoring the fact that abortion was a criminal offense (and had been since the 1870s), he suggested that if sterilization was difficult, abortion was the solution, since "it is very simple to perform and we could [use it] right away." Akagi disagreed and replied that the best approach would be to provide information about the dangers of mother-to-child transmission to those with the disease.[45]

Akagi's response to Chūma suggests that government bureaucrats did not believe that the goal of disease prevention trumped the rights of the biologically vulnerable. At the same time, the questions posed by Nakashima and Chūma and the divergent ideological positions they represent reveal the ambiguity at the heart of the new law. Was the intent of confinement to aid the sufferers of the disease by providing treatment and protecting their family from the threat of infection, or was its purpose to rid Japan of the scourge of leprosy? In other words, was the law primarily concerned with the obligation of citizens to the state, or the state to its citizens?

Akagi himself adopted a position somewhere in the middle and seems to have wanted a law that was similarly ambiguous. In his exchanges with Diet members, Akagi steadfastly refused to endorse the coercive transfer of patients to a sanitarium, even though he stated explicitly that the goal was to confine ten thousand people within ten years. If this could be accomplished, he argued, Japan would be leprosy-free within two decades. The goal of ten thousand could be met, he insisted, because leprosy sufferers would willingly enter a sanitarium. In his words, "The situation is that there is a very large number of patients who will step forward on their own and say that they hope to be allowed to enter a sanitarium."[46]

Under questioning by Diet members who noted the problems that the public sanitaria had faced with patient unrest, delinquency, and runaways, Akagi argued that the new sanitaria would be a different kind of institution, not only because of better funding but also because they would be populated by ordinary Japanese citizens, unlike the public sanitaria and their motley collection of vagrants and beggars. In the end, the tension between the language of the statute ("when the governmental authorities deem it necessary") and Akagi's hopeful vision of ten thousand happy "volunteers" entering the sanitaria went unresolved. Nor was there any effort to clarify the circumstances under which "a leprosy sufferer . . . can be made to enter a national sanitarium." The law, with its silences and contradictions left unaddressed, was passed by both houses of the Diet in April 1931.

Mobilizing the Public

From the vantage point of 1931–1932, Akagi's hope that leprosy sufferers would voluntarily seek admission to the sanitarium may well have seemed correct. According to the daily log of new admissions to Aiseien, 198 people applied directly for admission in 1931, surpassing the number of those who were transferred by prefectural authorities.[47] The demand from patients was so great that four months after its opening, Aiseien had reached its official capacity of 400 residents and the original aim of rehousing delinquent patients was abandoned. By the end of the year the new sanitarium was already over capacity.

Behind these rosy figures, however, lies a more complicated situation.[48] An application for voluntary admission came to be interpreted as a tacit declaration that the person applying posed a risk of infection, and this allowed volunteers to be cared for at public expense. An alternative was to be admitted as a paying patient. At Aiseien, for fifteen yen per month, one got slightly better housing but there were no other special provisions in terms of meals or medical care.[49] Fifteen yen was, however, not an insubstantial sum, and few paying patients stepped forward. What patients who sought voluntary admission may not have realized is that by entering the sanitarium under the "danger of propagation" clause, they were in fact agreeing to be confined indefinitely.

If the provision of free care and treatment encouraged people with leprosy to pursue admission, so, too, did the new public discourse that surrounded the disease. From the early 1930s leprosy sufferers who remained in their homes were the focus of an intense civic campaign that used the mass media and techniques of popular mobilization to promote the cause of "leprosy prevention." The most influential organization was the Leprosy Prevention Association (Rai Yobō Kyōkai; LPA), which in 1931 declared the start of a "national campaign to eradicate leprosy." Originally founded in 1928, the LPA took on the leadership of the campaign against leprosy after it received a donation of one hundred thousand yen from the former Taishō empress in 1931. This evidence of imperial approval encouraged other donors to step forward, and by the end of the year the LPA had considerable assets. Its membership, which included public health and other officials, journalists, teachers, doctors, and businessmen in every prefecture, grew rapidly, and with both funds and supporters it quickly became an influential civic organization, albeit one with close links to government at every level.[50]

One of the earliest initiatives of the LPA was the establishment of so-called counseling centers (sōdanjo) in various sites around the country, including on the grounds of Aiseien and the other sanitaria. Like the tuberculosis counseling centers created around the same time, those for leprosy offered free medical examinations for people with worrisome symptoms. If a diagnosis was made, center staff offered advice to patients and their families that, unsurprisingly, most often took the form of a recommendation of sanitarium admission, although some centers also provided medicines on an outpatient basis.[51] Patients were encouraged to consider a trial admission: for a fee of seven and a half yen per month they could enter a sanitarium for several months with the provision that they would then be free to leave.[52] But the staff of the centers had other duties as well. Using standardized forms, they also sought to obtain and record personal data from those they counseled, including where they lived and worked, their marital status, and the names of family members and whether they were infected, information that would have been useful for public health officers seeking to evoke the "danger of propagation" clause of the law.[53] Some of the counseling centers met with considerable success. By the late 1930s, the one on the grounds of the Kumamoto sanitarium was consulting with more than two hundred people each year, and about four out of five of those counseled agreed to enter the sanitarium.[54]

The LPA sought to reach patients and their families through other means as well. It published and distributed thousands of pamphlets with titles like A Conversation about Leprosy (Rai no hanashi, 1931), The Course of Leprosy Infection (Rai densen no keiro, 1935), and A Guide to Treatment (Ryōyō no tebiki, 1938). Typical of these works was the approach taken in A Conversation about Leprosy. Adopting an easy-to-understand question-and-answer format, the pamphlet explained that leprosy was an infectious disease, discussed possible paths of transmission, and described its various forms, but it also explicitly promoted admission to a sanitarium. In answer to the question "What should leprosy patients do?," the pamphlet informed readers that if faced with a diagnosis, "Don't despair or worry and don't rely upon the protection of the gods and Buddha. You should enter a sanitarium. If you do this, you will receive the best possible treatment and all your anxieties will be put to rest."[55]

Roughly a third of the fifteen-page booklet was devoted to explaining the benefits of sanitarium life. Reflecting the discourse on free convalescent zones, the institutions were described as "like villages of patients" that were "almost entirely self-governed" (a problematic claim, as we shall see), where life was organized around treatment, work, and recreation. Admission was open to all "without regard to assets or [the availability of] family support," and room, board, and treatment were provided at no cost. To be sure, the pamphlet also offered advice to "households with a leprosy patient." It outlined a regime that would have been onerous if not impossible for many. Patients were to be confined to a room separate from other family members and with separate bathing facilities; their clothing, linen, and dishes had to be washed separately with disinfectant and hot water; and the patient was to avoid contact with family members, particularly children.[56]

Suspected and confirmed leprosy patients and their families were by no means the LPA's only targets. Events such as Leprosy Prevention Day sought to educate the general public about the disease and its dangers through speeches, film screenings, discussions, and other means. Although there was always a national radio broadcast, most Leprosy Prevention Day celebrations were organized locally by regional chapters of the LPA, with the national organization providing literature for distribution, posters, and other support. The choice of June 25 for this event was not random. It was the birthday of the Taishō empress, whose donations to the sanitaria and leprosy relief organizations were well publicized. Leprosy Prevention Day was thus also a celebration of the imperial institution, whose concern for leprosy sufferers was held up as a model for the nation as a whole.

The campaign that most successfully mobilized public support for the sanitaria was the "ten-*tsubo* house movement" (*toppo jūtaku undō*). It began in 1932 as an attempt to expand the capacity of the sanitaria to accommodate the new wave of admissions. Although funding for the national and public sanitaria increased gradually each year in the 1930s, it never kept pace with the rapid growth of the patient population. Mitsuda pioneered a new and innovative strategy to resolve the budget crunch. He began to elicit private donations to construct new housing, targeting the general public for contributions to aid leprosy sufferers for the first time since the campaign to support Kihai Hospital more than four decades before. Inspired in part by the small patient cottages he had observed at Culion, Mitsuda conceived of what he called "ten-*tsubo* houses" (*toppo jūtaku*) and encouraged donations to construct them. The *tsubo* is a unit of measure equal to 3.3 square meters, and these small communal homes, each equipped with a kitchen and toilet, were intended to house between six and eight people in two small tatami rooms.

The campaign got under way with donations from the Taishō empress and the Imperial Household Agency as well as from corporations like Fujinnotomosha, publisher of a popular magazine for women. Adopting an approach much like that used by the US-based March of Dimes from the late 1930s, Mitsuda encouraged the participation of ordinary citizens in his campaign, calling upon each person to contribute ten sen towards the construction of a ten-*tsubo* residence, the cost of which was said to be 500 yen. Small coin banks in the shape of a ten-*tsubo* house, products of the pottery workshop at Aiseien, were placed in public places, and large envelopes that featured an image of a ten-*tsubo* house were distributed to volunteers, who canvassed for donations at schools, workplaces, temples and shrines, and on the streets.

Like the other leprosy-related campaigns of the era, the solicitation of donations, too, relied heavily on mass media. Over the course of the 1930s, a steady stream of newspaper and magazine articles, posters, and pamphlets encouraged people to participate by making or soliciting donations. These materials featured a complicated mix of rhetorical strategies that connected the emperor-centered ideology, national pride, public health concerns, and ideas about civic responsibility, while also playing upon long-standing stereotypes of the disease. For example, in a pamphlet produced by Aiseien, leprosy sufferers who remained outside the sanitarium were described as "pitiful," "living in darkness," and "in need of sympathy and support," but also as "foul smelling" and identifiable by their swollen and disfigured faces. Readers were asked to consider whether an infected person might be working in their local sweet shop or eatery and even now "extending the hand of unseen danger" towards them.[57]

The pamphlet provided a solution to this threat. Following the example of the imperial family, ordinary citizens could "combine their mutual strength and understanding" and raise money to house their "fellow citizens" (*dōhō*) within a sanitarium.[58] The term *dōhō* (literally "same womb") was a popular term to describe the citizenry in the 1930s. Implying that citizens were siblings referenced the ideas of Japan as a family-state headed by the patriarchal emperor and a "national body" (*kokutai*), both favored ideological tropes used to describe the organic union of the people, state, and emperor of Japan. The term "patriotic contribution" captures the new multilayered ideological significance of leprosy prevention: by contributing ten sen, one aided one's fellow citizens, protected one's self and the public, served the imperial will, and enhanced Japan's international prestige.[59]

The ten-*tsubo* house movement soon came to be closely connected to another public campaign, this one known as the "leprosy-free prefecture movement" (*muraiken undō*). Beginning in 1932, local chapters of the LPA and prefectural authorities in places such as Okayama, Aichi, Yamaguchi, and Tottori began to urge the residents of their prefectures to make donations to build ten-*tsubo* houses so that leprosy sufferers in their prefectures could be relocated to a sanitarium.[60] In Aichi and Yamaguchi such efforts were inspired by their relatively high rates of the disease: according to the 1921 survey of leprosy prevalence, Aichi had the fifth-highest rate of infection among Japan's forty-seven prefectures, following the Kyūshū prefectures and Okinawa, while Yamaguchi held eleventh place. In contrast, in Tottori leprosy was not particularly prevalent (neighboring Shimane had a far higher rate of infection), but an ambitious governor made the eradication of leprosy a personal cause. In Okayama, rates were lower yet, but the publicity surrounding Aiseien, which was located within the prefecture, contributed to a sense of heightened concern.[61]

While these efforts seem to have originally been independent local endeavors, regional newspapers began to suggest that prefectures were locked in competition to quickly achieve leprosy-free status. In 1936, the *Chūgoku shinbun* declared that "Aichi leads the country" because of its five-year plan to eradicate leprosy. Similarly in 1937, the local edition of the *Gōdō shinbun* declared that Tottori had "reached the top rank in the entire country" and was "leaping towards realizing [the status] of leprosy-free."[62] Sugiyama Hiroaki's careful study of the "movement" in Yamaguchi reveals the kinds of efforts that were used to promote the idea of a "leprosy-free prefecture."[63] Thousands of pamphlets were distributed, leprosy prevention posters were posted in public spaces around the prefecture, and public schools were required to hold assemblies where students heard speeches about the dangers of leprosy.

As this suggests, the leprosy-free prefecture movement quickly evolved from community-based efforts to expand the capacity of the sanitaria to a campaign to encourage the stricken to enter them. An anecdote related by Mitsuda suggests the impact of such efforts for leprosy sufferers who remained at home. In remarks intended to praise the dedication of a local policeman, Mitsuda described how an officer in Yamaguchi made more than twenty visits to a single leprosy sufferer until he finally consented to enter a sanitarium.[64] The ethos of voluntary admission notwithstanding, the line between coercion and volition was very thin.

The appeals to regional pride and local anxieties were clearly effective. In 1932 donations from Okayama residents were used to construct a Benevolent Okayama House (Jiokuryō) on the grounds of Aiseien; the following year, donations from Aichi were used to establish Atsuta House (Atsutaryō), named for the famous Atsuta Shrine in Nagoya. Over time, the landscapes of the national and public sanitaria were transformed by the construction of the ten-*tsubo* houses, which were rendered visible symbols of the support of people from all walks of life for leprosy sufferers and the ties that bound them to local communities and the nation. Like the residences associated with specific prefectures, those established with donations from the imperial family were also named in their honor and became known as "imperial gift houses" (*onshiryō*). Corporations were also recognized: for example, some houses were designated as Tomo Houses in honor of the contributions of Fujinnotomosha. Organizations that participated in fund-raising were also recognized. For example, a house established at Aiseien with funds from the Kyoto Christian Women's Association was called the Heian House, using the classical name for the old imperial city. But the most symbolically charged of all were the many units built by combining small donations that came to be known as "fellow citizen houses" (*dōhōryō*), which provided material evidence of the place of leprosy sufferers in the national polity.[65]

Patient Writing and Its Uses

Leprosy sufferers were not only the object of the public discourse on leprosy; they also contributed to it. In 1936, Hōjō Tamio (1914–1937), a patient at Zensei Hospital, won a major literary prize for his story "The First Night of My Life," which described a young man's induction into sanitarium life. Hōjō himself had entered Zensei Hospital in 1933 and quickly became involved in writing fiction there. He reached out by letter to the well-known author Kawabata Yasunari, who encouraged his efforts. Writing in the context of the national culture of leprosy, Hōjō became something of a sensation, and by the time of his death in 1937, his work had been published in a series of influential monthly magazines, including *Chūō Kōron*, *Kaizō*, and *Bungei shunju*. While Hōjō's work is notable for its publication in mainstream journals, it was only one part of a far larger culture of patient writing. In the early 1930s, the LPA and the sanitaria began to actively disseminate semiautobiographical fiction authored by patients in order to promote the cause of leprosy prevention. The effort to systematically encourage and publish patient writing created a body of "testimony" that was offered up to the reading public as evidence that leprosy patients were model citizens who suffered under the weight of popular prejudice and that the sanitaria system offered them protection and the possibility of a happy life.

Literary production within the sanitaria began at the initiative of the patients themselves. It was a social activity, a means of self-expression, and a way to gain recognition and perhaps a bit of pocket money. In 1909, haiku enthusiasts at Zensei Hospital organized a group they playfully called "Tarahara Kai" (literally "the Codfish Belly Society"), and within a few years similar organizations formed at other sanitaria as well. Patient interest in the composition of haiku, the brief poems consisting of three lines with five, seven, and five syllables, respectively, reflected its broad popularity in this period. The pioneer of so-called new haiku was Masaoka Shiki (1867–1902), a poet, critic, and journalist who argued that such poems were not just an amusing bit of wordplay, but in fact were a serious literary form—and one that was uniquely suited to the modern age because it was accessible to all. Masaoka himself wrote haiku that reflected upon, among other things, his declining health due to tuberculosis, the cause of his death at the age of thirty-four.[66]

Masaoka and his followers worked tirelessly to promote haiku composition, with considerable success. By the first decade of the twentieth century, newspapers and magazines were sponsoring haiku contests, encouraging its many new fans to submit their poems for scrutiny, with publication promised for the best. Patient interest in haiku composition was thus part of this larger cultural phenomenon. In his memoir, Sakurazawa Fusayoshi wrote of the success of one of his fellow patients at Zensei Hospital, who submitted his poems to such competitions and won the award of publication in a series of magazines and newspapers, often with the added benefit of a cash prize. His success encouraged others to try as well.[67]

In 1919 Zensei patients joined together to publish a literary magazine they called *Mountain Cherry* (*Yamazakura*). By this time, there were several club-type organizations at the hospital devoted to different poetic forms and short fiction. Initially, *Mountain Cherry* was a booklet of mimeographed handwritten pages that circulated only within Zensei Hospital, but later its editors began to send copies to the other sanitaria. In the preface of the first issue, the editors explained the origin of the journal, relating that some years before, Mitsuda had suggested to the patients that they "should try to make something like a newspaper that would record the good things that happen within the hospital."[68] The patients themselves were apparently not interested in a newsletter that celebrated the hospital; the preface states that they wanted a means to "provide solace for [our] feelings of loneliness and solitude." Its evocative title suggested that just as cherry trees blooming in the mountains went unnoticed, so, too, did patients writing within the sanitarium. *Mountain Cherry* was intended then to be a forum for patient self-expression, and its editors called for the submission of "discussions of religion, reflections on nature, essays, poetry, [examples of] dialect, and amusing stories."[69]

It did not take long for sanitarium administrators to recognize that patient writing might have other uses besides providing amusement and consolation. In the early 1920s, they began to explore its potential to shape both policy and perceptions outside of sanitarium walls. Takano's compilation of *Confessions of Leprosy Patients* was part of this turn; so, too, were the activities of Uchida Mamoru. A young doctor and an amateur poet, Uchida joined the staff of the Kumamoto Sanitarium in 1924 and quickly became involved with a patient club devoted to the composition of the classical poetic form known as tanka. In 1926, with Uchida's help, the group published their poems in a collection called *The Shadow of the Cypress* (*Hinoki no kage*). According to Uchida's preface, "Because of this literary work, society will know about the lives of leprosy sufferers and feel empathy for their suffering."[70] As word of its publication spread, amateur poets in other sanitaria around the country also began to create journals to showcase their work. At the Northern Area Rest Home, the smallest of the public institutions and one of the most poorly funded, patients began to organize poetry circles only in the late 1920s, but in spite of this late start, in 1930 they published (in mimeographed form) their own journal called *Fallen Leaves* (*Rakuyō*).[71]

With interest in patient writing growing, sanitarium authorities began to take steps to support it. In 1928, Zensei Hospital purchased a manual printing press and transformed *Mountain Cherry* from a coterie publication to an institutional journal. The work of the editorial board was redefined as a form of patient labor, and those involved were paid for their efforts. The new version of *Mountain Cherry* inspired similar efforts at the other sanitaria to create official publications. At the Northern Area Rest Home the director, Chūjō Suketoshi, decided to establish a sanitarium journal in 1930 with funds donated by the former Taishō empress. This official journal, called *At the Foot of Kōda* (*Kōda no suso*), a reference to the nearby Hakkōda Mountains, replaced the patient-driven *Fallen Leaves*. At Ōshima and Aiseien, it was staff rather than patients who took the lead in founding institutional journals. At Ōshima, the sanitarium pharmacist organized the publication of *Waterweeds* (*Moshiogusa*) in 1932 and headed its editorial board.[72] Aiseien's journal, *Aisei*, too, was primarily an administrative endeavor. It was edited by two staff members and had a distinctively institutional character, publishing not only patient works but also staff-authored essays on leprosy research, their travels to other sanitaria, and the like.

In 1931, Uchida summed up the thinking of sanitarium administrators about patient writing in an essay called "Leprosy Patients and the Literary Life" that was published in a special issue on leprosy in a social welfare journal. He suggested that just as the missionary institutions used religion to "guide patients" and "unify" them, the public sanitaria could do the same by encouraging patients to engage in literary production.[73] But patient writing had uses outside the sanitarium as well as within it. Uchida urged that it be used to further the goals of leprosy prevention. Literary works that described life in the sanitaria or expressed the "psychological condition" of patients could bridge the gap between the healthy and the sick and encourage the former not to forget "for a moment" the important task of eradicating the disease.[74] In other words, fostering awareness of the human dimension of life with leprosy could be used to inspire and sustain popular support for the policy of quarantine.

Within just a few years, two separate efforts to cultivate and diffuse patient writing were under way. In 1933, the editors of *Mountain Cherry* undertook a new endeavor, a "literary special issue" (*bungei tokushū*) that was to publish prizewinning works from an annual inter-sanitaria literary competition. The journal had sponsored such events in the past, beginning with a National Leprosy Patient Haiku Competition in 1920, but the literary special issue, which would be published annually until 1942, was a far more elaborate undertaking and one that would capture the interest of readers beyond the sanitaria. Prominent figures from outside the sanitaria were asked to serve as judges of specific categories of works, among them freestyle poems, tanka, haiku, children's stories, and short works of fiction. It is not clear who was responsible for choosing the judges, but they were an interesting group. For example, in 1934–1935, the evaluation of the short-story category was entrusted to Masaki Fujokyū, a physician employed at a TB sanitarium. Shikiba Ryūsaburō, who served as a judge in 1937, was a novelist and poet but also a psychiatrist and director of a psychiatric hospital. Kinoshita Mokutarō, the judge of the short-story category in 1939–1940, was an author, poet, and literary critic but also a professor in the medical school of Tokyo Imperial University and the author of a number of articles on leprosy.

The profile of the judges suggests that patient writing was evaluated not only, or perhaps even primarily, in terms of style, narrative technique, or some other literary criteria. At stake as well was the representation of sanitarium life. Typical of the prizewinning fiction in the early years of the competition was the short story that won second place in the 1934 competition, Tsubota Kimiko's "Seeking the Light."[75] It tells of a young woman named Akiko who was diagnosed with leprosy in her third year of high school, after a routine physical examination by the school physician. In order to conceal her condition, her wealthy and locally prominent family at first confined Akiko to her room, although a local doctor visited several times a week to provide treatment. As the disease continued to progress, Akiko was sent to Kusatsu, but after several months of treatment brought no improvement, she returned home. There she languished in seclusion until one day she came upon a magazine article about the public sanitaria. She then contacted the LPA for advice and was urged to enter a sanitarium "as soon as possible for your own good, the good of your family, and the good of the nation."[76]

The next section of the story takes place three years later. Akiko is about to leave the sanitarium, because after "appropriate exercise and the best possible treatment," she no longer poses a risk of infection. According to the narrator, "Everyone was overjoyed that Akiko had achieved a complete recovery, and they showered her with congratulations urging her to be careful about hygiene in the future and to continue to maintain her good health." Akiko responds by stating that while she will miss her friends within the institution, "every sanitarium is overcrowded and so someone who is non-infectious like me should not stay on, but should leave the hospital to make room for some poor patient who still suffers out in the world." Typical of the tone of the work overall is Akiko's declaration that "with the blessing of imperial mercy, I was able to receive treatment."[77]

This contrived little story, with its earnest young heroine and her quick cure within the happy sanitarium community courtesy of the imperial state, seems little more than a piece of propaganda for the Leprosy Prevention Law, but others were more compelling, exploring with considerable candor the stigma that continued to surround the disease. Shiba Tomotsu's "A Short-Term Home Visit" also appeared in the 1934 special issue. It tells of a boy in his teens named Yōzō, who after three years in the sanitarium is granted permission to go home for a two-week visit. He joyfully borrows nice clothing from fellow patients, considers carefully what gifts to bring to his younger siblings, and happily imagines a joyful welcome from his family when he returns in good health. What awaits him, however, is very different. His father greets him with anger, refuses to allow him to see his siblings, and confines him to the family storehouse, a thick-walled

windowless structure that stands separate from the main house. Designed
to protect valuables from fire, in fiction at least, storehouses were favored
sites for the confinement of troublesome family members, including leprosy sufferers, wayward children, and the mentally ill.

Sitting alone in darkness, Yōzō thinks, "Why did Dad put me in the
storehouse out of embarrassment, even though I had the hospital's permission [to return]? Is my sickness that terrible? . . . The hospital! It would
have been better if I had not come. Now I realize this for the first time.
. . . The hospital is the world that has been given to those who are sick."[78]
The story concludes with Yōzō returning to the sanitarium and resuming
life there. Thus, like "Seeking the Light," this story, too, represented the
sanitarium as a place of effective treatment, but it also offered an indict-
ment of the stigma of the disease that made it difficult for even those who
had recovered to return to ordinary life.

In the same year that the literary special issue got under way, the
LPA, too, began to solicit patient writing. It would eventually publish four
large volumes of short stories that were intended for the general public, in
1933, 1935, 1936, and 1937. Many of those who submitted works to the
Mountain Cherry literary competition also contributed to the LPA collections, and there is considerable overlap in themes, content, and style in
the stories they published. Positive accounts of sanitarium life abound,
as do exaggerated claims that successful treatment would lead to release
from the institutions. In fact, while the sanitaria were far more porous than
terms such as "absolute isolation" suggest, the requirements for release
were quite strict. According to data compiled in 1941 on eight institutions,
the percentage of the total patient population (cumulatively since 1909)
discharged as "recovered" was less than 5 percent, although there was
considerable variation from institution to institution.[79]

Although the stories in the LPA collections had much in common
with those published in the *Mountain Cherry* special issues, they also had a
number of distinctive elements that reflected the specific goals of the LPA.
"The Shining Sanitarium" by Uchida Shizuo is a good example. Born in
1922 in Ishikawa Prefecture, Uchida entered Zensei Hospital in 1930 and
died there in 1946. He was a prolific author whose poems, short stories, and
essays appeared often in *Mountain Cherry*, and in 1937, he was awarded
the grand prize in the fiction category of the annual competition.[80] "The
Shining Sanitarium," which appeared in the 1933 LPA publication, tells
the story of teenage boy named Ryōji who is growing up in a small fishing
village.[81] One day his childhood friend, a girl named Yōko, notices a small
lesion on his arm. When Ryōji consults a doctor, who diagnoses him with

leprosy, he realizes at once that he must have been infected as a child by a "vagrant leper," a man his compassionate parents had housed in their storehouse for several years. Ryōji and Yōko had befriended the man and even called him "uncle."

Ryōji's diagnosis devastates his family. His father at first refuses to believe it, because "our family is not part of a filthy lineage," but then is wracked with guilt when he learns the disease is actually infectious and that he exposed his son to it. His sister is abandoned by her fiancé, and his older brother and sister-in-law flee the family home. Ryōji turns to patent medicines, hot-spring treatments, prayers, and amulets in hopes of a cure, and then considers suicide. At last he decides his only option is to enter a sanitarium, a fate he contemplates with horror. He is surprised to discover after his admission that it is "an ideal village better than anything he could have imagined." He joins the young men's association, gets a job as a nurse, and spends his free time playing baseball and tennis and writing stories. When he is no longer infectious, Ryoji is allowed to return home to visit his family and quickly sets about educating family members and neighbors about the disease. Soon, his sister is reunited with her fiancé, his brother and sister-in-law move back in with his parents, and when Yōko, too, is discovered to be infected, she joins him in the sanitarium. The story ends with the two living happily in the sanitarium, and Ryōji declares, "Our happiness is because of the sacred love of the imperial family."

While there is little that is original in the basic plot of the "The Shining Sanitarium," it illuminates several motifs that figure prominently in the stories included in the LPA collections, especially when juxtaposed against the rejected stories, which are also extant. One thing that characterizes all of the successful stories is their attempt to confirm the infectious nature of the disease and disprove the still prevalent belief that it is hereditary. To that end, there is a strong emphasis on making the circumstances of infection crystal clear. As in Uchida's work, in story after story, the diagnosis leads to the discovery or recollection of the encounter that led to infection. In some cases, it is a parent who inexplicably disappeared years before who is revealed to be responsible, in others a nursemaid, in still others a casual acquaintance. Often, the risk of infection is exaggerated, with a single chance encounter leading to infection. In contrast, in the rejected stories, the path of transmission is often unexplored, and in some cases the central character engages in behavior that exposes others to the disease. For example, after the protagonist of a rejected story called "The Tortured Path" is diagnosed, he goes on a prolonged pilgrimage, staying on temple and shrine grounds where he mingles with others until he is finally picked up by the police.[82]

The appearance of the police in "The Tortured Path" may also have figured in its rejection. In the published stories, there is an overt emphasis on the voluntary nature of confinement and on correcting the negative image of the sanitaria. Like Ryōji, the characters within these stories initially express dismay at the idea of sanitarium admission, citing rumors that they are frightening, dangerous places, filled with vagrants and petty criminals. Upon arrival, the middle-class patients are quickly disabused of such notions and discover the sanitarium to be "a utopia," "a paradise," and even "a magnificent independent village." In contrast, many of the rejected stories make explicit mention of police involvement in the transfer to a sanitarium. In one, a leprosy sufferer staying at an inn is reported to the police by the innkeeper. In another, after a young girl is discovered to have leprous lesions during a school exam, the school reports her to the local police, who inform the prefectural authorities.[83]

Finally, the successful stories inevitably linked the experiences of their characters to broader ideological constructs, including the imperial state, the public good, and national prestige. Not all authors did this as overtly as Uchida, who ends his story with his characters bowing in the direction of the imperial place. A story called "On the Way towards a New Life" concludes with the central character, Hideaki, telling his family that he will enter the sanitarium to ensure that he will not "spread his poison around society."[84] Many successful stories also managed to work in explicit references to LPA initiatives. For example, a story called "The Evening of the Dance" tells of a young man named Yokichi who was discovered to have leprosy during the physical exam required of all conscripts. He lives in seclusion at home after it becomes clear that patent drugs and hot-spring treatments are useless. Then, on Leprosy Prevention Day he happens to hear a radio address by Mitsuda Kensuke and decides at once to set out for Aiseien.[85]

The stories selected for publication in both the LPA volumes and *Mountain Cherry* were clearly intended to shore up the official leprosy policy. For this reason, historians and literary scholars have tended to ignore or dismiss this body of work as nothing more than propaganda. Arai Yūki, the author of *Kakuri no bungaku* (The Literature of Isolation), has argued that the works from the 1930s are evidence that "the internal life of the patients was completely controlled."[86] Others ignore the great bulk of patient writing as propaganda but valorize a handful of authors who are said to represent the true voice of the patients.[87] It is undeniable that the patient-authored works that made their way into the LPA collections and the sanitarium journals were mediated in various ways. The sanitaria and the LPA provided an incentive to write by establishing competitions, funding publication, and rewarding patients who became authors with recognition. But rather than trying to distinguish authentic self-expression from propaganda, it is more useful to view all patient writing as reflecting both the agency of the authors and the web of constraints that shaped their lives. Stories like "Seeking the Light" and "The Shining Sanitarium" reveal that sanitarium patients, no less than their fellow citizens, framed their lives and experiences in light of the imperial ideology of the day, and they also offer a window into why many came to feel that voluntary confinement offered their best chance of a meaningful life.

The Many Meanings of Leprosy

Leprosy patients were not the only ones writing stories about the disease in the early 1930s. As the mass campaigns got under way, leprosy became a favored plot device within both mass and highbrow fiction authored by those who did not suffer from the disease and had no interest in public health, the LPA, or the sanitaria. Given the new status of leprosy in national culture, its frequent appearance in diverse genres of fiction, with distinctive if overlapping readerships, is perhaps not surprising, but authors who referenced the disease did not simply echo themes found in patient writing. Instead, they complicated the discourse on leprosy that emanated from official sources.

One site where stories about leprosy proliferated was the mass-circulation magazines, such as *New Youth* (*Shinseinen*) and *Profile* (*Purufuiru*), that published detective and mystery fiction. Such stories were associated with so-called *ero guro* culture, a Japanese term coined from "erotic grotesque nonsense" that was used to describe fiction, art, and film that challenged orthodox values with an ironic sensibility. Stories about perverse sexuality, morbid secrets, and science gone bad filled the pages of *New Youth* and its competitors. "The Storehouse," published in *Profile* in 1935, is typical of the stories in which leprosy figures.[88] Its author, Nishio Tadashi, had become notorious the year before when his first published work, also in *Profile*, caught the eye of the censors, which resulted in the entire issue being banned.

Nishio's title suggests the intersection between patient writing and mass fiction. As we have seen, the storehouse was a favored motif in the patient-authored stories and was associated with familial responses to leprosy. The plot of "The Storehouse" unfolds gradually through a series of letters written by a young man, his mother, a doctor, and others in the style of an epistolary novel. They describe how the young man fell in love with a foreign woman while vacationing in a resort town popular with Western residents of Japan. Eventually the two become intimate, but the relationship ends when the girl and her family abruptly disappear one day. Rumors then begin to circulate that she was suffering from an unnamed but terrible disease. When he hears this, the young man becomes concerned and seeks out an examination by a physician, who diagnoses him with leprosy. He immediately decides to commit suicide but before his death writes to his mother explaining the circumstances that led him to this act. Upon reading her son's final letter, his mother, too, commits suicide but like her son leaves a note behind. It relates that it was not the foreign woman who gave the boy leprosy, but his putative father, who has been confined secretly within the family storehouse for more than a decade. According to the mother's letter, her son was actually the product of an illicit love affair, and when her husband discovered this, he purposefully infected the boy when he was a child.

With its plot points of illicit sex, revenge, and suicide, "The Storehouse" is in many ways a stereotypical mystery story of the time, except for the fact that the mystery at its center, and at the center of all the mystery stories that take up leprosy, is the question of "Who infected whom?" This was, as we have seen, the question that animated many of the stories in the LPA collections as well. But the secret at the center of the mystery stories is always the surprising identity of the "infector." In "The Storehouse," it was not the seductive foreign woman or a nameless vagrant who was responsible for infecting the boy but his supposed father and by extension his adulterous mother. The story thus manipulates the themes of the leprosy prevention campaigns to imply that everyone is potentially a leprosy sufferer and every relationship carries with it the possibility of infection. In this dystopian world, suicide, not the sanitarium, is the only possible resolution.

Leprosy also figured thematically in works of a different nature, fiction of the sort Japanese literary historians like to classify as "pure literature" (*jun bungaku*), that is, highbrow fiction written for an educated audience. The modernist writer Yokomitsu Riichi, whose wife suffered from tuberculosis, had made that disease a theme of some of his earlier work, but leprosy is at the center of "The Carriage" (Basha), which was published in *Kaizō*, an influential journal of literature and criticism, in 1932. The story describes the experiences of Yura, a young man from Tokyo who is suffering from neurasthenia, a diverse collection of physical and psychological symptoms associated with the stress of modern life that plagued many

Japanese intellectuals in this era. Seeking relief, Yura travels to a hot-spring resort (clearly modeled on Kusatsu), where he becomes acquainted with a middle-aged man. Obsessed with fortune-telling, the man speaks at length about the intricacies of different methods of divination. Eventually it is revealed that after his daughter, a beautiful young woman, was diagnosed with leprosy, he had forced her to live in the "leper village" adjacent to the hot-spring resort. Some years later an examination by another physician re-vealed that the girl had been misdiagnosed, and she was actually free from the disease. However, she chose to remain in the leper village rather than return to her father, and the knowledge of his role in making her a "leper" is the cause of the father's breakdown and his fixation on understanding fate.

Yura himself soon becomes obsessed with the leper village and the man's beautiful daughter. He begins to daydream about the village, "imag-ining to himself what kind of life those wretched people might live." The village is called Yumedono (literally "Dream Hall"), but it is described as remarkably ordinary: "There were shops, inns, workers; there was even a brass band . . . and one could see fresh young children running about." As Yura's attraction to the girl deepens, he begins to wonder if it is his fate to marry her and to enter the leper village himself. At the same time, he is appalled by this idea and resolves to return to Tokyo. His determination, however, is cut short when he unexpectedly encounters the young woman, and he "realized fully at last that he might struggle as hard as he pleased but it seemed unlikely that he would ever be able to part from her now."[89]

As this summary suggests, Yokomitsu used leprosy to explore the relationship between fate and free will, science and belief, but he also refer-enced the official discourse of leprosy prevention that celebrated sanitarium life. The serenity of the daughter and the other inhabitants of the leper village stands in sharp contrast to the psychological turmoil of both Yura and the father. In the end, Yokomitsu suggests that life in the leper village might be preferable to the world outside and that those deemed healthy are actually the sick.

The works by Nishio and Yokomitsu are just two of the many works of fiction in this era that deployed leprosy and the figure of the leprosy sufferer. While they clearly reflect the rise of the discourse of leprosy pre-vention, they do not simply reiterate it. Instead, leprosy as a trope became a means to criticize contemporary social norms, modernity, and the official discourse on the disease. Nishio's story can be read as a parody of the up-lifting tales the LPA was circulating: it was not the "vagrant leper" who was dangerous but a cuckolded husband. Yokomitsu's work exaggerated the claims of the leprosy prevention campaigns by portraying leper villages, the object of so much laudatory rhetoric, as an ideal world that even the uninfected should aspire to enter.

The establishment of Japan's first national sanitarium and the passage of the 1931 Leprosy Prevention Law ushered in a new moment in the long history of leprosy in Japan. At the outset, Mitsuda and his colleagues were committed to creating a new kind of sanitarium, one that would serve the interest of the patients and the nation, providing a model for the rest of the world. Central to this vision was the idea that patients would not be coercively confined but would accept quarantine for both their own good and that of the wider public. As "colonizers" they would participate fully in Japanese national life, albeit from within the confines of the sanitarium.

As officials, civic organizations, and ordinary citizens joined forces to promote sanitarium admission as the solution to Japan's leprosy "problem," those with the disease came under new and intense pressure. Mitsuda's anecdote of the heroic policeman reveals the kind of social coercion "patients in the home" faced, but it also implies that they could still refuse to enter a sanitarium. Patient-authored fiction suggests that for some the sanitarium offered the possibility of a life less constrained than that outside, allowing them to work, marry, and recover. It reveals as well that some patients were active consumers and producers of the imperial ideology of the day. But as the public discourse on leprosy unfolded, shaped by multiple voices and differing agendas, it became a complicated mix of competing claims. Were leprosy sufferers dangerous others or "born of the same womb"? Should they be feared, pitied, or celebrated? Was the world of the sanitarium a mirror image of that outside, something worse, or something better? In the next chapter, we turn to explore how these issues shaped the evolution of the sanitarium system in national life in the darkest chapter of Japan's modern history.

Chapter 7

The Sanitaria in the Time of National Emergency

O n August 13, 1936, a group of patients at Aiseien made their way to the highest point on the island. Known as the Shining Hill, it was the site of the Bell of Mercy (Megumi no Kane). Purchased with a donation from Nishi-Honganji Temple in Kyoto, the bell was inscribed with a poem written by the Taishō empress for Japan's leprosy sufferers that stated, "Although I think of you often, I cannot be there to comfort you, so I send this in my place." In 1934, staff and patients working together had built a tower to house the bell, which was rung on the twenty-second day of each month as patients and staff stood at attention to commemorate the opening of Aiseien.[1] On this hot August day, however, the young men who made their way to the bell had another purpose in mind. They wanted to call their fellow patients to an emergency meeting to protest sanitarium policies. However, whether intentionally or by happenstance, their vigorous ringing of the bell resulted in a large crack. The patient protest, which was to last almost two weeks and draw national attention, was quickly dubbed the "Nagashima Incident" by the Japanese press, a designation that aligned it with other recent "incidents" of unrest, like the failed coup d'état of six months before in Tokyo. Accounts of the incident made much of the cracked bell, claiming that subversive patients had attacked this symbol of imperial compassion, religious largesse, and institutional unity.

This chapter explores the rise of patient activism in the 1930s in relation to both the national culture of leprosy explored in the last chapter and the demise of Japan's fragile experiment with "imperial democracy" that followed the military takeover of Manchuria and the outbreak of the second Sino-Japanese War.[2] I argue that the efforts by patients to force the institutions to make good on their promises of autonomy and self-government created an ideological crisis in what was declared to be "a time of national emergency," as Japan's military involvement in China deepened. Patient activism called into question the image of the organic "national body" and the inclusiveness of Japanese society that the sanitaria had been used to signify at a time when the state had a greater stake than ever in this vision of the nation. In the wake of the patient protest, there was a fundamental reorganization of the sanitaria system—one that transformed patients from "colonizers" who had a powerful place in national culture to the inhabitants of internal colonies.

Institutions under Stress

As we saw in chapter 6, the campaigns of the early 1930s sought to encourage patients to step forward and apply for sanitarium admission. To what degree these efforts influenced any single patient is, of course, impossible to measure, but within a few years Aiseien and several of the public sanitaria were facing serious overcrowding. In December 1934, the official capacity of Aiseien was 732, but the actual patient population reached 1,000. This figure included 78 patients who had been relocated from the sanitarium at Sotojima after it was destroyed in 1934 by a typhoon that killed 187 patients and staff. The 400 survivors of the disaster were divided up among the various sanitaria. The absorption of the new patients strained several institutions. Zensei Hospital, for example, was about a hundred patients over capacity in this period, most of whom were refugees from Sotojima.[3]

The situation was particularly acute at Aiseien, which was almost 40 percent over capacity by 1936, the result of Mitsuda's policy of turning no potential patient away, even though government funding was based on official capacity and did not increase automatically as patient numbers climbed. To make ends meet, Mitsuda began to reduce patient wages as well as expenditures for meals and medical care. At one point, the Ministry of Finance intervened, instructing Mitsuda to stop admitting new patients because his requests for additional funding could not be met. According to Mitsuda, he refused on the grounds that "infectious disease doesn't recognize quotas." He also justified his stance on humanitarian grounds, stating that refusing to admit patients who had stepped forward led some to take desperate measures, including suicide.[4]

There is, however, more to this story. Even after Aiseien was seriously overcrowded, Mitsuda continued to aggressively encourage new admissions. One of his efforts was the production of a glossy pamphlet called

A Guide to Nagashima (*Nagashima annai*). Richly illustrated with photographs of Aiseien's impressive facilities, it included directions on how to travel to the sanitarium from all parts of the country.[5] He also dispatched Aiseien staff to rural areas to directly recruit patients, an endeavor that came to the public's attention with the publication of the 1937 best seller *Spring on a Small Island* (*Kojima no haru*) by Ogawa Masako, a young female physician who joined the staff of Aiseien in 1932.[6] Between 1934 and 1936, Ogawa made several trips to rural Shikoku, where she worked with the local authorities to persuade leprosy sufferers to leave their homes and enter Aiseien. Ogawa was an enthusiastic amateur poet and in her book she interspersed her account of interactions with leprosy patients with a series of evocative poems composed in the classical style. The work captured the popular imagination and made Ogawa a heroine in the minds of many.

As Mitsuda's defiant response to the Ministry of Finance suggests, the directors of the sanitarium continued to have a good deal of freedom to manage their institutions as they saw fit. Not every director agreed with Mitsuda's position that overcrowding was necessary to further the project of leprosy prevention. The public sanitarium in Kumamoto was under capacity throughout the 1930s, even though Kyūshū continued to be known for its high rates of the disease. In Kumamoto itself, a large community of leprosy sufferers continued to live in makeshift housing in an area adjacent to Honmyōji Temple, where its members openly begged for alms. This situation so enraged Mitsuda that he publicly criticized Miyazaki Matsuki, the director of the Kumamoto sanitarium, at a meeting of sanitarium directors and Home Ministry officials. At one point Mitsuda wrote directly to the Kumamoto prefectural government to criticize Miyazaki's inaction, offering to house Kumamoto's leprosy sufferers at Aiseien.[7] The under-capacity status of the Kyūshū Sanitarium did not reflect Miyazaki's opposition to the policy of confinement, but rather his concern about provoking patient unrest. In 1932, the sanitarium had been the site of an embarrassing incident when hundreds of patients walked out to protest the dismissal of a popular staff member. Following the pattern of patient protest already noted, their intention was to make their way to the prefectural governor's office to lodge a complaint, but before they could follow through with this plan the police quickly intervened and returned them to the sanitarium.[8]

In spite of the Home Ministry's stated aim of confining ten thousand people within ten years and the growing problem of overcrowding, only three new sanitaria were constructed before 1935. In 1931, Miyakojima became the site of Okinawa's prefectural sanitarium, known as Nanseien (Southern Peace Sanitarium). Then, the following year a second national sanitarium, known as Rakusen'en (Happy Hot Spring Sanitarium) was established outside of Kusatsu. A much-anticipated attempt to implement the kind of "free convalescent zone" that had elicited so much discussion, Rakusen'en had a unique structure. Half of the area of the institution, known as the "official zone" (*kanku*), was organized on the model of the public sanitaria, with communal residences, medical facilities, and a meeting hall. The other half was designated as the "free zone" (*jiyūku*). Intended primarily to appeal to the affluent residents of Yunosawa, the free zone offered them the opportunity to build a private residence (at their own expense) on the sanitarium's grounds. Those who resided in the free zone were to live independently, although for a fee they could also receive meals prepared in the sanitarium's kitchen. Medical care was to be provided at no cost at the sanitarium clinic, and residents would also have access to its bathhouse, which featured the hot sulfurous waters for which Kusatsu was famous. Rakusen'en administrators were so eager to promote relocation from Yunosawa that they de-emphasized the danger of infection that figured so prominently in the leprosy prevention campaigns of the time, assuring potential residents that they could both employ "healthy attendants" (*kenkō tsukisoenin*) and reside with their uninfected spouses. Uninfected children, however, were required to live in an on-site childcare center.[9]

At the time of its official opening, Rakusen'en was still under construction and had a capacity of only fifteen patients, but by the end of 1933 it housed ninety-five people, eighty-four of whom had relocated from Yunosawa. When ninety-eight survivors of the Sotojima disaster arrived in 1934, there was no available housing and the refugees were forced to reside in tents for several months. However, to the disappointment of the advocates of the free convalescent zones, those who moved from Yunosawa were not wealthy property owners but poorer members of the community who may have found the sanitarium an appealing alternative to the "semi-monastic" atmosphere offered by St. Barnabas. Two years after Rakusen'en opened, there were only twenty-some residences in the free zone, while Yunosawa had a population of about eight hundred people.[10] In the face of this failure, interest in the free convalescent zone concept began to wane, and the third national sanitarium, Keiaien, established in Kagoshima in 1935, was a conventional institution.

Although the attempt to create a free zone met with little success, Rakusen'en is significant for another, albeit largely unacknowledged reason. Responding to the continuing presence of a large population of leprosy sufferers in relative proximity to the sanitarium, the medical staff began to offer treatment on an outpatient basis, and this soon became one of the important functions of the new institution. In 1933, the sanitarium saw 1,301 patients on an outpatient basis, and in 1934, 1,811 patients.[11] The potential of this kind of approach—that is, the publicly funded outpatient treatment of leprosy, which would have allowed leprosy sufferers to live at home—went unrecognized amidst the frenzied efforts to promote confinement.

The Emergence of Patient Activism

The ten-*tsubo* house movement was intended to ease the housing crisis in the sanitaria, while the leprosy-free prefecture movement aimed to encourage new admissions. As a result of these contradictory endeavors, there was no quick resolution to the problem of overcrowding, and as patients flowed into Aiseien after 1933, they confronted a reality that had little in common with either Mitsuda's original vision of "an ideal separate world" or the portrayal of sanitarium life offered up in publications like *A Guide to Nagashima*. Rooms designed to house six patients housed eight, even nine, and meals consisted largely of poor-quality rice cooked with other grains to produce a mixture many regarded as inedible.

Patient frustration was growing, but Mitsuda was either unaware or unconcerned. When the number of patients reached one thousand, he organized a celebration at Aiseien, one aspect of which was to be the publication of a commemorative volume of patient writings. The project had to be abandoned, however, when only about 15 percent of patients responded, and almost half of their submissions were critical of the sanitarium. Many of these focused on issues of food, housing, and medical care. One patient supplied only two terse sentences: "These days the food is terrible. Please do something." But others took note of growing tensions within the institution, not only between patients and staff, but also among the patients. According to one patient, "Recently many new rules have been issued, telling us 'this is not allowed,' and 'that is not allowed.' We know such things without being constantly cautioned [by the staff]. Moreover, those who try to follow the rules to the letter and do exactly as instructed are mocked by others who say, 'Look, it's a bootlicker, sucking up to the staff.'"[12]

The minutes of the Council of Residence Heads offer a window into patient frustration in these years. The ostensible purpose of the council, a forum of patient representatives who met regularly with Mitsuda and his senior staff, was to allow for patient involvement in the administration of the sanitarium, but the rules governing its membership seemed designed to ensure that it would not pose a challenge to the director's authority. Under the system devised by Mitsuda, each of the communal residences was allowed to put forth the names of three candidates based upon internal elections, one of whom was chosen by Mitsuda to join the council. Mitsuda also selected two additional members who were meant to represent the patient population at large.[13]

Although the council was made up of Mitsuda's appointees, they took their role as the representatives of the patients seriously. Even before over-crowding became a serious issue, council members had begun to convey patient frustration with the constraints of institutional life. They reported that patients resented that small, useful personal items such as razors and pocketknives were confiscated when they entered the sanitarium, that staff monitored conversations with visiting family members, and that they had no access to a telephone.[14] As the budgetary crisis became acute in 1934–1935, the list of complaints grew, with patients expressing dissatisfaction with the quality of the food and medical care they were offered, the reduc-tion of their wages, and the lack of adequate clothing, toothbrushes, soap, and even thongs for their wooden clogs.[15] Mitsuda showed little sympathy, insisting that conditions at Aiseien were no worse than at other institutions and that patients should be willing to tolerate deprivation so that their fel-low sufferers could be admitted as soon as possible.[16]

The top-down structure of the council aimed to maintain Mitsuda's authority, but it also reflected the institutional ideology of Aiseien. Al-though he had advocated for a self-governing colony throughout the 1920s, after Aiseien opened Mitsuda showed little interest in actually creating one, a choice that reflected both the political climate of the 1930s and his personal ambitions. Aiseien, he proclaimed, was "a great family" in which patients and staff were united by the shared ideals of mutual responsibility, harmony, self-sacrificial service, and a desire to expand the sanitarium. Every family needs a father, and that was his role—and just as Japan's civil code gave fathers considerable authority over their children, including the right to discipline them when necessary, so he was endowed with similar authority over patients.[17]

Mitsuda's conception of what he called "familyism" (*kazokushugi*) was directed both at patients inside the sanitarium and at the larger society outside, and it mirrored one of the most powerful political metaphors of the day, the notion of Japan as a "family-state," with the emperor as the father of his subjects. Mitsuda would make the case throughout the 1930s that the organization of Aiseien reflected the proper social and political order of Japanese society. The support of the imperial family for Aiseien offered legitimacy to Mitsuda's insistence that affective ties, rather than politi-cal rights, should order relations within Aiseien. Members of the imperial family provided not only a steady stream of donations but also poems they authored, pieces of calligraphy, and other tokens of imperial favor and concern. Even gifts that did not come directly from the imperial family, such as the Bell of Mercy, were used to signify the special relationship of the sanitarium and the imperial institution.

The concepts of mutual responsibility and self-sacrifice associated with familyism were not simply useful and timely moral platitudes. They were also instantiated in various ways in institutional life. For example, as at other institutions, Aiseien patients were paid for their work within the sanitarium, but Mitsuda established the rule that any wages that exceeded three yen per month must be contributed to a fund administered by the Comfort Association (Iankai), a group of patients and staff who, in addition to organizing funerals, celebrations, and other events, also provided a small allowance to seriously ill and disabled patients who were unable to work.[18] To Mitsuda's dismay, to avoid the mandatory contribution, some patients simply limited how much they worked, a choice that reflected less a lack of sympathy for their fellow patients than resentment that they should be compelled to shoulder this burden out of their meager wages. Mitsuda resolved this issue by requiring all working patients to contribute one yen per month regardless of their total income.[19] This tendency to put ideology over practical concerns continued even as conditions declined. For example, Mitsuda repeatedly rejected the suggestion of council members that patients should be allowed to grow vegetables on small individual plots to supplement the meager sanitarium meals, arguing that granting private plots would undermine the principle of mutual responsibility that was exemplified in cooperative agricultural labor in communal fields.[20]

Sanitarium directors and Home Ministry bureaucrats had explained the problems that plagued the early public sanitaria as the result of the moral failures of their patients, the "vagrant lepers" who lacked the sense of civic duty that animated proper Japanese citizens. They now discovered that the patients who entered in the 1930s, often better educated and more politically conscious than the first generation of patients, were even less receptive to the authoritarian paternalism of the sanitaria and their powerful directors. Some of the new patients may also have recognized their newly ambiguous political status. From the time of the first elections in 1890, suffrage was both limited to men and tied to the payment of a certain amount of tax, with the result that only a small fraction of the adult male population was qualified to vote. In 1925, after considerable debate, the Diet finally voted to extend the right of suffrage to all adult men over the age of twenty-five, but there continued to be a strong sentiment that full citizenship required contributing to the national economy. In 1926, the privy council sponsored an amendment to the electoral law that denied both the vote and the right to stand for election to anyone receiving public or private relief (*kōshi kyūjutsu*). Although this revision did not specifically target sanitarium patients, they were among those who were disenfranchised under its provisions.

Unlike unhappy patients in the 1910s and 1920s, who had most often attempted to speak with their feet, this new generation of patients began to explicitly raise the question of their place in the nation. One frustrated patient no doubt spoke for many when he wrote in 1934 in response to the call for submissions for the planned commemorative volume that he had entered Aiseien voluntarily, "believing wholeheartedly that this was a national project," only to find that even basic needs of the patients went unmet.[21] As the gap between the ideology and reality of sanitarium life became apparent, some patients turned away from mainstream politics. Aiseien was not the first sanitarium to see patients embrace ideas the government viewed as subversive. In 1932, a group of patients at Sotojima Rest Home established the first explicitly socialist organization for the biologically vulnerable when they organized the Japanese Proletarian League for the Liberation of Leprosy Sufferers and began to publicize an ambitious agenda for change. They wanted the freedom to go in and out of the sanitarium, better working conditions and higher wages, improved medical care, better care for the seriously ill, and the end of punishment, censorship, and restrictions on freedom of speech and association. They also called for social change outside the sanitarium walls, in particular an end to social discrimination against leprosy sufferers and their families.[22]

The director of Sotojima at this time was Murata Masataka (1884–1974), and the emergence of political activism under his watch would end his career in the civil service. Trained in the medical faculty of Tokyo Imperial University, Murata had joined the Home Ministry after graduation and was appointed director of Sotojima in 1927. Widely regarded at the time as one of the worst of the public sanitaria, Sotojima had long been plagued by staff problems, runaway patients, and poor conditions. Murata quickly set about changing things. He doubled the amount spent on patient meals, hired new staff, created a baseball team and a library, and most significantly, established a system of what he called autonomous self-government (*jishu jichi*) that gave the patients' elected representatives control over many aspects of daily life, from running the sanitarium store to determining punishments for those who broke sanitarium rules. The Ōshima and Northern Area sanitaria also established forms of limited self-government around this time, but Murata went further than anyone else, even promising the patient leaders that he would tear down Sotojima's walls and guard stations, if they could bring problems such as gambling and abscondments under control.[23]

While Murata's efforts to reform Sotojima won him the respect and affection of his patients, they also caught the eye of the Special Higher Police, created in 1911 in the aftermath of the discovery of a plot to assassinate the emperor. The authority of the Special Higher Police expanded dramatically after the passage of the 1925 Peace Preservation Law, which aimed to combat the growing political influence of socialism, communism, and anarchism. Not long after the establishment of the Japanese Proletarian League for the Liberation of Leprosy Sufferers, the Osaka branch of the Special Higher Police began to investigate rumors of "red" activities at Sotojima.[24] Beginning in August 1933, local newspapers began to portray Sotojima as a veritable hotbed of leftist political activity, with one headline declaring: "Red and the Leprosy Bacteria: The Battle against the Spread of a Double-Threat."[25] It was reported that communist sympathizers among the staff were involved in organizing patients, who were in turn attempting to organize the day workers employed by the sanitarium.[26] In other words, leftist ideas were spreading like an infection.

As questioning of the staff and patients got under way, Murata attempted to resolve the situation by quietly discharging the leaders of the activist patients from the sanitarium one evening. This was a legitimate exercise of his authority as director under the guidelines for disciplinary actions approved by the Diet, which allowed him to expel recalcitrant patients. However, when this came to light, Murata, too, came under suspicion. Newspapers reported that he had abetted the "escape" of politically dangerous patients, and much was made of the fact that rather than releasing the activists penniless, he had given them some money out of his own pocket to help them on their way. It was implied that Murata himself had leftist leanings, and his support of patient self-government, interest in Esperanto, and purchase of works by Marx for the sanitarium's library were offered up as evidence of his personal politics.[27] After weeks of attack, Murata resigned as director in 1933, to the dismay of his patients. He would never again hold an official position.

The Nagashima Incident
Three years after Murata left Sotojima, newspapers around the country were again reporting that "red" patients were creating unrest in a

sanitarium, but this time the stakes were much higher. The unrest was at Aiseien, the first national sanitarium, an institution celebrated as "the best sanitarium in the world" and much favored by the imperial family. As the protest unfolded over two weeks in August, there was widespread shock among those who believed it to be a model institution, filled with happy patients and headed by a visionary director. Explanations of what sparked the uprising are varied. One patient in a letter to Mitsuda dismissed the uprising as nothing more than a "food fight" that resulted from patient frustration with the poor meals they were offered.[28] Another explanation, this one from a staff member, was that patients became angry after an attempted escape was foiled and the would-be runaways were confined in the sanitarium's jail.[29] Sasaki Mamoru, vice chairman of the patients' "executive committee" during the protests, offered yet another explanation. According to his account, after a cut in wages that reduced them by almost half was announced, some patients refused to work. This led to an angry clash with staff, who reportedly taunted the patients, stating, "Three of us can do the work of more than ten of you."[30]

Whatever sparked the protest, on the evening of August 13, in response to the ringing of the Bell of Mercy, a large number of patients gathered and voted to call a general strike in order to pressure for reforms. They wanted the resignation of Mitsuda and other senior staff, an end to overcrowding, improvement of living conditions, direct communication with the Home Ministry, and the establishment of self-government. By the following morning, the sanitarium walls were plastered with handwritten posters with slogans such as "Off with the Director's Head!," "Nagashima Is Hell!," and "Comrades! Let's Fight Together to the End!"[31] Soon there were incidents of violence on both sides. Staff members turned firefighting hoses on patients, and when Mitsuda tried to negotiate with the protesters, some responded by throwing their wooden clogs at him. Police and officials soon began to arrive on the island, local police officers first, followed by the chief of the Okayama Prefectural Police Bureau, a member of the Special Higher Police, representatives of the Home Ministry, and even Murata Masataka, who was brought in to negotiate with the former Sotojima residents who had joined the protest.

All indications are that the police took an evenhanded approach, listening to the concerns of the patient representatives and treating the protest as within the limits of the law.[32] The representative of the Special Higher Police, a man named Horibe, played a particularly important role by acting as a mediator between the members of the patients' executive committee and Mitsuda.[33] The members of the executive committee, organized to coordinate the protest, had all held influential positions before it began, as members of the Council of Residence Heads or as the leaders of various work teams. Eighteen of the nineteen men (all of whom Mitsuda would subsequently accuse of "thought crimes") were between the ages of twenty-five and thirty-nine, and most had entered Aiseien after 1933. Thus, they had been fully enfranchised citizens before they entered the sanitarium. The petition they addressed to Home Minister Ushio Shigenosuke made it clear that while they resented the label of "pathetic cripples," their complaint was not with the policy of confinement itself. Rather, they wanted the sanitarium to live up to its own promises, and they held Mitsuda responsible for the poor conditions at Aiseien. In their words, he "goes about trying to make a name for himself while ignoring our human needs."[34] Whatever the politics of those involved in the protest, their target was not the Japanese state but Mitsuda.

Over the course of the sixteen days of the protest, Horibe met repeatedly with the members of the executive committee and Mitsuda. The process of the negotiations was carefully chronicled in the newspapers of western Japan, including the *Ōsaka mainichi shinbun*, *Ōsaka asahi shinbun*, *Chūgoku minpō*, and *San'yō minpō*. A report published in the *Ōsaka asahi* quoted Horibe's praise for the protest's leaders: "The attitude of the representatives is calm and very serious and [the negotiations] have a friendly atmosphere." Several reports contrasted Murata's stance on self-government with Mitsuda's approach, with one headline declaring, "Self-Government or Familyism? Leprosy Relief Is at a Crossroad." The *Ōsaka mainichi* published a carefully composed letter by Kimoto Iwao, one member of the executive committee, who suggested that patients were advocating for something between the approaches of Murata and Mitsuda. In his view, both were problematic. The self-government system at Soto-jima had failed "to control patients," while Mitsuda's familyism had treated the patients' quite reasonable frustration as akin to a toddler's tantrum. According to Kimoto, what patients were seeking—"self-government under the protective supervision of the sanitarium director"—was not in any way subversive.[35]

As the days dragged on, the executive committee tried another desperate strategy, declaring a hunger strike for all but the sickest patients. But gradually support for the protest began to wane. After the Home Ministry agreed to increase funding to cover the excess number of patients, some felt that continuing to protest in the face of this concession would lead to a backlash.[36] They had reason to be worried. The *Asahi shinbun* reported that those it termed "red elements" and "the extreme left" were leading the protest and that the Home Ministry had decided to "suppress" it.[37] A few days later, the staff of the sanitarium issued their own joint declaration, charging that the protest was "a plot by a group of patients who hold left-leaning ideas and should not be considered a part of our national polity."[38] On the twenty-third, a majority of the patients (984 to 42) voted to abandon their demand for the resignation of Mitsuda and the other staff.

The only remaining point of contention on the table was the issue of self-government, and Horibe, the Special Police officer, and Murata, the disgraced former director, became unlikely allies. Both urged Mitsuda to accept a greater level of patient involvement in the administration of Aiseien.[39] With working systems of self-government in place in other sanitaria and the failure of familyism evident, Mitsuda had little option but to agree. The executive committee, too, had to compromise. It had initially demanded control of thirty different aspects of sanitarium life, including a role in staffing, educational policy, food, wages, and other issues that were central to patient life, but the Home Ministry refused, arguing that it could not hand over authority over matters involving government funds (*kokuhi*). In the end, patients settled for the right to manage the sanitarium store and some forms of sanitarium labor.[40]

The Special Hospital Ward

The Nagashima Incident sent shock waves through Japanese society. An editorial in the *Ōsaka mainichi* summed up the reaction of many: "We happily imagined that the leprosy sanitarium was a separate world free of the concerns of mundane life, where the staff and patients united by love and gratitude enjoyed a peaceful life, and so it is difficult to learn of a general strike, a hunger strike, and other kinds of disturbing violence."[41] Although the course of negotiations and its outcome seemed to imply a recognition of the patients' rights and political agency, in the aftermath of the incident sanitarium directors and Home Ministry officials worked to ensure that no similar event would emerge to call into question the ideological work performed by leprosy prevention. Less than two weeks after the end of the protest, the Kansai Branch of the Japan Mission to Lepers convened a roundtable to discuss the events at Nagashima and invited politicians, social welfare advocates, journalists, judges, academics, and public health officials to participate. Much of the discussion centered on the patients who had led the protest. The perspective that now prevailed was that embraced by Mitsuda and his allies, with the result that activist patients were newly cast as gangster-like criminal elements or as left-leaning activists who had terrorized and misled their fellow patients.[42]

Not everyone subscribed to this view. Diet member Kawamura Yasutarō, who had a long history of labor activism, blamed Mitsuda's familyism for the protest, arguing that it was natural for patients to have felt "oppressed" since "as humans" they wanted some degree of freedom within the sanitarium.[43] The most outspoken critic, however, was Miura Sangendō, an editor of the progressive Kyoto-based Buddhist newspaper *Chūgai nippō*. He challenged his fellow panel members, asking, "Why do you want to say that 'reds' are responsible? I don't see how this will help at all to improve the situation at Aiseien."[44] *Chūgai nippō*'s coverage of the protest had been sympathetic to the patients, and a week before this meeting, Miura had written a scathing two-part editorial that had enraged Mitsuda's supporters. He quoted "someone connected to a sanitarium"— presumably, a patient—who reportedly told him, "Those within the sanitaria today don't believe they were established for our benefit; no, rather they were established for the benefit of the healthy general population. In other words, we have sacrificed ourselves and endure the cramped life of the sanitarium for all of you. Therefore, the society and state owe us at the very least treatment that makes it possible to enjoy a satisfactory everyday life." According to Miura, when he heard this statement he immediately recognized the truth of it.[45] At the MTL meeting, he suggested that the Nagashima protest should prompt the public to recognize that the government had failed to adequately provide for those within the sanitaria.

If Miura hoped to provoke a discussion of confinement, patient rights, and state responsibility, he failed miserably. His remarks fell flat at the MTL meeting, and in the weeks that followed, the view that the Nagashima Incident was the fault of the patients quickly coalesced, precluding a real interrogation of what went wrong at Aiseien. As a result, when the directors of the public and national sanitaria met with Bureau of Hygiene officials in Tokyo in October, there was no postmortem of the protest, no discussion of self-government or patients' rights.[46] The cause of the events at Aiseien was treated as a settled question: "bad apples" in the patient population were responsible. The question then was what to do with them.

By the 1930s, all but two of the sanitaria, the Northern Area and Miyakojima institutions, had some kind of facility for disciplining patients who failed to adhere to sanitarium regulations. These differed only slightly in form. For example, Zensei Hospital had three very small rooms for solitary confinement and three rooms that could house multiple patients, while

Aiseien had five rooms for solitary confinement and three larger rooms.[47] To this point, the breaking of sanitarium rules was still treated as bad behavior rather than a criminal act. Under the regulations approved by the Diet in 1916, sanitarium directors had been allowed to confine a patient to the sanitarium jail for a period of no more than thirty days. In 1931, the Diet extended the period of confinement to up to two months. In fact, however, there were few instances of serious crime in the sanitaria. At Aiseien, even in 1935 as conditions worsened dramatically, only twenty-three patients were placed in detention, nine of them for attempting to escape. The others were punished for acts such as vandalism, gambling, theft, smuggling, and "corruption of public morality."[48] However, after the Nagashima Incident, sanitarium directors were quick to conclude that their patient populations included criminals for whom harsher punishments were necessary.

An important participant in the discussions at the October meeting was Suwa Masasue, who headed the colonial sanitarium in Korea. Located on Sorokdo Island (J. Shōrokutō), it was known as Kōseien (literally "Rebirth Sanitarium"). The confinement of leprosy sufferers on Sorokdo dated from 1916, when the colonial government had established a small sanitarium there with a capacity of one hundred patients. Leprosy policy in Korea at the time was modeled on Japan's 1907 law and required the confinement only of indigent sufferers of the disease. In 1934, however, the governor-general had promulgated the Leprosy Prevention Act, which, like the 1931 law in Japan, authorized the confinement of any leprosy sufferer who posed a danger to public health. Japan's other colony, Taiwan, too, had a leprosy sanitarium. In December 1930, the colonial government had established Rakuseien (Ch. Losheng; literally "Happy Life Sanitarium") outside of Taipei. It too was intended to house indigent people with leprosy and had a capacity of only one hundred patients.[49]

Suwa's involvement in the post–Nagashima Incident meeting of sanitarium directors reflects more than just the aim of integrating the metropolitan and colonial institutions. He had a dual role on Sorokdo; he was director not only of Kōseien but also of a prison that stood adjacent to it. The latter housed not only leprosy sufferers who had committed crimes while unconfined but also patients who had violated sanitarium rules. In other words, in this institution the distinction between "delinquency" and "criminality" was effectively erased. In his remarks at the meeting, Suwa described the relationship of these two institutions, but he also noted that "[the colony] is different from the metropole (*naichi*)," implying that citizens of Japan could not be treated in the same manner as colonial subjects. His metropolitan colleagues did not share his scruples. In the wake of the

Nagashima Incident, patients who did not comply with sanitarium rules were newly described as "political patients" (*shisō kanja*), a term that implied they had committed "thought crimes" (*shisōhan*).[50]

Over the course of two days, those at the 1936 meeting debated the pros and cons of the "Sorokdo solution." Not everyone was convinced that a separate prison for leprosy patients was the answer. Alternatives discussed included a "special sanitarium" for problem patients on an isolated island, an idea that had been considered since the 1920s, and some kind of detention center that would have stricter rules and fewer amenities than a sanitarium. There was also considerable disagreement over the necessary capacity of any such a facility: the director of the Ōshima Sanitarium proposed fifty people; the director of Rakusen'en, one hundred. Mitsuda suggested it should be able to house three hundred, since "just because you have leprosy doesn't mean you don't commit crimes."[51] Significantly, in this debate, there was no consideration of the legality or ethicality of treating patients as criminals or of giving sanitarium directors the authority to act as both prosecutor and judge. In the end, the Sorokdo approach of adjacent institutions was adopted.

The turn towards a colonial institution for a solution to a metropolitan problem suggests how much ideas about leprosy had changed over the course of less than a decade. Mitsuda and his colleagues had sought to build a sanitarium that would be a model for the rest of the world, one that would demonstrate Japan's progressive approach to its stricken citizens. In keeping with this vision, the first patients of Aiseien had been celebrated as "colonizers" whose achievements were part and parcel of Japan's national and imperial projects. But by the late 1930s, public health authorities had begun to regard sanitarium patients as potentially dangerous others who had to be controlled and contained. Adding to the sad irony of this outcome was the location of what became known as the Special Hospital Ward (Tokubetsu Byōshitsu), the institution to which "criminal" patients could be transferred at the discretion of a sanitarium director, without recourse to due process. Constructed on the grounds of Rakusen'en, it stood not far from the free convalescent zone, where patients were promised a normal life.

For the nine years of its existence (1938–1947), the Special Hospital Ward was shrouded in secrecy. Few records were kept, and only a handful of patients and staff at Rakusen'en ever had access to it. In 2013, however, the site of this facility was excavated and the former prison gradually gave up its secrets. The Special Hospital Ward was a peculiar institution, one that bore little resemblance to other penal facilities in Japan, and the "hospital" in its name notwithstanding, it was in no sense oriented by medical concerns. It consisted of eight isolation cells, which were separated from each other by multiple walls to ensure that escape was impossible and that patients would have no contact with one another (figure 7.1). The windowless cells themselves were only about 14.8 square meters in area, unheated in a region where winter temperatures could reach twenty degrees below zero Celsius and heavy snowfall is common. Meager meals of rice and pickles were provided through a small opening in the cell door, and provisions for sanitation consisted of a bucket in a corner.

Over the course of its existence, at least ninety-three patients were confined in the ward, twenty-three of whom died in custody. The most common "crimes" cited in available records were morphine addiction, gambling, theft, and attempting to run away, but some patients were removed out of concern that they were troublemakers. Ten percent of those confined were former members of the community at Honmyōji Temple in Kumamoto, who were jailed because they were regarded as "leaders"

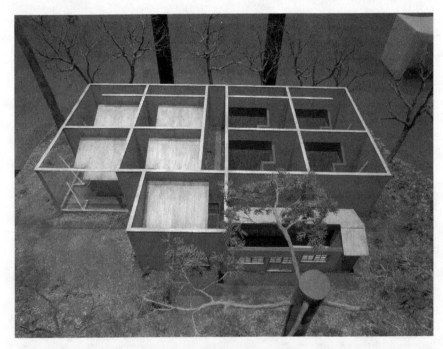

FIGURE 7.1. Model of the Special Hospital Ward on display at the Jyu-kanbo National Museum of Detention for Hansen's Disease (Kusatsu, Gunma Prefecture). Photograph by the author.

(*yakunin*) of a group that had refused voluntary confinement; the surnames of another 10 percent suggest that they were ethnic Koreans. One man was confined because he was mentally ill; one woman was confined because her husband was labeled disruptive after he refused to work.[52]

Most of the documented transfers to the Special Hospital Ward took place between 1940 and 1942, as Japanese society was mobilized for total war. The denial of basic civil rights to sanitarium patients reflected the larger transformation of Japanese society in this period, as the government came under the control of militarists and their allies acting in the name of the emperor. In this period the limited forms of self-government in place in the sanitaria came to an end as well. In 1941, for example, the patients at Aiseien voted to end the forms of self-government for which they had fought so hard only five years before. The announcement that followed this decision described self-government as "inappropriate for these times" and declared the intention of the patients "for the good of the nation as a whole" to follow the orders of their director.[53]

From Volition to Coercion

The authoritarian turn that led to the founding of the Special Hospital Ward also propelled the rapid expansion of the sanitarium system in the late 1930s. New national sanitaria were established in Miyagi (1937) and Okinawa (1938), and the zone three sanitarium that had once stood at Sotojima was reconstructed on an undeveloped part of Nagashima and renamed Kōmyōen in honor of the Kōmyō empress. Then in 1941, the five public institutions were nationalized, bringing them under central control for the first time and ending the era of autonomy and experimentation once and for all. Institution building continued even as the war progressed. In 1943 a sanitarium was established on one of the Amami Islands that lies between Okinawa and Kyūshū. Japan's national sanitarium system was completed in December 1944, less than a year before the surrender, when the final sanitarium was established in Suruga at the foot of Mount Fuji. Its mission was to house soldiers who were diagnosed with leprosy during their military service.

As the sanitarium system expanded, the ethos of voluntary admission began to give way to a new willingness to coercively confine people with leprosy who remained outside the sanitarium. The turning point was 1940. In July of that year, prefectural officials, elaborately clothed in what would now be termed hazmat suits, swept into the slum adjacent to Honmyōji Temple and began to remove the leprosy sufferers who still lived there.

In the end 157 people were divided among sanitaria around the country, an approach taken out of concern that the Honmyōji group might form a powerful and dangerous clique if placed within any single institution.[54]

The following year the transfer of Yunosawa residents got under way, bringing an end to the celebrated community that had endured for sixty years. Unlike those at Honmyōji, who were confined as a danger to public health, the residents of Yunosawa required different handling. They were property owners who were already living in a segregated community, making it difficult to simply force them into confinement. In the end, the dismantlement of Yunosawa was facilitated by the decision on the part of its trustees to close the St. Barnabas Mission. Over the years, the mission's financial situation had grown increasingly precarious. Cornwallis-Legh, by this time elderly and in poor health, had retired in 1939, and international support for her mission had declined as criticism of Japan had grown. Without the safety net of St. Barnabas's services, poorer residents had little choice but to accept transfer to Rakusen'en, and under pressure from local authorities, those of means agreed to cooperate with what was described as the "peaceful and orderly" dissolution of the community, which required them to sell off their property. In total, 350 people left Yunosawa for Rakusen'en: seventy-five took up residence in the free zone, while the remainder entered the sanitarium proper.[55]

St. Barnabas was not the only missionary sanitarium to encounter hard times as the war progressed. Donations, the lifeblood of these institutions, declined dramatically as tensions between Japan and the United States and Britain increased. At the same time, the foreign nationals and Japanese Christians who ran the institutions were subjected to growing degrees of police surveillance and harassment. Jingo Tobimatsu, the Japanese administrator of Kaishun Hospital, spent three months in police detention in 1940. Under economic and political pressure, the hospital closed on February 3, 1941, and its patients were transferred to the Kumamoto sanitarium, now known as Keifūen.[56] Ihaien survived until August 1942, when its patients were transferred to Zenshōen, as Zensei Hospital had been renamed when it was nationalized. The Catholic institutions fared a bit better. Fukusei Hospital continued to operate during the war years, although in much diminished form. At the end of the 1930s, it housed 150 patients, but five years later the patient population was less than half that number, an attrition that reflected not only a policy of reducing patient numbers but also an increasing number of patient deaths due to lack of food and medicines. Tairōin in Kumamoto, too, managed to hang on. In 1941, the ten European nuns who worked at the institution were transferred to a camp for enemy aliens, but their Japanese counterparts persevered through the end of the war.[57]

The nationalization of the public sanitaria and dissolution of many of the missionary institutions were part of a larger government effort to centralize its control over the public health administration as part of war-time mobilization. In 1938, the government created a new ministry, the Ministry of Health and Welfare (Kōseisho), with the aim of centralizing the health and social welfare administrations. The new ministry absorbed the responsibilities of the Home Ministry's Bureau of Hygiene and took control of physical education and school hygiene from the Ministry of Education. The intent of the reorganization was to improve the health of the citizenry overall, but especially that of potential conscripts, who would be needed to fight an extended war.

It was under the new ministry that a new and aggressive policy to-wards tuberculosis was adopted, driven by the discovery of high rates of the disease among conscripts. In 1939, the ministry established a Tuberculosis Section, which spearheaded efforts at prevention, early detection, and treatment. Innovative new policies included mass screenings using tuberculin tests and X-rays, government funding for improvements to housing, and the establishment of a system of health centers (*hokenjo*) to treat people in the early stages of the disease. In addition, new sanitaria were established for those whose conditions were more advanced and for soldiers infected with the disease. In 1943, these efforts were supplemented by a new policy of mass inoculation with the BCG vaccine.[58]

These developments stand in sharp contrast to policy towards leprosy, which saw few if any changes, in part because, unlike for tuberculosis, there were no breakthroughs in screening, treatment, or prevention. Indeed, as the war continued, conditions within the sanitaria worsened. Like the rest of the civilian population, patients in the sanitaria suffered from a lack of food, medicines, clothing, and other basic commodities. At Aiseien, all available land was given over to agriculture in order to supplement the insufficient supply of rationed foods, and patients were forced to reduce the number of pigs they were raising. In these straitened times, there was no food for livestock. According to the *Aiseien Annual Report* for 1945, patients were receiving only about fourteen hundred calories per day. Under these conditions, the health of many patients declined dramatically.[59] Between 1931 and 1937, patient deaths averaged about 5.3 percent of the total population per year. In contrast, in 1945, the death rate was 22 percent.

In these conditions, some desperate patients chose to escape rather than await death in confinement. Between 1942 and 1945, more than four hundred patients fled Aiseien.[60]

Reproductive Policy in the Wartime Sanitaria

The intense concern for promoting the health of the citizenry in the late 1930s also emboldened proponents of eugenics, who had been gaining influence since the 1910s. In 1935, Aragawa Gorō and Ikeda Hideo, two members of the Constitutional Democratic Party, jointly sponsored a eugenics law in the lower house, the first attempt to write eugenic theory into statute. Known as the Racial Eugenics Protection Law, it would have legalized the compulsory sterilization of those suffering not only from hereditary disorders but also from infectious diseases such as leprosy, syphilis, and tuberculosis, as well as alcoholics and some criminals. The bill went nowhere, nor did a second draft law, submitted in 1936, which would have legalized the sterilization of the mentally ill, violent criminals, alcoholics, and leprosy sufferers, with their consent or that of their families.

Following a wave of criticism about the intended use of sterilization for nonhereditary conditions, another draft law limited its use to those who suffered from hereditary forms of mental illness, blindness, and physical deformities, but criticism continued. Some opposed the bill on an ideological basis, arguing that legalized sterilization was antithetical to the Japanese family-state and to the widely publicized reproductive ideology of "give birth and multiply"; others, from the position of science, noted that there was no evidence that such measures would actually improve the genetic pool or that the diseases in question were truly hereditary. As a result, the National Eugenics Law that finally passed in 1940 was stripped of many of the earlier provisions. It allowed for sterilization only in cases of hereditary mental disease and effectively only with the consent of the patient or his or her legal guardian.[61]

As the debate over a eugenics law was unfolding, the use of vasectomy continued within the sanitaria. In 1936, just months before the protests at Aiseien began, an article by Mitsuda appeared in the sanitarium's house journal, *Aisei*. Entitled "Twenty Years of Vasectomy," it celebrated the use of vasectomy in the sanitaria. The first patients to receive the procedure were "now men of 40 or 50, in middle-age, and the fact that they are even now healthy and active shows that [vasectomy] is the secret key to allowing the world's leprosy patients of both sexes to live together and flourish together."[62]

Mitsuda was not the only one writing on vasectomy in this period. Between 1936 and 1942, at least seven reports on the use of vasectomy on leprosy patients were published in Japanese medical journals, evidence of the new interest in verifying the effectiveness and safety of this method of sterilization. Typical of these was the study published by Tamamura Kōzō and Yajima Ryōichi, two doctors on the staff of Rakusen'en, in a public health journal in 1942. They reported on the outcome of 140 surgeries they performed between 1935 and 1941, most on patients of the sanitarium, although five men from Yunosawa were also among their patients. The presence of the Yunosawa residents is significant. Since they were not under the authority of the sanitarium, the procedure could only have been performed at their request. Tamamura and Yajima stressed that in the sanitarium, too, vasectomy was only performed when men requested it, out of concern for the effects of pregnancy on their partner or because they "did not think they could bear the psychological burdens that would follow a birth." They noted that the number of men seeking out the operation had increased gradually over the years, that there were no significant side effects, and that "most patients were pleased with the outcome because their anxiety was lessened."[63]

This rosy picture of the use of sterilization in the sanitarium stands in sharp contrast to recent scholarly work and public discourse on the sanitaria in which no issue looms larger than the claim that male patients were routinely, coercively, and unnecessarily sterilized, while women who became pregnant were forced to undergo abortions, sometimes in the final months of their pregnancies. Fujino Yutaka has likened the use of vasectomy in the sanitaria to the Nazi policy of sterilization and made it a powerful symbol of the Japanese fascist state, as he characterizes the prewar and wartime governments. He paints a horrific picture of reproductive policy towards leprosy patients in this period: physicians and their untrained surrogates performed medical procedures on unwilling patients with no regard for their rights, dignity, or well-being and adversely affected their physical and mental health.[64]

The situation was more complicated than the position of either complete volition or complete coercion allows. Even after the passage of the National Eugenics Law, there were those who continued to believe that people with leprosy should not be allowed to reproduce. Diet member Yoshida Shigeru (a bureaucrat turned politician, not the famous diplomat) introduced a revision to the Leprosy Prevention Law that would have made the sterilization of leprosy sufferers and the use of abortion to terminate pregnancies compulsory. He argued that although leprosy is not hereditary, it is "a disease of a special nature," a reference to the long-standing theory that some people were more susceptible to infection than others.[65] In his 1936 article on vasectomy, Mitsuda had offered up his own theory on susceptibility. He argued that the testicles were "favored by" *M. leprae*, which reproduced rapidly within them and damaged the sperm they produced. A pregnancy that resulted from "diseased sperm" (*byōteki seieki*) produced a "weak fetus" and one that would then be susceptible to infection.[66] This claim is baseless. While leprosy can affect the testicles, causing low sperm counts and weak sperm motility, thus compromising fertility, it does not produce "diseased sperm." To be sure, Mitsuda was not the only physician speculating about susceptibility in these years. In the 1930s it was widely theorized that individual physiology, a history of beriberi or rickets, or some other factor might be involved in determining who, among those exposed, would actually be infected.[67]

The members of the lower house committee to which Yoshida presented this proposal were not receptive, even though all concerned acknowledged that vasectomy was routinely used within the sanitaria. Takano Rokurō, the official who had overseen the *Confessions* project two decades before, reminded Diet members, "As you know, in cases of leprosy sterilization has been going on for a long time," noting that it took place on a voluntary basis among patients who "strongly wished to live together as couples without having children." Tanaka Yōtatsu, an obstetrician who operated a lying-in hospital in Shiga Prefecture, was the most outspoken critic of the proposed revision. He noted that the government had spent considerable energy trying to educate the populace that the disease was, in fact, infectious. To legalize sterilization would "profoundly contradict" that stance and encourage the problematic view that leprosy was hereditary in nature, thus contributing to the stigma of the disease, which continued to burden families. Another member of the committee agreed: hadn't they taken great pains to delimit the new eugenics law to only hereditary diseases? To revise the leprosy law in this way would undermine these efforts. Still another member pointed out that research on leprosy was ongoing and that sufferers who might yet be cured should not be sterilized against their will.[68]

In the end, the attempted revision of the Leprosy Prevention Law was abandoned. But the apparent consensus among the Diet members—that sterilization and abortion on a consensual basis posed no issue—left unexamined the crucial question of the status of "consent" in the context of the sanitaria. As with other issues of policy, the sanitaria took different approaches to reproductive issues. At Amami Wakōen, neither sterilization nor abortion was used, apparently because a significant number of patients and staff were Roman Catholics. There is anecdotal evidence that some patients at other sanitaria who became pregnant and wished to have the child requested transfer to Wakōen. In other cases, women who became pregnant were either released from the sanitarium or after delivery were required to turn the child over to family members or to sanitarium nurseries.[69]

Although the sanitarium doctors insisted that consent was the rule, a small number of documentary sources and a larger body of patient testimony suggest that the sanitarium actively sought to encourage sterilization, most often by requiring men who wished to marry or live with a female partner to undergo vasectomy. A file of records related to the "housing of married couples" preserved at Aiseien includes requests from patients for shared accommodation in which a staff person had noted whether the male partner had undergone sterilization.[70] Pointing to this kind of evidence, Fujino and others have argued that coerced sterilization and abortion were the norm within the sanitaria.

This was the position that guided the research undertaken by the Japan Law Federation (Nichibenren Hōmu Kenkyū Zaidan; JLF) in the aftermath of the Kumamoto suit, during which patients had offered vivid testimony of forced abortion and sterilization. In 2004, the JLF surveyed Japan's former leprosy sufferers, seeking to gain information about "the real damage" caused by Japan's leprosy policy to be used in negotiating reparations with the government. "Eugenics policy," the term applied to reproductive issues, was one of the nine topics of the survey. Others included the circumstances of admission to a sanitarium, relations with family members, treatment, work, daily life, and punishment within the sanitaria. The 3,566 people who still resided in national sanitaria were invited to participate, and roughly a fifth (758) responded. In relation to reproduction, participants were asked whether they had had a child while in a sanitarium. Those who replied negatively (95 percent of those interviewed) were then asked to explain their decision by choosing from the following options: (1) did not marry within the sanitarium (23 percent); (2) due to vasectomy, abortion, or (female) sterilization (49 percent); (3) failed to conceive (8.8 percent); (4) avoided because of Hansen's disease (8.8 percent); (5) other (12.5 percent).[71] (Percentages have been rounded.) What is significant here is that patients were not asked to explicitly comment on whether they had consented to "vasectomy, abortion, or sterilization." The unspoken assumption was that these procedures could only have been coerced.

But the supplemental statements offered by the patients who participated in the survey suggest that they understood reproductive decisions in terms different from the assumption of coercion that underlay the survey.

According to a female patient who entered a sanitarium in 1938, "In the first place, it was a mistake for patients who married to have children. We were in a sanitarium. I thought it was the proper thing for the husband to have a vasectomy when patients married here." A man who entered a sanitarium in 1944 responded, "After my wife fell pregnant, I had a vasectomy and she had an abortion. At the time we did this because we consented. It was all we could do to manage our own lives and we didn't feel confident about raising a child. . . . I don't think the sanitarium is to blame. And I don't feel that I was coerced." A woman who entered a sanitarium in 1939 related, "Vasectomy was required in order to marry. I thought that was reasonable. And I personally didn't feel that I wanted to have a child. I was worried that I would infect a child, and I would never want my child to experience the pain that I have suffered." A male patient who had a vasectomy stated, "I was infected by my mother and I thought that I would not want to infect my own child. My wife felt the same."[72]

Interviews carried out by Yamamoto Sumiko and Katō Naoko between 2002 and 2006 at Keiaien in Kagoshima provide further evidence that the binary of coercion/volition does not capture the complex interplay between institutional power and intensely personal concerns that led to a decision to accept or refuse sterilization or abortion. Their work focused primarily on female patients, and in contrast to the survey method adopted by the Japan Law Federation, they took an ethnographic approach, interviewing a small group of women over a four-year period. According to Yamamoto and Katō, only two of their nine primary informants characterized the sterilization of their husbands or the use of abortion as the result of coercion. The others described the fact that they had not had a child as "unavoidable" (shikata ga nai), given their illness, the constraints of sanitarium life, and anxiety over transmitting the disease.[73] One woman, when asked if she had wanted a child, replied, "Well, of course, my illness was very advanced. Ordinary healthy people, I'm sure they want children. But in our case there was the rule that you absolutely shouldn't have them, and so we didn't really think about having them. To want to have a child, that was something we couldn't aspire to, and so I didn't want one."[74]

This statement, like those of the patients interviewed by Japan Law Federation researchers, provides evidence of how sanitarium regulations mediated patients' reproductive choices by valorizing the decision *not* to reproduce as normative and ethical. Given that the reproductive ideology of the 1930s encouraged Japanese citizens to think of procreation as both a civic and a familial obligation, one that sustained the family-state and the expanding empire, it might be argued that denial of the right to procreate became, in effect, yet another means of denying leprosy patients a place in the civil society. But patient writing from the wartime years defies such a facile interpretation by offering a window into the hope, guilt, and shame that accompanied the decision to have a child.

A case in point is a story called "The Leprous Family" (Rai Kazoku) by Hōjō Tamio, the best-known author of "leprosy literature." Published not long after "The First Night of My Life," the work that established Hōjō's reputation, "The Leprous Family" explores the tensions between a man and his adult children. We gradually learn that although the father in question was already showing signs of leprosy at the time of his marriage, he chose first to ignore his symptoms and later to conceal them from his wife, and the couple went on to have three children, two sons and a daughter. The man's disease continued to progress, however, and it later became apparent that his daughter, by this time in her teens, had also developed the disease. Father and daughter entered the sanitarium together and for a time all seemed well. But then it became apparent that the eldest son was infected as well, and he, too, entered the sanitarium, where his condition worsened rapidly. Confined to a hospital bed, the son is bitter and sullen and blames his father for deceiving his mother into marriage and ruining the lives of his sister and himself. Into this complicated situation a letter arrives that relates that the youngest child of the family, too, has been diagnosed with leprosy and will soon be arriving at the sanitarium. The story ends with the father overcome by guilt and regret as he contemplates the ruin of the family for which he had longed.[75]

If "The Leprous Family" explores the complicated emotions that resulted from intrafamilial infection, another story by Hōjō, "Conception in the Leprosarium," offers a window into why patients might choose to risk a pregnancy.[76] At the center of the story is a female patient who discovers she is pregnant by her lover, a young man who is in the early stages of the disease and who longs to escape the sanitarium. The story unfolds as those around her contemplate whether she should terminate the pregnancy. Her brother, a patient whose disease is advanced, at first suggests she should have an abortion. He speculates that the blood of their old and distinguished family has grown "weak" and "muddy" and thus susceptible to infection. Her lover, who can't bear the thought of bringing a child into the confined world of the sanitarium, hangs himself, leaving the decision of whether to continue the pregnancy to the woman. Meanwhile, a mutual friend of all three is alternately disgusted and fascinated by the idea that love, sex, and

desire are possible for those whose bodies are slowly being consumed by
the disease. In the end, the brother has a change of heart. He tells her she
must have the baby and give it their family's surname.

Both stories suggest that for patients, reproductive decisions were not
simply or even primarily about compliance with or resistance to sanitarium
policy. The decision to accept sterilization, to abort, or to continue a pregnancy required patients to reconcile their desire for children, informed as
it was by socially prescribed ideas of marriage and family, with the reality
of life constrained not only by the sanitarium but also by a chronic and disabling disease. Hōjō's work is important for another reason as well: it alerts
us to how reproduction in the sanitarium—in the 1930s, no less than the
present—has largely been framed as an issue of male reproductive rights.
In the "Leprous Family," the husband's desire for a family led him to ignore
the interests of both his wife and his future children, and in "Conception in
the Leprosarium," it is the male gaze on the pregnant woman's body that
drives the story. Ironically, then, Fujino's outrage at the use of sterilization
in the sanitarium reflects the reproductive ideology of the very state he
seeks to critique, one that could conceive only of procreative sex, one that
privileged male sexual and procreative desires over women's health.

By the end of the 1930s, the sanitaria had been transformed, but this went
largely unnoticed and unexamined by the public. Perhaps the best evidence
of the continuing embrace of the sanitarium system by the Japanese people
is the immense popularity of the film adaptation of Ogawa Masako's *Spring
on a Small Island*, which was released in 1940. Directed by Toyada Shirō,
who adopted a faux documentary style, it featured the popular actress
Natsugawa Shizue as Ogawa. Filmed as though perpetually bathed in light,
she is depicted sympathetically as she works with local officials and police
to convince leprosy sufferers to enter a sanitarium. The film ends as one
unwilling patient finally agrees to leave his home. Although the patient
and his family have been ostracized by their neighbors and his young son
bullied, now the whole village turns out to see him off in a show of public
support that seemingly excuses their behavior to this point.

The film adaptation of *Spring on a Small Island* made the sanitarium
an emblem of national unity, but like so much of wartime propaganda it
concealed a darker reality. In the context of a growing sense of "national
emergency," patient activism came to be viewed as a threat to the order
and security not only of the sanitaria but also of the nation-state itself.
Mitsuda's familyism sought to make the sanitaria an emblem of the imperial
family-state, but it was challenged by patients who accepted confinement

but wanted some measure of independence and a role in shaping the institutions that were their homes. Thus, the patient protests at Aiseien, while successful in the short run, ultimately propelled a new stage in Japan's leprosy policy, bringing an end to the reliance on voluntary confinement and giving rise to a new willingness to treat problematic patients as criminals rather than citizens. While leprosy policy evolved in relation to the formation of the wartime state, I disagree with attempts to draw simplistic parallels with the eugenics policy of Nazi Germany. The final section of the chapter argued that while the sanitarium policy of promoting sterilization undeniably came to mediate the sexual and procreative lives of patients, for some it offered the possibility of reproductive choice, an option denied those outside the institutions.

Chapter 8

Leprosy in Postwar Japan

Biological Citizenship and Democratization

In July and August 1953, an unprecedented series of events unfolded in Nagatachō, the area of central Tokyo where the National Diet, the government ministries, and the headquarters of the various political parties are located. On July 2 a group of about 50 leprosy patients gathered in front of one of the entrances to the Diet building. They had come to protest a draft bill revising the 1931 Leprosy Prevention Law that included none of the changes patients had requested through the recently organized National Conference of Sanitarium Patients (NCSP, later renamed as the National Council of Sanitarium Residents). Within a few days, the number of protesters swelled to more than 150. In the sanitaria, too, patients expressed their outrage by organizing hunger strikes and work stoppages. For the next week, the group in Nagatachō remained in place, sheltering in tents and holding up signs inscribed with slogans such as "Don't Treat Leprosy Patients as Prisoners!" and "Freedom and Human Rights for Leprosy Patients!" All the while, representatives of the Ministry of Health and Welfare and the Tokyo metropolitan government pleaded with them to return to the sanitarium. They finally agreed, but only after members of the Health and Welfare Committee of the lower house publicly announced that they would give careful consideration to the patients' demands. So it was with a sense of betrayal that the patients learned a few weeks later that the bill sent to the upper house was unchanged. In protest, patients descended again upon central Tokyo.[1]

The new forms of patient organization and activism that fueled these protests and others were part of a concerted effort by patients to renegotiate their place in the body politic in the wake of Japan's defeat in 1945 and the occupation-led program of "democratization." As we have noted, patient protests had long involved attempts to engage directly with the government, but it was only with the formation of the NCSP in 1951 that they were able to lay claim to a unified voice. By this time, Promin, the sulfone drug that proved effective in treating leprosy, was in use in all of the national sanitaria, and some patients had already been released. Nonetheless, in the struggle over the revision of Japan's leprosy policy, neither patients nor those in government called for the dissolution of the sanitaria. Rather, the question was what form they should take given the rights and protections guaranteed to all citizens under the 1947 constitution and the fact that leprosy was now a treatable disease. This chapter explores the preservation of the sanitarium system in spite of these new developments and the transformation of "patients" into "residents" that resulted.

Occupation-Era Reforms and the Sanitaria

By the time of Japan's surrender in 1945, the national sanitaria had been stressed to the breaking point. The two institutions in Okinawa had suffered damage during the US invasion, and Wakōen on Amami had been all but destroyed by US bombing in 1944.[2] Even institutions that escaped the direct effects of warfare struggled to deal with the profound shortages of food, medicine, and fuel that shaped life on the home front. With Japan's defeat, SCAP (as the occupation administration headed by General Douglas MacArthur was known) assumed direct control of the two sanitaria in Okinawa and Amami Wakōen, while the others remained under the control of the Ministry of Health and Welfare (MHW), now newly accountable to SCAP's Public Health and Welfare Administrative Section.[3]

SCAP targeted Japan's constitution, educational system, economy, military, and mass media for reform, but for the most part it found little fault with its approach to public health, and officials consistently affirmed both the policy of leprosy prevention and the management of the sanitaria. A civilian physician on the staff of SCAP who visited Ōshima in 1947 reported that "the institution was well equipped with laboratory material and laboratory facilities" and that "the social welfare of the people is cared for quite adequately." Two years later, a staff officer visited both Ōshima and Nagashima, and he, too, submitted a positive report, describing Ōshima as "well operated" and Nagashima as "unusually well operated."[4] Brigadier General Crawford Sams, who headed up the military's medical unit, noted approvingly in 1950 that the ministry planned to expand the sanitarium system by two thousand beds.[5] Perhaps the best indication of SCAP's endorsement of Japan's leprosy policy is that it initially emulated it; in 1947 the US military announced the policy of required quarantine for all leprosy sufferers on the Amami Islands.[6] It was not until the 1960s that the US military began to establish outpatient clinics in Okinawa, control of which reverted to Japan only in 1972.

Although SCAP made no direct efforts to reform Japan's approach to leprosy prevention, the policies it sponsored soon had an impact nonetheless. In 1946, in response to SCAP prompting, the Diet passed the Livelihood Protection Law (Seikatsu Hogohō), which guaranteed a minimum standard of living for those who found themselves on the edge of poverty after the surrender. As a result, sanitarium residents began to receive monthly payments of 150 yen in 1947, a small amount but one that vastly improved the situation of patients, especially those who were too infirm to work. Important for those outside the sanitaria was the passage in 1947 of a new public health law, also at the urging of SCAP. The establishment of the MHW in 1938 had removed the medical and public health administration from the Home Ministry, but enforcement had remained in the hands of the police. The 1947 law ended police involvement in public health matters and put local governments in charge of public health centers.[7]

By any measure, it was the political reforms championed by SCAP that had the most immediate impact upon the sanitaria. In December 1945, the Diet passed a bill extending the right to vote to women and lowering the voting age to twenty. Subsequent legislation brought an end to the denial of the vote to recipients of aid. In some sanitaria, polling booths were established as early as the 1946 elections for the lower house.[8] The revival of the left-leaning political parties was important as well. Organizers associated with the Japanese Communist Party soon reached out to patient activists at several sanitaria. But nothing was as significant as the promulgation of the 1947 constitution in prompting many patients to begin to reconceptualize their relationship with the Japanese state. The new guarantees of "life, liberty, and the pursuit of happiness," public education, due process, and a minimum standard of living defined citizenship in terms of "rights" rather than obligations to the state for the first time. In light of this, aspects of sanitarium life that had long been the object of criticism—the disciplinary power bestowed upon the directors, low wages for sanitarium work, lack of provisions for education, and restrictions on patients' movement—were now defined as infringements on patients' civil rights. In the words of the authors of one sanitarium history, in the postwar era "in the sanitaria too, political consciousness grew rapidly."[9]

The first indications of this new political consciousness were efforts to revive the patient self-government organizations, most of which had been suspended in the early 1940s. At Aiseien, patients held a general election for seats on a patient council in October 1945, although Mitsuda Kensuke refused to recognize the organization for almost two years.[10] In 1947 patients at Zenshōen organized the Alliance for the Protection of Everyday Life (Seikatsu Yōgo Dōmei), which took as its goal "the realization of a system of complete patient self-government." Although Hayashi Yoshinobu, Zenshōen's director, was willing to tolerate a self-government organization that functioned under his direction, as the prewar patient council had done, patients now wanted more. The "complete self-government" they envisioned would leave medical care in the hands of administrators but put all other matters related to patients' daily life in the hands of an elected patient government.[11] At Rakusen'en, a patient council had continued to meet during the war years, but its members were despised by many of their fellow patients as toadies of the sanitarium administration. When elections were held in 1946, a new reform-minded council was voted in.[12]

The revival of the patient councils at these and the other sanitaria was accompanied by a new development. Patient activists began to establish inter-sanitarium organizations that were intended to overcome the considerable insularity (one encouraged by sanitarium directors) of the institution in order to allow patients to speak directly and with a unified voice to bureaucrats and politicians in Tokyo. In July 1947, patients at Keiaien in Kagoshima proposed the formation of a National Alliance of Leprosy Patients for the Support of Everyday Life (Zenkoku Raikanja Seikatsu Yōgo Dōmei) and sent a carefully composed declaration of intent to the patient councils of the other institutions asking them to participate. The declaration, signed by "the patients of Keiaien in unity," denied any affiliation with a specific political party and acknowledged the "love and understanding of the entire nation" for leprosy sufferers but called for "the democratization of the leprosy administration," including the closure of the Special Hospital Ward at Kusatsu and improvements in food, medical care, and wages.[13] The disavowal of radical intent and the appeal to nationalism were strategic. As we saw in chapter 7, since the early 1930s, patient activism within the sanitaria had been viewed with suspicion, and with organizers from the Japanese Communist Party working with patients at some of the sanitaria, there was growing concern on the part of sanitarium administrators that patients were being radicalized.

Although designed to stress the conservative nature of the new organization, the petition was rebuffed by some patients. Nakazuka Kenzō, writing for "the patients of Ōshima Seishōen in unity," refused outright to join the proposed alliance. In his words, "we trust our director completely," and he informed the organizers of the proposed national alliance that all discussion of reforms must include the director.[14] As this suggests, the political cultures of the sanitaria varied greatly in these early years. In contrast to Ōshima, where the patient council was content to acknowledge the authority of the director, those at Rakusen'en, Zenshōen, Keifūen, and Keiaien were dominated by activists who called for "complete self-government," while at Aiseien there continued to be considerable tension between patients who embraced Mitsuda's paternalism and those who did not. Even so, patient-led attempts to establish forms of inter-sanitarium cooperation met with some success. By 1948, three alliances had taken form: patients at the three Seto Inland Sea institutions had come together to form a "conference," those at Rakusen'en and Zenshōen had an ad hoc policy of cooperation, and the patient leaders at the three Kyūshū sanitaria and the two in Tōhoku had created the "Five Sanitaria League."[15]

Patient activists soon developed effective strategies to overcome the constraints on movement and communication that continued to define sanitarium life. Town hall–style meetings that drew large crowds became exercises in direct democracy in these years, and handwritten and mimeographed newsletters were utilized to exchange information both within and among the sanitaria. The sanitarium literary journals, too, became a medium for political expression. The haiku, *waka*, and short stories that had long filled their pages did not disappear completely, but now the journals also included passionate opinion pieces on a range of issues. Patient-authors often addressed each other directly in these works, at times offering cutting refutations of the opinions expressed by others. The new patient political-ity that breached the boundaries of the individual sanitarium also found expression in newly coined terms of affiliation: in newsletters, speeches, essays, and declarations, patients consistently referred to each other as "comrades in sickness" (*byōyū*) and "sanitarium comrades" (*ryōyū*).

The sanitaria were profoundly impacted by another occupation-era reform, one that originated in the Diet rather than with SCAP. In 1948, the postwar Diet passed the Eugenics Protection Law, which replaced the National Eugenics Law of 1940. Drafted by Taniguchi Yasaburō, an ob-stetrician turned politician and upper house member, it revised an earlier bill authored by members of the socialist party in the lower house. The socialists' bill would have legalized contraception, voluntary sterilization, and abortion, but it also included provisions for the compulsory steriliza-tion of some criminals and those with serious mental illnesses. In the words of Tina Lorgren, it was "a strange mixture of progressive humanitarian measures and repressive, retrograde eugenic measures."[16]

Taniguchi's version of the bill excluded several of the "progressive humanitarian measures," including the provisions for promoting contraception and the legalization of abortion and sterilization in cases of financial hardship. In the new bill, abortion was permitted only in instances of rape, genetic disease or disability, or when pregnancy posed a danger to the life of the mother. Moreover, both procedures required not only the consent of the spouse but also that of newly established local Eugenic Protection Committees, made up of doctors and local officials. This bill, too, included provisions for compulsory sterilization in cases of genetic disease or disability. The process outlined required consultation with the spouse, parent, or guardian of the person involved and the approval of prefectural-level Eugenic Protection Committees. Notably, in a bill concerned primarily with hereditary diseases and disabilities, leprosy is mentioned specifically. The provisions for voluntary sterilization and abortion allowed both procedures when either a man or a woman was infected with leprosy and "feared their descendants would be infected."[17]

It has been argued that the passage of this law reflected the survival of prewar notions of racial purity into the postwar era, but Matsubara Yōko has convincingly argued that it was intimately tied to occupation-era concerns. Not only had population swelled as settlers and soldiers returned from Japan's far-flung empire, straining the resources of the devastated country, but there was also a strong sense among many in government that the best of a generation of young men had been lost on the battlefield, leaving only those unfit for service, because of physical or psychological "weakness," alive to procreate. Reflecting this concern, Taniguchi's bill opened by declaring that it was necessary to "prevent the birth of undesirable offspring."[18]

By this time, (male) sterilization had been in use in the sanitaria for three decades, but its explicit legalization gave rise to heated debate that spilled into the pages of the sanitarium journals. A case in point was the contentious back-and-forth that followed the publication of an essay entitled "What I Want to Say to You," by Toyota Kazuo in *Aisei* in 1953. Born in Hiroshima in 1926, Toyota entered Aiseien in 1944 and would live there for almost six decades. Addressing "those of you who keep saying that [leprosy's] infectiousness is mild," he mounted a passionate defense of sterilization, citing his own personal history. His father, who had died of leprosy only a year after his birth, had infected not only Toyota himself but also three of his five older siblings, two of whom had died of the disease. Toyota held his parents responsible for this tragic outcome, referring to his father only as "the selfish person" (*wagamama mono*) and describing his mother as "ignorant."[19] In a follow-up essay published in 1954, Toyota would relate that when he learned as a teenager that both he and sister had been conceived when his father's disease was advanced, he had gone to his grave site and urinated upon the gravestone as a gesture of his anger and disdain.[20]

In Toyota's view, choosing to have children one might infect was "akin to murder" and thus sterilization was a rational choice for those with leprosy. He noted as well that in the wake of the Eugenics Protection Law even healthy people were choosing sterilization in order to control the size of their families.[21] Most of the published responses were critical of Toyota. Hoshi Seiji, a patient in the Aomori sanitarium, expressed pity for what he characterized as Toyota's "obsequiousness, sense of inferiority, and anxiety" and asserted that Toyota knew little of either leprosy or democracy.[22] Kai Hachirō, writing in Rakusen'en's journal, was slightly more conciliatory. He wrote that rather than blaming his parents for having children, Toyota should understand the social forces that compelled this, specifically the "traditional Japanese idea of family."[23]

It is notable that all the respondents were men. Their rejection of Toyota's stance signaled a growing willingness among male patients to reject vasectomy. Within the sanitaria no less than outside them, the effect of the Eugenics Protection Bill was to shift responsibility for the control of reproduction onto the female body. After the revision of the bill to allow for termination of pregnancy on the grounds of economic hardship, rates of abortion soared outside the sanitaria, from about 250,000 in 1949 to well over a million in 1953, when 34 percent of reported pregnancies ended in a legal abortion.[24] Within the sanitaria, too, the routine use of vasectomy gave way to a new reliance on female sterilization and abortion, even though tubal ligation is a far more invasive procedure and one that requires general anesthesia. In 1955, for example, only 14 men underwent a vasectomy, while 115 women were sterilized and 303 abortions were performed.[25]

These figures are particularly startling given that in the postwar sanitaria, as in those of the prewar period, male patients continued to outnumber women. With the passage of time, the trend of preserving male fertility at the expense of female patients became even more pronounced: between 1960 and 1970, only 31 vasectomies in total were performed, while 266 women were sterilized and 1,389 abortions were performed.[26] The willingness of sanitarium doctors to abandon the procedure they had pioneered and the safety of which they had demonstrated in multiple studies is puzzling, but it coincided with a new development—the introduction of the drug

Promin, which made it possible for patients to envision the possibility of a cure and a release from the sanitarium. In this context, male patients (with the cooperation of sanitarium doctors) became less willing to compromise their reproductive potential. In his 1954 essay, Toyota noted that his fellow patients who were quick to label vasectomy "an abuse of human rights" seemed untroubled by the rising number of abortions.[27]

The "Promin for All" Campaign

The evolving reproductive politics within the sanitaria is just one indication of how Promin profoundly altered social relations within these institutions, in Japan and around the world. The drug was initially tested as a treatment for tuberculosis, but Guy Henry Faget, a physician on the staff of the US National Leprosarium in Carville, Louisiana, thought that it might be effective for leprosy as well since the mycobacteria that cause the two diseases are similar. In 1941, he began testing Promin on a small group of patient volunteers at Carville, many of whom saw immediate and dramatic improvement of their symptoms. By 1943 reports on Promin were appearing in the international medical press, but information on the new treatment took some time to reach Japan. Ishidate Morizō, a professor of pharmacology at Tokyo Imperial University, eventually learned of Faget's work from an article in a Swiss medical journal, and he quickly began work on synthesizing the drug. After he succeeded in producing a small amount in March 1946, Ishidate contacted Hayashi at Zenshōen to get his cooperation in carrying out a small trial there. Three volunteers, all with advanced cases of lepromatous leprosy, received injections of Promin on alternate days for sixty days, and all showed improvement, something that quickly caught the attention of their fellow patients. Soon other small trials were under way, using Promin acquired from the United States through SCAP.[28]

In 1948 Yoshitomi Pharmaceuticals, a manufacturer based in Osaka, began to produce Promin, albeit initially only in sufficient quantities to carry out further trials (still with pools of only thirty to thirty-five patients) at several sanitaria, including Ōshima, Keifūen, and Zenshōen. At Zenshōen, where patients had firsthand knowledge of the drug's effects, volunteers were so numerous that a lottery system had to be employed to select participants. Elsewhere, the initial reaction was less enthusiastic. A patient at Ōshima later recalled that the first volunteers in Promin trials were mocked for their willingness to serve as "guinea pigs."[29] Skepticism quickly gave way to hope, and hope to frustration, as the trials progressed. With clear evidence that Promin, at the very least, brought a rapid improvement in symptoms, patients vied with one another for access to the small quantities available. When a small amount of Promin was delivered to Zenshōen in March 1948, more than six hundred people lined up in hope of getting an injection.[30]

Frustrated by their lack of access to the drug, in October 1948, patients at Zenshōen formed a Promin Treatment Promotion Committee. Its members wrote to the self-government committees at other sanitaria asking them to join the movement "to protect our lives and establish sanitaria that are filled with hope." Within months, a sophisticated campaign was under way. Taking as its slogan "Promin for All" (*Dare ni mo puromin wo*), the Promin Treatment Promotion Committee encouraged the self-government committees to organize campaigns within their individual institutions. At Rakusen'en and Zenshōen, some patients organized hunger strikes and work strikes as a demonstration of their frustration. At Aiseien, patients wrote a petition to the staff pleading for Promin not only for their own benefit but also, in a savvy appropriation of the language of leprosy prevention, to achieve the goal of "a leprosy-free Japan in the future."[31]

Significantly, the Promin campaign was not only aimed at sanitarium authorities. It targeted as well those in government and the general public. The Promin Treatment Promotion Committee produced a booklet that was sent to Diet members and other prominent public figures to publicize the effects of the drug and the patients' desire for treatment. It included statements by Ishidate and other doctors, a translation of one of Faget's articles, and first-person accounts of the effects of Promin by participants in the trials. But the most moving parts of this publication were the statements of patients who had not yet had access to the drug but had heard of its effects. A young woman wrote that since she had learned of the drug, "I am like someone infected with Promin fever. Whether I am asleep or awake, [Promin] occupies my entire brain." According to another patient, "Promin has brought hope to leprosy patients who, having given up their dreams and lost hope and strength, have fallen into a deep sleep of despair and indolence."[32]

In fact, the MHW shared the goal of "Promin for All." The delay in providing it was the result of an inability to secure an adequate supply. But it is also true that mass Promin treatment was not the priority of everyone in government. In 1949, the ministry requested six hundred million yen with the aim of extending treatment by Promin to every patient. In the final budget, however, that request was reduced by one-sixth. The influence of the patients' campaign is clear from the reaction of one Diet member. Matsudaira Tsuneo, former ambassador to the United States and Great Britain and onetime head of the Imperial Household Agency, wrote to

Prime Minister Yoshida Shigeru to protest the cut in funding. Referencing a petition authored by patients at Rakusen'en, he described it "as akin to asking patients to commit suicide."[33] In actuality, when patients learned of the reduction in funds for Promin, they responded not with despair but with outrage. At Zenshōen, hundreds of patients attended a meeting where they voted to write in protest to MacArthur, Yoshida, and the ministers of Finance and Health and Welfare. At Rakusen'en, 140 patients joined a hunger strike, footage of which was included in a newsreel produced by Nippon Eigasha.[34] In the end, market forces worked their magic. The production of Promin increased, its price fell, and even with the reduced budget the ministry was able to acquire enough of the drug to begin treating all patients in 1950.

Even if the patients' campaign for Promin did not actually hasten its general adoption, the impact was profound. This first attempt at unified action helped patients to develop a repertoire of strategies that could be used to shape public opinion, and it spurred new interest in creating a national organization to represent patient interests. In 1951, the leaders of the Five Sanitaria League asked the patients at Zenshōen to join them. In response, the Zenshōen group proposed creating a national organization, and in 1951 the National Conference of Sanitarium Patients was formed. The first general meeting of representatives elected by the patients of each institution was held in May 1952 at Zenshōen. On the agenda were the reform of the Leprosy Prevention Law and the possibility of redefining the place of leprosy patients in Japan's postwar democracy.

Revising the Leprosy Prevention Law

SCAP sources reveal that as early as 1949 Japanese officials were already contemplating the revision of the Leprosy Prevention Law, and to that end they requested a copy of the rules and regulations for leprosy then in effect in Hawaii.[35] It is unclear what, if any, information made its way into Japanese hands, but patients and public health officials alike would have been surprised to learn that in both the US territory and the US mainland, the era of effective treatment did not bring quick legislative change. At Carville, patients won the right to vote only in 1946, the same year as their Japanese compatriots, and the barbed wire that had surrounded the US National Sanitarium since its founding was not removed until 1948.[36] Frustrated by the slow pace of reform, patients at Carville established the United Patients Committee and drew up a petition that was submitted to Congress. Signed by all of the more than three hundred patients confined at the time, it called for the end of mandatory confinement, funding for outpatient treatment, financial support for families, vocational training, and a national campaign to address the stigma of the disease. Their efforts found support not only from longtime supporters of improved social welfare measures but also from advocates for military veterans, who were sympathetic to the plight of the thirty-two veterans confined at Carville.[37]

A National Leprosy Act that reflected patient demands was quickly drafted in 1948, only to die in committee. The following year, public hearings were held on a revised version of the bill, which would have repealed the requirement of quarantine. Supporters argued that quarantine destroyed lives, was against democratic principles, and was simply ineffective, encouraging sufferers to hide their disease rather than seek treatment, but medical opinion was split. Faget, for one, believed that treatment should take place in a sanitarium setting, although other doctors argued that outpatient treatment was a reasonable option. The US Public Health Service spoke out against the bill, arguing that the bill's proposed system of outpatient centers, which were to be funded by different agencies, would be ineffective, that singling out the sufferers of a single disease for special attention would set a bad precedent, and that government funds would be better spent on diseases such as cancer that affected many more Americans.[38] In the end, critics prevailed, and the bill was never passed. Instead, reforms came not via new legislation but as the result of administrative policies adopted gradually by the national sanitarium. In the 1950s patients who were no longer infectious began to be routinely discharged if they could demonstrate that they had adequate financial resources for their support and agreed not to live in close contact with children. The last case of compulsory confinement was reportedly in 1960.[39]

On Moloka'i, things unfolded very differently. According to Michelle Moran, "The war . . . effectively drew the territorial administration's attention away from the settlement and reinforced among many Kalaupapa residents a strong sense of community and Hawaiian identity."[40] The introduction of Promin, which began in 1945, challenged that sense of community. In 1948, a group of seventeen patients who had received treatment with Promin tested negative for the presence of *M. leprae*. Because territorial law required only that active cases remain quarantined, members of this group applied for and received permission to leave Moloka'i. Others soon followed. Within a few years, legislators were seizing upon the rising number of inactive cases to call for a new policy that would require all of those who were free of the disease to leave the colony. As the first step towards the goal of closing the colony, the legislature ended clothing and health allowances for those who tested negative but chose to stay at Kalaupapa. Such measures ignored the desire of many to stay on after treatment, either because they had a family member in residence or because they had no life to which they could return. As efforts to compel them to leave the colony got under way, patients began to organize to resist.[41]

As in the United States, in Japan, too, potential reform of the legal structure of quarantine was a subject of intense concern for patients. Many were outraged by an event that became known as "the testimony of the three sanitarium directors" (san'enchō shōgen). In 1951 the Committee on Health and Welfare of the upper house invited the directors of Zenshōen (Hayashi), Aiseien (Mitsuda), and Keifūen (Miyazaki) to participate in a hearing on social welfare issues. Asked to address the possible reform of the Leprosy Prevention Law, all three offered their endorsement of mandatory confinement, with Mitsuda famously declaring that people should be confined in a sanitarium for their own good even if it required "putting them in handcuffs." He also expressed concern about sanitarium order, arguing that patients had "misunderstood democracy" and thought it licensed their defiance of the sanitarium administrators and staff. In light of this, he argued that sanitarium directors needed more authority to suppress patient activism. Although Hayashi and Miyazaki offered their views in slightly less hyperbolic terms, they, too, supported the continuation of the policy of quarantine.[42]

News of the directors' stance reached the sanitaria after members of the NCSP distributed a copy of their testimony to representatives of each of the sanitaria. In the face of the groundswell of fury that resulted, Mitsuda, Hayashi, and Miyazaki were quick to step back from their opinions. Mitsuda, for one, explained that he thought he was to be questioned only about medical matters and had spoken off the cuff about policy in terms that "lacked preparation and were unsatisfactory and which did not adequately convey my views."[43] However, such efforts at fence mending did little to appease angry patients, and from mid-1952, discussion of the reform of the 1931 law filled the pages of the NCSP's newsletter, the Zenrai kankyō nyūzu. In September, a group called the Strategy Committee for the Revision of the Leprosy Prevention Law issued a preliminary list of patient demands that included an end to coerced confinement and the disciplinary power of the directors, the protection of patients' civil rights, financial aid for families, better wages for sanitarium labor, and opportunities for vocational training for recovered patients.[44]

The new political clout of the patients is clear from the events that followed. In December a group of Diet members visited Zenshōen and met with patient leaders. Their numbers included Hasegawa Tamotsu (1903–1994), a Christian and member of the Socialist Party, with long-standing interest in social welfare issues. In the 1930s he had founded a "sanitarium farm" for impoverished sufferers of tuberculosis in his home prefecture of Shizuoka that had garnered a sizeable donation from the emperor. Subsequently, Hasegawa and other Socialist Party members took the lead in pressing the government for the revision of the 1931 law. It was not only Diet members who were visiting the sanitaria in this period. MHW bureaucrats, too, were newly attentive to patient sentiment. Omura Takehisa, who headed the national sanitarium administration, made several visits to Zenshōen in this period for what were described as "friendly chats" with patient leaders.[45]

Given such evidence of new interest and support, patient-activists were perhaps unprepared for the draft revision that became public in March 1953. It began promisingly enough: the opening articles stated that the intent of the law was not only to prevent the spread of the disease but also to provide for the treatment and social welfare of its victims, and it specifically forbade discrimination against people with leprosy. Other articles included requirements for the protection of patient privacy, the extension of public education to the sanitaria, and provisions for the financial support of family members and dependents. But on most other issues the draft bill was a refutation of the NCSP demands. For one, the law required confinement of any patient who posed a risk of infection, stating that prefectural officials should "encourage" patients to accept admission but allowing them to "order" patients to enter an institution if persuasion failed. It also allowed local public health officials to intervene to prevent leprosy sufferers from working in occupations that might facilitate the spread of the disease, required anyone suspected of being infected to undergo a medical examination, and mandated the creation of a patient registry. Finally, the law confirmed the authority of sanitarium directors to "maintain order" by punishing patients, although it newly required the involvement of a disciplinary committee and specified that patients must be allowed to mount a defense before the committee.[46] In the Diet debates that followed, MHW officials defended the draft law strenuously, arguing, in essence, that any perceived similarity between the 1931 law and this one was misleading. In the age of Promin, the primary intent of the new law was to provide treatment to patients as soon as possible, before the disease had led to irreversible impairment.

In the weeks and months that followed, the NCSP mounted a campaign against the new law, which it argued simply legalized the continued abuse of their civil rights. Patients made use of a variety of tactics to protest it, including public declarations, petitions, work stoppages, hunger strikes, and letter-writing campaigns to prominent public figures, among them Eleanor Roosevelt, who was visiting Japan in June 1953. (She politely refused the invitation for a meeting, citing a packed schedule.)[47] As the campaign progressed, so, too, did the demands of the patient activists. By summer 1953, the NCSP was calling for a radically different kind of sanitarium system, one in which admission was to be completely voluntary, where patients would be free to come and go as they chose. In addition, it rejected the requirement for screening examinations and demanded compensation for patients and their families, for lost wages, closed businesses, and the like. At the same time, the NCSP wanted, conversely, for new powers to be conveyed to the sanitaria in order to detach leprosy sufferers from the larger structure of public health and social welfare. It demanded that local public health centers not be involved in the examination or treatment of suspected patients and that families of leprosy sufferers not be subject to the same scrutiny that was required by law of others seeking welfare benefits. In both cases, the NCSP argued that the involvement of local authorities would expose leprosy sufferers and their families to possible discrimination.[48]

In a phrase that evoked the status of *rai* sufferers in the early modern period, patient representatives argued that the draft law, if passed, would render leprosy sufferers "outcasts" (*hinin*) by singling out their disease for a set of peculiarly restrictive measures. This stance, however, ignored the considerable similarity between the draft bill and the Tuberculosis Prevention Law of 1951. Like leprosy, tuberculosis, too, was newly treatable. The antibiotic streptomycin, which had been discovered by an American researcher in 1944, was introduced to Japan in 1948, and its effectiveness spurred government efforts to bring the disease under control. The 1951 law required mandatory reporting by doctors, created a national patient registry, allowed prefectural governments to require sufferers to enter a sanitarium, and authorized mass mandatory screening for the disease in schools, factories, and offices. To encourage patients to seek treatment, the government assumed the total cost of in-patient care and offered partial funding to support the construction of public and private sanitaria. These provisions propelled the rapid establishment of TB sanitaria around the country, making sanitarium-based care widely available for the first time. In 1947, there were only about 53,000 beds in total for tuberculosis patients in public, private, and national sanitaria. By 1956, Japan had a total of 713 TB sanitaria with 260,000 beds, 95 percent of which were occupied.[49] One important difference between the 1951 Tuberculosis Prevention Law and the proposed leprosy law was that the former allowed for outpatient treatment, although in this case patients had to bear a portion of the cost and submit to careful monitoring by local public health authorities, something that the NCSP rejected on privacy grounds.[50]

The Japanese government never seriously considered the option of outpatient treatment for leprosy. MHW bureaucrats argued that sanitarium-based treatment was necessary given that it was still unclear whether Promin was, in fact, a "cure." This was a valid concern. By 1950 doctors at Carville were reporting that 25 percent of those released as "arrested" after receiving treatment for a period of between thirty-nine and forty-nine months subsequently relapsed.[51] Amidst discussion of whether Promin offered a real "cure" or simply temporary improvement, public health officials and sanitarium directors insisted that the controlled environment of the sanitarium was the best means to monitor treatment and assess recovery.[52]

As the refusal to countenance the involvement of the public health authorities suggests, there was a central contradiction in the stance of the NCSP. While it criticized the government for singling out leprosy sufferers for special requirements, the organization also insisted that its members were in fact a special category of citizens because of the historical status of leprosy as a stigmatized disease. It was on this basis that the organization lobbied for special entitlements for its members. The issue of the Livelihood Protection Law is a case in point. While the government's stance was that the families of leprosy sufferers should, like other citizens in economic difficulty, apply for aid under the guidelines of that law, it also tried to address patient concerns about privacy by authorizing sanitarium directors to appoint a staff member to mediate between family members and the local public health authorities. Sanitarium activists wanted more. They argued for specific provisions for support within the leprosy law—a stance that was at odds with the guiding principle of postwar welfare reform (one that originated with SCAP), which sought to dismantle the prewar system of offering preferential treatment to some groups (most notably, military veterans and their families.)[53]

Some patients recognized the contradictions in the NCSP's stance. Perhaps the most pointed criticism came from Shima Hiroshi, who four decades later would be credited with initiating the lawsuit that resulted in the Kumamoto judgment for compensation. Trained as a biologist, Shima was diagnosed with leprosy while teaching at the Tokyo College of Forestry. He initially entered Ōshima Seishōen, which was located in his home prefecture of Kagawa, in 1947, but soon applied for transfer to Keiaien in Kagoshima, an institution known for patient activism. Shima was no fan of the postwar government, which he described as "becoming fascist," and he argued that the disciplinary power the draft law would convey upon sanitarium directors was a violation of the right to due process guaranteed by the new constitution, but he also rejected the NCSP's stance on confinement. Characterizing citizenship as based on the interplay between rights and duties, he argued that patients were able to lay claim to public aid for themselves and their families precisely because they agreed to confinement to protect the health of their fellow citizens. To insist that the sanitarium system (with its provision of treatment and support at no cost) be maintained, while at the same time asserting the freedom of patients to choose or reject confinement and to leave the sanitarium at any time, was to ignore the reciprocal nature of this implicit bargain. According to Shima, if patients wanted to reject the requirement of confinement, they must be prepared to assume the expense of their own treatment and for the support of their families.[54]

Shima's view was an unpopular one—one critic took note of the "poverty" of his political consciousness—but it neatly captured the logic at play in leprosy prevention, tuberculosis prevention, and arguably the postwar system of social welfare as a whole.[55] In the case of tuberculosis, the bargain struck between the government and afflicted citizens (the provision of free treatment and social welfare benefits for compliance) worked as intended. The combination of vaccination and effective treatment with new antibiotics drove TB rates steadily downward, and by the mid-1960s, sanitaria were closing their doors. By 1986, only twenty-one sanitaria remained in operation.[56] In contrast, the final passage of the new Leprosy Prevention Bill into law on August 15, 1953, did not usher in the end of the leprosy sanitaria.

Debating "Returning to Society"

In 1956, Mori Mikio, a twenty-three-year-old member of the staff of Kōmyōen, set off a storm of debate when a brief essay he authored, entitled "A New Sanitarium for a New Era," was published in the sanitarium's journal. In a much-referenced passage, Mori wrote, "Now in the sanitarium, there are quite a few mildly impaired patients (*keishōsha*) who have the energy and strength to devote themselves to energetic competitions in baseball and volleyball, who go to the movies once or twice a week, and who sit in front of the television even before the sun goes down." He compared such patients, whom he described as "people who are idle because of excessive assistance," to productive citizens who worked up a sweat at a factory job or doing some other kind of work. In Mori's view, recovered patients who lingered on in the sanitarium were in violation of the 1953 Leprosy Prevention Law. In his words, "according to article 6, patients who pose a danger of infection are supposed to enter a sanitarium for the period necessary for leprosy prevention. On the other hand, there is no requirement that those for whom confinement is not necessary for leprosy prevention stay in the sanitarium. These patients should leave as soon as possible. I find it very curious that these people who are not required to be confined and yet stay on do not complain about the violation of their fundamental human rights."[57]

Mori's essay, with its image of the sanitarium as recreation center and its sly dig at patients' frequent recourse to the language of "human rights," seems intended to provoke—and it did. But it also brought new attention to the changing nature of the institutions in the era of Promin. Prompted by both the requirements of the new law and the promise of effective treatment, the sanitarium population swelled after 1953, reaching a peak of more than twelve thousand in 1955. Mori wrote as growing numbers of patients were beginning to test negative for the disease. In contrast to the prewar period, when only about 5 percent of patients were discharged, sanitarium doctors were initially quick to release those who had repeated negative skin smears. The first patient to recover with the benefit of Promin therapy was released from Keiaien in 1949, and a photograph of the occasion shows him dressed in a suit and surrounded by a crowd of patients and staff as he makes his triumphant farewell.[58]

Initially, each sanitarium director was able to set his own criteria for the discharge of patients, but in 1956 the MHW issued new guidelines. Patients with lepromatous leprosy whose lesions had entirely disappeared were required to undergo testing (skin smears from multiple sites on the body) at two-month intervals and to show no evidence of the presence of *M. lepra* for six tests, a policy similar to that employed at Carville at this time. In addition, however, the MHW's guidelines required the bimonthly administration of the lepromin test. Pioneered by Mitsuda in the 1920s, this involved injecting a small amount of inactive *M. leprae* into a patient to test for an immune reaction. According to the MHW guidelines, the test had to produce a reaction (known internationally as the "Mitsuda reaction") in the form of a nodule at least six millimeters in diameter. For cases of tuberculoid leprosy, patients were required to test clear of *M. leprae* for three successive bimonthly tests and to have a lepromin reaction of at least ten millimeters. The ministry departed from the Carville protocol in another way as well. In making a decision about discharge, physicians were allowed to consider the patient's readiness to leave the sanitarium, a judgment that was to reflect not only the patient's adjustment to any physical disabilities but also his or her psychological readiness.[59]

It has been charged that the Japanese sanitaria retained patients far longer than necessary, something that the subjective decision about social adjustment certainly made possible. To be sure, many patients, perhaps unaware of the possibility of relapse and of drug resistance, felt that doctors delayed their release unnecessarily. As the visible signs of the disease disappeared, some patients simply left the sanitarium without waiting for official approval, a path that came to be known as "self-discharge." In response, sanitarium doctors began to discharge people on a "temporary" (*ichji kisei*) or "long-term" (*chōki kisei*) basis, designations that stopped short of full discharge and that allowed them to stipulate requirements for follow-up. These forms of discharge also benefited patients, since they could continue to receive drugs and medical supplies without cost, undergo regular exams for signs of relapse, and reenter the sanitarium at will.

But if patients initially chafed at the rigorous and lengthy process of release, by the time Mori wrote, a new pattern had become evident. Patients who were deemed recovered were remaining within the sanitarium. One patient activist, writing in 1960, estimated that 70 percent of those confined were no longer infectious and could apply for release.[60] The number of those who attempted what was described as "returning to society" (*shakai fukki*) was far smaller than those who qualified for release. According to data compiled by the NCSP, between 1949 and 1975, a total of 2,128 patients were officially discharged, with the number peaking in 1961–1962 and declining steadily thereafter. By the 1970s the number of discharges had slowed to a trickle. The low point came in 1974, when only twelve patients were released from the ten sanitaria located outside Okinawa.[61] Equally disconcerting was that some who seemed to have successfully transitioned out of the sanitarium began to return.[62]

That patients were staying on in the sanitarium after recovery was the subject of considerable concern for patients, administrators, and public health officials alike, and a series of studies were carried out to try to discern why. They reveal that a complicated set of factors shaped a patient's willingness to pursue release. Those who entered the sanitarium while in the early stages of the disease and who responded to treatment quickly were far more likely to seek discharge than those who were left with any degree of impairment. This meant that patients who entered in the 1950s and were immediately treated with Promin were more likely to leave the sanitarium than those who entered earlier. All the surveys were in agreement that patients who had been confined for more than ten years, no matter what their physical condition, tended not to seek release. But age, physical condition, and length of confinement were not the only variables in play. Patients who had been employed before they were confined and thus had skills and work experience were more likely to pursue discharge than those who had entered a sanitarium as a child or a teenager. Those who remained in contact with family and friends were more likely to pursue release than those who had not. Patients who had married within the sanitarium had less interest in seeking discharge than those who were single. Generally, women—even those who were relatively young and without serious disability—were less interested in leaving than men, perhaps because in a society where few women were able to support themselves, they had legitimate concerns about their chances for either marriage or employment.[63]

Mori's suggestion that the sanitaria offered a life of ease ignored how legitimate concerns encouraged patients to choose the known if constrained world of the sanitarium over the uncertainties of life outside, and the response of patients to his essay was immediate and angry. Patients wrote in the NCSP newsletter and the sanitarium journals, objecting to the characterization of those who had recovered as "idle." Those who had suffered through the difficult war years in quarantine were particularly incensed. Morita Takeji (1910–1977), who was first admitted to the Kumamoto sanitarium in 1932, ran away in 1941, and then entered Aiseien in 1942, wrote that Mori's characterization of patients was simply one of many insults directed at leprosy sufferers over the years. He argued that those Mori deemed "idle" were the historical product of a sanitarium system that had sought to render patients passive and compliant. The policy of encouraging patients to marry was singled out for particular criticism: "It played the greatest role in making patients give up hope [of leaving the sanitarium]." Evoking the patriarchal perspective on reproduction examined in chapter 7, Morita suggested that "ordinary citizens" worked primarily to provide for their children, and patients who had been robbed of their reproductive potential thus had no reason to embrace the ethos of work.[64]

Sawada Gorō (1930–2007), who had entered Rakusen'en in 1941, attacked Mori from a different perspective, arguing that, far from being idle, "mildly impaired patients" were an important part of the sanitarium economy, which relied upon their low-paid work as nurses and aides to those who were disabled or bedridden.[65] Sasakawa Makoto, a patient at Keifūen, suggested that the question of whether a patient was "recovered" could not be reduced to a series of negative skin smears. Many of those who were judged to be only mildly impaired in fact suffered from various kinds of invisible disabilities, not only physical symptoms such as neuralgia and neuropathy but also psychological damage as a result of their long confinement, the discrimination they had faced, and in some cases profound anxiety over their disfigurement or disability. This kind of damage was, he said, "a gaping wound that is still bleeding in their hearts."[66] Although Sasakawa did not use the terms, others described the psychological condition of long-term patients as "institution sickness" and "hospitalism" and argued that many long-term patients suffered from a sense of inferiority and a lack of confidence that made leaving the sanitarium difficult.

In contrast, Morioka Ryōji (1911–1995) suggested that patients were, in fact, not so different from those outside the sanitaria, who, in the aftermath of war, defeat, and recovery, wanted nothing more than the "bourgeois pleasures" of going to the movies, playing baseball, and watching pro wrestling on TV.[67] Morioka had entered Zensei Hospital in 1932, leaving his life as a student of philosophy at Tokyo Imperial University behind. Although a critic of the policy of leprosy prevention, he also looked back on the pre-Promin era with nostalgia. According to Morioka, "The prewar view of the sanitarium as a community" had no meaning for those who entered with the view that "I have come for treatment." This new generation of patients was not interested in serving on the self-government council, nor did they involve themselves in the serious literary pursuits that had sustained earlier generations of patients. For Morioka, then, the sanitaria were simply a mirror that reflected the postwar mass culture.

In fact, his provocative description of "idle patients" notwithstanding, Mori (who went on to have a long and distinguished career in social welfare) was overtly critical of the policy of quarantine and recognized the ill effects of prolonged confinement. The primary intent of his essay was to spark a discussion about how to reform the sanitarium system in order to better meet the evolving needs of its patients. He outlined an ambitious plan for the "division and reorganization" of the sanitaria that was intended to promote the discharge of recovered patients. Mori argued that the sanitaria had come to house three distinct and incompatible populations: (1) recovered patients, some with minor degrees of impairment; (2) those who had recovered but had been left seriously disabled; and (3) those who were still in treatment. He proposed that each group should be reassigned to a different sanitarium that had been redesigned with their particular needs in mind. Those who were actively in treatment should be in a thoroughly medicalized institution devoted to promoting a fast recovery; as their condition stabilized they should be transferred to a different part of the facility, where they would gradually transition into a more "normal" life of work and independent living. Patients who had recovered but were impaired should be in an institution organized around vocational training and other help designed to encourage them to develop the "willpower" (*kiryoku*) to rejoin ordinary life. In contrast, those whose disabilities made it impossible for them live independently should be transferred into an institution organized for their long-term care, although they should be encouraged to engage in handicraft production or other work, to the degree they were able.

At the heart of Mori's essay was an economics of citizenship. He believed that the sanitaria should be reserved for those in treatment or truly unable to work. All others should join the workforce. He was by no means alone in this view. As Sheldon Garon has written, "in Japan's darkest hour, economic nationalism . . . came to define the post-war national mission."[68] Hard work, frugality, and saving had long been important social values, but now they came to be understood as patriotic behavior in a country stripped of the colonial possessions and military power that had been a focus of popular pride for half a century. Successive governments encouraged citizens to participate in rebuilding the nation's shattered economy and to regard Japan's economic growth as a point of personal pride. Mori's contemptuous reference to daytime television viewing within the sanitarium was an implicit comparison with the normative Japanese (male) citizen, for whom such pleasures were reserved for the evening hours. Mori was not alone in his concern about the creation of an entitlement culture in the sanitaria. In his 1958 memoir, Mitsuda Kensuke wrote that as a result of increases in so-called comfort funds and the aid they received under the Livelihood Protection Law, patients had become reluctant to perform work in the sanitarium, even though wages had increased dramatically. According to Mitsuda, the prevailing view among patients was that "it was natural that pitiful sufferers of leprosy and their families should be supported by the nation."[69]

It is undeniable that sanitarium life improved dramatically in the 1950s. In addition to the payments mentioned by Mitsuda, in 1958 patients became eligible for support under the provisions for disability in Japan's new national pension law, and in 1960 about 40 percent of patients began receiving stipends. A survey undertaken by the NCSP in 1956 estimated that even before the national pension law was passed patients had on average about fifteen hundred yen of income per month, the total of the various benefits they received plus wages from sanitarium jobs. In an era in which a full-time female factory worker often earned less than ten thousand yen per month, this was not an insignificant amount, given that basic needs such as food, lodging, and medical care were provided within the sanitaria.[70] As Mori suggested, new kinds of leisure activities, including sports, television, and movies, were now available in the sanitaria. Aiseien even got its own on-site pachinko parlor in 1954. Patients also enjoyed what they called *basureku* (bus recreation), excursions in sanitarium buses to scenic areas and local sites. One particularly memorable trip for Zenshōen patients was an outing to central Tokyo to see the neon lights of Ginza.[71]

But as many of those who responded to Mori accurately pointed out, while the welfare benefits patients received provided for a comfortable life within the sanitarium, they were not sufficient to allow them to live independently. Japan's welfare system was still premised on the availability of considerable family support for those unable to work, support that many recovered patients lacked. It was not only leprosy patients who found the welfare provisions available insufficient for independent living. In the 1950s, many of Japan's sixty thousand disabled and maimed veterans also suffered from insufficient aid that left them and their families in poverty. In desperation, some turned to public begging to survive, wearing distinctive white robes (*hakui*), derived from hospital gowns, as evidence of their disabled veteran status. In the 1950s and 1960s, these "white-robed heroes" came to be termed "white-robed beggars" by some and were the subject of considerable criticism by politicians and the general public, who called for them to "rehabilitate themselves" rather than rely on charity.[72] Mori's criticism of the recovered leprosy patients reflected the new anxiety over the expansion of social welfare and the belief that it threatened to undermine national recovery.

Patients, for the most part, harshly rejected the equation of benefits with charity. Yokoyama Ishitori was one of many who argued that the problem was not that leprosy sufferers were getting too much aid but that they were not getting enough. Born in 1925, Yokoyama had entered Rakusen'en in 1947, after developing symptoms of leprosy while recovering from injuries incurred while in the navy's air service. He soon became an activist; he was one of the sanitarium's representatives to the National Conference of Sanitarium Patients in the tumultuous period of 1952–1953. Then, in 1966, at the age of fifty-six and after almost twenty years in the sanitarium, Yokoyama successfully "returned to society," breaking the pattern of "early in, quickly out" that characterized those who reintegrated into life outside the sanitarium. He went on to establish a local monthly newspaper and served on the Kusatsu Board of Education.[73]

In his 1957 essay "Obstacles to Returning to Society" published in Rakusen'en's journal, Yokoyama urged his readers not to simply dismiss Mori as either ill informed or mean-spirited, although he noted sharply that the receipt of social welfare benefits did not require the abandonment of one's civil rights. Yokoyama argued that the limited level of aid essentially trapped recovered leprosy sufferers in the sanitarium: "If we are discharged, it is just as if we are naked. We don't have capital to start a business, and we don't have the means to make a living. During our long confinement, we have grown distant from our relatives upon whom we should be able to rely. We can't even borrow money to get by." Analyzing figures from the national budget, he argued that collectively leprosy patients received far less aid than other disadvantaged groups in Japanese society, including tuberculosis patients, the unemployed, and the families of the war dead. Given this situation, Yokoyama called for robust financial support for those seeking to reenter society, a onetime lump payment of thirty thousand yen to help them rebuild their lives plus five thousand yen per month for the first six months after their discharge. In addition, there should be special provisions to allow former patients to borrow money to start a small business.[74]

Like Yokoyama, other patients, too, essentially embraced the economics of citizenship that oriented Mori's work. Arguing that recovered patients wanted to reenter society as working, tax-paying citizens, they demanded that the government take responsibility for aiding them in this transition. One bold suggestion was that since it cost the ministry one hundred thousand yen per annum to house a patient within the sanitarium, this amount should simply be turned over to recovered patients who agreed to be discharged.[75] Others called for a program of housing subsidies and the funding of vocational training. This became the official stance of the NCSP, which consistently lobbied the government for more benefits for leprosy sufferers and, like Yokoyama, sought to draw attention to the disparity between the aid its constituents received and that bestowed upon disabled veterans and others.

By 1960, however, some patients were questioning this kind of clientist approach to social welfare, which put them in competition with other disadvantaged groups for scarce aid. Yokoyama, for one, began to openly criticize the patient movement for a lack of "principle," arguing that the heads of the self-government councils and the National Council had fallen into a pattern of "please-give-us-ism" (onegaishugi) in relation to the government. According to Yokoyama, rather than bargaining for concessions, leprosy patients should make common cause with others who also suffered under Japan's inadequate social welfare system. He wrote, "The movement of Hansen's disease patients should go forward as one wing of class warfare. Then, for the first time, it will be clear that in relation to the larger fight for social welfare the special circumstances of the Hansen's disease sufferers aren't special at all."[76] Honma Kiyoshi, like Yokoyama a patient of Rakusen'en, made a similar point, albeit without the Marxist framing: "I think we need to stop asking for special treatment on the basis that because we have Hansen's disease we need special benefits. . . . People who have recovered and are not disabled should register at the employment centers like everyone else. Then from that position we can make the case that our social welfare system is too weak."[77]

Such calls notwithstanding, the NCSP never abandoned its interest-group approach to lobbying government, nor did other disadvantaged groups within Japanese society. Attempts to forge such an alliance might have been difficult to achieve given the considerable discrimination leprosy patients continued to face well into the postwar era. We can recall the outraged reaction of the Buraku Liberation League in 1969 to Kobayashi Keiichirō's statement that leprosy sufferers were among those considered "base" in the early modern period. And indeed some patients argued passionately that the special historical circumstances under which leprosy patients labored meant that they did in fact deserve specific accommodation. Sasakawa Makoto, who advocated for special provisions for leprosy patients, objected to the new anti-clientist clamor: "Now there is a thunder of voices who say [to sanitarium patients], you are in violation of the spirit of social welfare that requires 'reasonable accommodation.' Like everyone else, you should enter an appropriate facility or get what you are due under the Livelihood Protection Law and leave the sanitarium."[78] He noted that there was growing anxiety among patients that the Ministry of Health and Welfare would adopt the policy in place in the TB sanitaria, which required patients to leave once they tested negative, even if they resisted. Ironically, then, less than a decade after the 1953 law was promulgated, concern had turned from forcible confinement to the possibility of forcible discharge.

Colonies Revisited

As the debate over "returning to society" unfolded, there was renewed interest in the idea of establishing separate communities for leprosy patients that would buffer them from discrimination while allowing for fuller participation in civic life. In the 1953 debates on the revision of the Leprosy Prevention Law, there had already been discussion of founding "colonies" for recovered patients in order to aid them in transitioning back to life outside the sanitarium. Mori had employed the term "colony" in his 1956 essay, using it to describe a new kind of institution for permanently disabled patients. Patients, too, quickly seized upon the term and began to use it to imagine the possibility of post-sanitarium life. Those who advocated for colonies ignored not only the prewar discourse on "colonies" and "free zones" that had emanated from the prewar advocates of quarantine but also the irony of proposing the creation of "colonies" within the new post-imperial and democratic Japan.

Sano Reishin, a patient of the Shinseien in Miyagi Prefecture, offered up his vision of such a colony by describing an imaginary community seven years after its founding. He called his colony Shining Town (Hikari No Machi) and situated it about an hour's bus ride from a major railway station in a pleasantly rural area not far from an established village. Shining Town had a population of about four hundred people, most of whom worked in agriculture, although others were employed in a variety of industries including garment production, canning, furniture making, and bamboo craft. The goods they produced were sold to public facilities, such as prisons and nursing homes. Other residents operated small businesses, repairing bicycles, radios, and shoes and providing services such as bookkeeping for community members and people in the neighboring village. People were free to stay indefinitely, but some chose to move on after they acquired the skills they needed to rebuild their lives elsewhere. While the community still had a professional director, "colonists" looked forward to a time when they would be absorbed into the nearby village, fully assimilated into national life.[79]

Sano's imaginary Shining Town offers a window into the aspirations for the communities termed "colonies." Unlike the solitary endeavor of "returning to society," the proposed "colonies" had the aim of keeping sanitarium communities intact. Indeed, one of the most popular ideas floated in this period was that recovered patients, with training, could gradually replace the able-bodied (kenjōsha) staff members as regular employees who were paid standard wages, transforming the sanitaria into therapeutic communities entirely staffed by former leprosy sufferers.[80] This was Mitsuda's vision of leprosy colonies based on mutual aid, reinterpreted for the era of Promin and democracy. Sano's imagined community represented a different model of the colony. Like the free zones that many had championed in the prewar period, it was to be a productive community of (former) leprosy sufferers that, while ostensibly operating like an ordinary village, would require government involvement and planning. The presence of a professional director and the provision of favorable contracts with institutions within the social welfare sector were to aid the community until an unspecified moment when it could function without support.

The embrace of what were generally imagined as permeable but separate communities is clearly at odds with the goal of full citizenship that had animated the patient activism in the early 1950s. The stance of patient activist Shima Hiroshi towards proposals for "colonies" is revealing of how many came to accept them as the best path out of the sanitarium. Writing in 1953, Shima had rejected the idea that the sanitaria could be turned into self-governing productive colonies, an idea already in circulation. These, he argued, would only perpetuate the stigma of leprosy, by isolating those who had recovered from the larger society.[81] Three years later, Shima had changed his mind. Writing in Rakusen'en's journal in 1956, he called for the establishment of a colony that had much in common with Sano's imagined Shining Town. It would employ former sanitarium residents in a variety of independent businesses and community enterprises, and they would be free to go or stay as they wished. The one substantial difference was that Shima wanted the community to be open as well to settlement by those he termed "healthy people." Shima explained his rejection of the goal of "returning to society" individually in favor of collective resettlement in semi-segregated communities by arguing that the latter would not only alleviate the anxiety that prevented many patients from seeking discharge, they would also be a way of countering popular prejudice towards the disease by demonstrating visibly and dramatically that former patients "had recovered and were building their lives." In his words, "In order to take that difficult path towards our dream, we must do it arm in arm. Firmly united, let's take the first step towards establishing a colony."[82]

If the enthusiasm for colonies reflected the difficulty of "returning to society," the belief that the creation of new communities specifically for recovered patients could be a path towards social integration was surely misguided. As Jane Kim has discussed, in the 1950s the South Korean government adopted such a policy, and by the late 1970s almost a hundred so-called resettlement villages for recovered leprosy sufferers had been created, most on abandoned land far from population centers that lacked basic infrastructure, including running water, provisions for sewage and electricity, and medical care. Children from the resettlement villages were generally denied admission to local public schools. When Dr. Dharmendra, renowned Indian leprologist and follower of Gandhi, visited South Korea in 1966 as a representative of the World Health Organization, he harshly criticized the resettlement villages as simply another form of segregation. He was right. The residents of these communities and their descendants continue to face considerable social discrimination five decades later.[83]

It is fortunate, then, that Japanese bureaucrats showed little inclination for the kind of social experimentation that would have been required to create "colonies" of any type. Instead, the MHW and sanitarium administrators responded to the problem of recovered patients with a program of limited and piecemeal support. In 1958, the sanitaria got new funding to aid recovered patients in transitioning out of the sanitaria. This took the form of small grants of "preparation money" that were capped at fifteen thousand yen. In the same year, the ministry began offering a greater level of support through grants administered by an organization known as Wisteria Wind Society (Tofū Kyōkai), the successor to the prewar Leprosy Prevention Association. The stated mission of the new organization, created in 1952 and headed by Prince Takamatsu, the emperor's younger brother, was to counter popular prejudice by educating the public and to provide support to patients and those who had recovered. In 1958, the society offered funding in the form of "household re-establishment funds." In 1964, these were transformed into "occupational capital grants," which paid thirty thousand yen until 1970, when that amount was raised to fifty thousand yen. In this period, the number of those who received funding tracked closely with the number of those who were discharged, suggesting that most people applied for and received funding. Patients could also apply for training grants, and in the 1970s these, too, seemed to be awarded routinely.[84]

Recognizing that patients would have to quickly find work after their release, the sanitaria tried to offer patients vocational training. Courses were offered in sewing and dressmaking, typing, *soroban* (abacus), hairdressing, and driving the then popular three-wheeled vehicles. At Aiseien, a "piecework club" was created to help patients earn and save money with an eye to possible discharge. In 1961, the sanitaria adopted the policy of allowing patients to seek work outside while they continued to live in the sanitarium. This appears to have worked especially well at Rakusen'en, where the inns and eateries in the nearby spa town offered ready employment, but enterprising patients elsewhere also benefited. Wakibayashi Kiyoshi entered the sanitarium on Ōshima in 1948 at the age of seventeen. Although the disease left him with partially paralyzed hands, with intensive rehabilitation he recovered enough to leave the sanitarium in 1964. He journeyed to Tokyo, where he enrolled in a technical college and became qualified to repair small electronics. However, after two years in the capital he elected to return to Ōshima. He did not, however, give up on his profession. Instead, he negotiated an arrangement with a home electronics shop in Takamatsu, a short ferry ride away from Ōshima. The owner brought him televisions, radios, and vacuum cleaners that needed fixing, and Wakibayashi would sometimes travel to Takamatsu to make repairs in the shop. To Wakibayashi, it seems, the sanitarium had ceased to be an institution; it was home.[85]

Even as the sanitaria were being redefined in this way, efforts to encourage recovered patients to leave continued throughout the 1960s. Staples of the sanitarium journals in this period were essays and round-tables that painted an attractive picture of life after "returning to society." For example, in an essay entitled "My Life after the Sanitarium," a former female patient called Yamamoto Yoriko described how she "achieved the joy of working and freedom" by getting a job in a factory.[86] But as recovered patients left the sanitarium and the admission of new cases slowed to a trickle, the complicated mix of different kinds of patients that had troubled many in the mid-1950s gradually gave way to stable populations of long-term residents, all of whom were essentially cured. By the late 1960s, in a pattern similar to that at Carville, change in administrative policies, not statutes, transformed the sanitaria. Most of them no longer restricted patient movement, and the requirement for sanitaria admission for those newly diagnosed was quietly abandoned in favor of outpatient treatment, in part because sanitarium directors recognized that newcomers challenged the cohesion of sanitarium communities.

The contraction of the institutions was not only a matter of patient numbers. Many of the things that had long defined sanitarium life were gradually abandoned. The use of patients as nursing staff and aides for disabled patients gave way to the employment of a fully professional medical staff. Patient dormitories were torn down and in their place tidy rows of small cottages were constructed, each with its own small garden plot, allowing the so-called mildly impaired to live independently. Patient work, too, came to an end, and sanitarium fields were allowed to grow fallow, livestock was sold off, and tasks like printing the sanitarium journals were outsourced. Even the hard-won right of self-government, for which patients had labored so long, proved hard to sustain. In 1966, at Zenshōen, the center of patient activism in the early 1950s, the self-government council collapsed when no one stood for election.[87] Elsewhere, positions on the council came to rotate among a small group of residents.[88]

Japan's long fight with leprosy was essentially over by 1975, when the number of new cases of the disease fell below one hundred for the first time. Even so, more than eight thousand people continued to live in the sanitaria and the 1953 Leprosy Prevention Law remained in place, propping up the shell of a system created to treat and prevent a disease that no longer constituted any kind of a threat. While the NCSP at times proposed revising the law, it never advocated for the abolition of the sanitaria. In point of fact, the preservation of the law on the part of the government was benign in its indifference, since leaving it in place provided for those for whom the sanitaria had become home. Discussion of revocation came only in the 1990s, when Ōtani Fujio, a former Ministry of Health and Welfare bureaucrat turned director of the Wisteria Wind Society, took the lead in calling for its official end. Mediating between the government and the patient organization and with the support of the Association of the Sanitarium Directors and the Japanese Leprosy Association, he brokered a deal that guaranteed the preservation of the sanitaria. In 1996, the Diet voted to abolish the 1953 law and passed the Law in Relation to the Revocation of the Leprosy Prevention Law, which officially declared the patients to be "residents" and ensured the preservation of the sanitaria.

This chapter has explored the politics of leprosy prevention in the postwar era. I have argued that the preservation of the sanitarium system in the age of effective treatment resulted from a complex of factors, medical, social, and political. While patients, empowered by the postwar ethos of democratization and civil rights, pushed for a new kind of sanitarium system, one that would reflect the special status of leprosy as disease and social phenomenon, politicians and bureaucrats ultimately approved a different plan, one that was premised upon new approaches to social welfare and public health and the new economic nationalism of the postwar period. No longer privileged icons of the national community, for those in government, leprosy patients became just one more interest group lobbying for better benefits. In fact, patient activists were correct. The long tradition of stigma and the physical and psychological aftereffects of the disease and quarantine meant that many of those who had recovered needed greater levels of support than they received. The burst of enthusiasm for colonies in the late 1950s and 1960s reflects the growing desperation of those who were unable or unwilling to abandon the communities they had built within sanitarium walls. But this bleak assessment does not do justice to the meaningful lives patients managed to craft against significant odds. Yokoyama Ishitori's "return to society" after twenty years in the sanitarium and Wakibayashi Kiyoshi's decision to pursue a career in electronics repair within the institution remind us that patients were powerful agents in their own right.

Conclusion

Biological Citizenship and the
Afterlife of Quarantine

This book has explored the social, political, and medical dimensions of Japan's leprosy policy. In contrast to the "denunciatory history" that holds that the modern Japanese state purposefully and systematically created policies designed to oppress leprosy sufferers and encouraged discrimination at the hands of their fellow citizens, I have argued for a more complicated and nuanced understanding of how the policy of quarantine took form, one that acknowledges the long premodern history of the disease and the powerful role of civic actors and international norms in the late nineteenth century, one that sees the Japanese state as less a cohesive agent than a collection of competing interests, and one that rejects the conclusion that the desire to eradicate a disease equates to a desire to eradicate those who suffer from it. As we have seen, long before the Japanese government took up the problem of defining a national policy, leprosy was already profoundly marked by ethical and political concerns, associated with sin, pollution, heredity, and outcast status in the premodern period, and with new concepts of race and civilization from the 1870s.

After 1900, a clamor of voices, domestic and international, called for the Japanese government to quarantine all sufferers of the disease. However, Japan's first leprosy law, which remained in place until 1931, was fundamentally a poverty law motivated by a new commitment to social welfare that sought to aid, if also to "manage," indigent sufferers of the disease. The passage of the law, marked as it was by classist assumptions about the poor and paternalistic conceptions of state benevolence, ushered in a long period of contestation and experimentation that centered on the status of leprosy sufferers as citizens of the nation and their rights within and outside the sanitaria. At the center of the ongoing debate on leprosy was the question that troubles every public health policy: how to balance the rights of the individual against the health and safety of the larger society. To be sure, bureaucrats and politicians in Tokyo took the lead in attempting to forge a solution, but others were involved as well, including local officials, directors and staff of the sanitaria, foreign missionaries, and, most important, people who suffered from leprosy.

As we have seen, singularly and together, leprosy sufferers played a powerful role in shaping the sanitaria, the policies of leprosy prevention, and ultimately ideas about citizenship itself, when, against considerable odds, they used the options available to them to define their place in Japanese society. The tactics they deployed included individual and coordinated acts of abscondment, organized protests, and the creation of representative bodies that allowed them to speak with a unified voice to sanitarium directors and government officials. An early example of patient action, and one that would profoundly shape the sanitaria, was the refusal to accept institutional efforts to enforce sexual abstinence, a policy that had shaped the physical design of the early sanitaria. In the end, in the face of ongoing patient resistance, sanitarium directors and Bureau of Hygiene officials ended their efforts to maintain a sexual divide.

It is undeniable, however, that the efforts and aims of people with leprosy were always mediated by wider discourses of citizenship in both the prewar and postwar periods. Before 1945, Japan's imperial democracy made sacrifice for and contributions to the national good prerequisites for full participation in civic life. Thus, public health officials and patients alike struggled to define an institutional form that would fully integrate the sick into the nation. When leprosy sufferers spoke of "a perfect separate world" and politicians debated the merits of "free zones," they were attempting to imagine institutions that would eradicate leprosy while also allowing patients to live as productive citizens.

Whatever form they took, Japan's leprosy sanitaria did not mesh neatly with "the camp" as Agamben defines it. Over the course of the 1910s and 1920s, the public sanitaria were transformed into complex communities of work and cultural production that engaged with the world "outside," even as they were also sites of research and treatment. In the 1930s, far from being marginalized or excluded, sanitarium patients were celebrated as representing the organic unity of the Japanese nation, a nation in which citizens were bound together not by the rule of law but by affective ties and an ethos of mutual aid and responsibility. It is undeniable that many people with leprosy embraced this vision of the nation, and as Bureau of Hygiene officials predicted, they voluntarily chose confinement within a sanitarium.

But this shared vision of citizenship was challenged as conditions in the sanitaria declined as a result of overcrowding and underfunding, and patients refused to accept that self-sacrifice was their primary role in the body politic. A crackdown on all forms of "subversion," suspected and real, accompanied the mobilization for total war, and patient unrest made it possible to sanction both coerced confinement and the transfer of those deemed troublesome to the notorious Special Hospital Ward.

Japan's defeat and the SCAP-led program of democratization that followed inspired patients to renegotiate their place within the nation. The desire of patient-activists to retain the sanitaria system, seek new entitlements, and demand full recognition of their civil rights ran counter to both the new economic nationalism and the proclaimed egalitarian structure of the postwar state—but in the end, patients succeeded in laying claim to a special place within Japan's postwar welfare system. What other scholars have failed to acknowledge is that, as at Moloka'i, the preservation of the sanitaria in the age of effective treatment resulted in part because patients fought not only for the right to leave the sanitaria but also for the right to stay.

My account of Japan's leprosy policy and the sanitaria is likely to anger some readers, including, to my regret, some sanitarium residents and the staff of the museums devoted to leprosy who have showed me great kindness during the long years of work on this project. In particular, my assertions that the reproductive policy of the sanitaria offered reproductive choice challenges the narrative of forced sterilization that has ossified in the wake of the Kumamoto court's judgment. Ultimately, the intertwined juridical imperatives of determining responsibility and calculating reparations that ordered this lawsuit and the judgment cannot do justice to the difficult decisions made by those living with a disabling, chronic, and at the time incurable disease. The pattern of intrafamilial infection baffled researchers, but it was a specter that haunted patients, many of whom knew all too well that to have a child was to gamble with *M. leprae.*

If the framing of Japan's leprosy policy within the denunciatory narrative has obscured the agency of patients, their powerful role in shaping policy and institutions, and their difficult choices, it has also failed to explore the ways in which leprosy policy intersected with and departed from public policy towards those who suffered from other chronic diseases, most notably tuberculosis and mental illness. Japanese scholars have argued that leprosy prevention policies stigmatized people with leprosy, but this ignores the fact that they were also singled out for aid within a political economy that made few provisions for the biologically vulnerable. Was life in a public sanitarium, which offered community and medical care but required submission to the disciplinary authority of the director, better or worse than years of solitude in "home confinement," ill clothed, ill fed, and without access to treatment? Would the working-class sufferer of tuberculosis, who was unable to work and without the means to seek medical care, have preferred life in a sanitarium even at the expense of his liberty? These questions, for which there are no easy answers, have gone unacknowledged in the flood of books, films, and documentaries that have relentlessly but also myopically documented the history of leprosy.

Now, more than a century after its founding, the sanitarium system is entering its final phase. As of May 2018 the number of residents has fallen to 1,333, and with an average age of eighty-five many are infirm and bedbound. When I walked the grounds of Zenshōen and Aiseien in the spring of 2016, I encountered not a single resident, a very different situation from the lively communities I discovered when I began this project. In 1999, I first traveled to Zenshōen to visit the small museum patients had constructed there. I was accompanied by my then four-year-old daughter, who unsurprisingly had little interest in the exhibits. Several former patients who were working as volunteer guides stepped forward to amuse her with offers of sweets and crayons, so that I could tour the museum with one of their colleagues, and now almost twenty years later I can still recollect the intense pride of my guide as we made our way through the jumble of artifacts donated from sanitaria around Japan.

As the number of residents has fallen, the fate of the sanitaria is now under debate once again. At Ōshima, where fewer than sixty patients remain, the director has spoken openly of the need to consider relocating patients to another facility, although the agreement forged between the residents and the government after the Kumamoto judgment requires the sanitaria to continue to operate as long as even one long-term resident chooses to remain. Others have begun to contemplate what will follow once that commitment has been met. One proposal that has considerable support is to turn the former sanitaria into heritage sites that will use the history of leprosy to encourage reflection on discrimination, human rights, and social justice.

In actuality, the process of museumization has already begun. As I noted in the introduction, five of the sanitaria now house museums of various sizes and sophistication. Their staff devotes considerable energy to organizing events designed to educate visitors about the quarantine system. Several years ago, the curator of Aiseien's museum began to organize summer boat tours that allow visitors to reimagine the course taken by patients who arrived by boat to enter the "separate world" they had been promised and the "colony" they were charged with building. Others, including Zenshōen, have created walking tours that guide visitors around notable sites in the sanitarium, although unfortunately few structures of historical interest remain. Most of the buildings that stand today are built in the dull institutional style of postwar public buildings, and there is little that is visually interesting or inspiring—with one notable exception. The tour at Zenshōen takes visitors to the columbarium, where the cremated remains of those who died in quarantine are housed. This, at least, is a powerful material trace of lives lived and lost within the narrow confines of the institutions. In some of the sanitarium museums, residents have played a role in shaping the exhibitions. For example, in contrast to the National Hansen's Disease Museum on the grounds of Zenshōen, where the practice of sterilization is the subject of a central exhibit, the use of vasectomy goes unmentioned at Aiseien's museum, in spite of this sanitarium's close association with Mitsuda Kensuke, who pioneered the practice and enthusiastically promoted it. This, I was told, was at the request of the patients, who declined to invite the public to scrutinize this most personal of decisions.

But as leprosy recedes, first from lived experience and then from memory, we need to consider what stories the silent and empty shells of the places that once housed its victims will be made to tell, who will tell them, and to what end. Kusatsu is a case in point. The hot-spring town where Yunosawa once stood now houses two museums devoted to leprosy. One was established by the members of St. Barnabas Church and celebrates the work of Mary Cornwallis-Legh. Its hagiographic depiction of the mission she built makes no mention of the regime of sexual segregation she insisted on, her reliance on support from the Japanese state, or the questionable quality of care she offered those who turned to the mission for help. The other, far grander in scale, is the government-funded Jyu-kanbo National Museum of Detention of Hansen's Disease Patients. It features a reconstruction of the Special Hospital Ward that illuminates the terrible conditions endured by confinees, but it fails to explore its connections with the larger wartime culture of political oppression and thus renders it symbolic of Japan's leprosy policy as a whole. What goes completely unmemorialized is the lively community of Yunosawa itself, the independent community of leprosy sufferers over which so much ink was spilled, to which so many journeyed in hope of a cure, and which inspired the concept of the "free zone" with its promise of a normal life that endured even into the postwar era. Yunosawa finds no mention in any guidebook and no placard marks its site, which is now occupied by a grand public spa facility. Town officials prefer that this aspect of local history be forgotten. As a result, the crowds of domestic and international visitors who flock to Kusatsu in search of relaxation and a quintessential Japanese experience leave with no knowledge of this remarkable community.

The erasure of Yunosawa from the landscape of Kusatsu is emblematic of the larger erasures that shape the now ossified history of leprosy in Japan. These include the failure to acknowledge the role of civil society, elected officials, and ordinary people in making and perpetuating a culture of discrimination and the unwillingness to recognize that even seemingly compassionate aims and acts—the provision of aid to the impoverished and the sick, for example—can lead to oppressive policies. The story of the evil Japanese state, its collaborators, and its victims is an appealing one, precisely because it allows well-intentioned people to ignore their culpability in the system that emerged and their role in obscuring its history. If the museumization of the sanitaria is to be meaningful, it must grapple with the questions of how to represent this complex history and how to make it meaningful to those who know little of the terrible toll of leprosy. Acknowledging that leprosy policy unfolded as part of the larger citizenship project of modern Japan may, I hope, provide the means to link this important part of Japan's history to the still important and unresolved question of the place of the biologically vulnerable in Japanese society and elsewhere.

Notes

Abbreviations
Archives and document collections frequently cited in the notes:

FYB-Keiō	Fujikawa Yū Bunko, Keiō University Library
FYB-Kyoto	Fujikawa Yū Bunko, Kyoto University Library
HBZ	Ōka Makoto, Otani Fujio, Kaga Otohiko, Tsurumi Shunsuke, and Taguchi Mugihiko, eds. *Hansenbyō bungaku zenshū*. 10 vols. Tokyo: Koseisha, 2002–2010.
HSA	Hawai'i State Archives
KKIS	Otsuka Yoshinori and Yakazu Dōmei, eds. *Kinsei kanpō igakusho shūsei*, vols. 1–116. Tokyo: Meicho Shuppan, 1979–1984.
KNHMSS	Fujino Yutaka, ed. *Kingendai Nihon Hansenbyō mondai shiryō shūsei*. 20 vols. Tokyo: Fuji Shuppan, 2003.
NAJ	National Archives of Japan
NDL-Digital	National Diet Library, Digital Collection
NHK	Okayama-ken Hansenbyō Mondai Kanren Shiryō Chōsa Iinkai, ed. *Nagashima ha kataru: Okayama-ken Hansenbyō kankei shiryōshū*. 2 vols. Okayama: Okayama-ken Hansenbyō Mondai Kanren Shiryō Chōsa Iinkai, 2007–2009.
TMA	Tokyo Metropolitan Archives
USNA	United States National Archives (College Park)

Introduction
1. As of May 2018 the number of residents of the national sanitaria was 1,333, according to the official website of Kagawa Prefecture, http://www.pref.kagawa.lg.jp/content/etc/subsite/kansenshoujouhou/upfiles/skhqet151211224415_f03.pdf, accessed July 23, 2018.

2. Nikolas Rose and Carlos Nova, "Biological Citizenship," in *Global Assemblages: Technology, Politics, and Ethics as Anthropological Problems*, ed. Aihwa Ong and Stephen J. Collier, 439–463 (Malden, MA: Blackwell Publishing, 2005); a revised version of the same article is in Nikolas Rose, *The Politics of Life Itself: Biomedicine, Power, and Subjectivity in the Twenty-First Century* (Princeton, NJ: Princeton University Press, 2007), 131.

3. Recent films include *Ai suru* (1997), *Suna no utsuwa* (2004), *Shin atsui kabe* (2007), and *An* (2015). The collection of documents is Fujino Yutaka, ed., *Kingendai Nihon Hansenbyō mondai shiryō shūsei*, vols. 1–20 (Tokyo: Fuji Shuppan, 2003). The collection of patient writing is Ōka Makoto, Otani Fujio, Kaga Otohiko, Tsurumi Shunsuke, and Taguchi Mugihiko, eds., *Hansenbyō bungaku zenshū*, vols. 1–10 (Tokyo: Koseisha, 2002–2010). The journal is *Hansenbyō shimin gakkai nenpō*.

4. The five museums are the National Hansen's Disease Museum on the grounds of Tama Zenshōen (Tokyo), the Jyu-kanbo National Museum of Detention for Hansen's Disease Patients (Kusatsu, Gunma), and smaller museums on the grounds of Nagashima Aiseien (Okayama), Kikuchi Keifūen (Kumamoto), and Okinawa Airakuen (Okinawa).

5. See, for example, Sakurai Hōsaku, *Kyūrai no chichi Mitsuda Kensuke no omoide* (Kyoto: Rugārusha, 1974). Ogawa's book, *Kojima no haru*, was published in 1938 and went through many editions. The film adaptation was released in 1940.

6. On this first museum, see Susan L. Burns, "History, Testimony, and the Afterlife of Quarantine: The National Hansen's Disease Museum of Japan," in *Quarantine: Local and Global Histories*, ed. Alison Bashford, 210–229 (London: Palgrave, 2016).

7. Yamamoto Shun'ichi, *Nihon raishi* (Tokyo: Tokyo Daigaku Shuppankai, 1993); Sawano Masaki, *Raisha no sei: Bunmei kaika no jōken toshite no* (Tokyo: Seikyūsha, 1994); and Fujino Yutaka, *Nihon fashizumu to iryō: Hansenbyō wo meguru jisshōteki kenkyū* (Tokyo: Iwanami Shoten, 1993).

8. Hirokawa Waka, *Kindai Nihon no Hansenbyō mondai to chiiki shakai* (Osaka: Osaka Daigaku Shuppankai, 2011), 7–8.

9. Fujino Yutaka, *"Inochi" no kindaishi: "Minzoku jōka" no na no motoni hakugai sareta Hansenbyō kanja* (Kyoto: Kamogawa Shuppan, 2001), 296.

10. Ibid., 301–319. Hirokawa, *Kindai Nihon no Hansenbyō mondai to chiiki shakai*, 189–192.

11. The plaintiffs' lawyers have authored a history of the case. See Hansenbyō Iken Kokubai Soshō Bengodan, ed., *Hirakareta tobira: Hansenbyō saiban wo tatakatta hitotachi* (Tokyo: Kōdansha, 2003).

12. This figure swelled dramatically in the wake of the Kumamoto court's ruling on May 11, 2001; in the space of a few weeks, an additional thousand people joined the three suits. See ibid., 378.

13. Ibid., 132–180.

14. Major sections of the judgment have been published in book form. See Kaihō Shuppansha, ed., *Hansenbyō kokubai soshō hanketsu: Kumamoto chisai dai ichiji daiyoji* (Osaka: Kaihō Shuppansha, 2001).

15. Igarashi Masahiro, "Nihon no 'sengo hoshō saiban' to kokusaihō," *Kokusaihō gaikō zasshi* 1, no. 12 (2006): 1–28.

16. For an account of Sakaguchi's apology at one of the sanitaria, see "Kagawa de Sakaguchi kōrōsō Hansenbyō seisaku de shazai," *Asahi shinbun*, July 5, 2001, morning edition, 29.

17. Kokuritsu Hansenbyō Shiryōkan, eds., *Kokuritsu Hansenbyō Shiryōkan kaikan kinenshi* (Higashimurayama: Kokuritsu Hansenbyō Shiryōkan, 2007), 9.

18. Nichibenren Hōmu Kenkyū Zaidan, *Hansenbyō mondai ni kansuru kenshō kaigi saishū hōkokusho*, vol. 1 (Tokyo: Akashi Shoten, 2007), 7.

19. James Orr, *Victim as Hero: Ideologies of Peace and National Identity in Postwar Japan* (Honolulu: University of Hawai'i Press, 2001).

20. On the national museum, see Burns, "History, Testimony, and the Afterlife of Quarantine."

21. "Kokuritsu Hansenbyō Shiryōkan saikaikan," *Shiryōkan tayori* 55 (April 2007): 1.

22. See, for example, the blog posts by Yabumoto Masako, a former newscaster for Nihon TV, "Fukakai. Kokuritsu Hansenbyō Shiryōkan," *Yabumoto Masako no burogu*, September 26, 2007, http://ameblo.jp/yabumoto /entry-10048721209.html, and by Ogata Masahiro, an elementary schoolteacher, "Kokuritsu Hansenbyō Shiryōkan to Tama Zenshōen no kengaku," *Suzu tanoshii jugyō no kai*, July 18, 2009, http://www2.nsknet .or.jp/~mshr/report/hansensiryoukan.htm, both accessed October 26, 2017.

23. Prasenjit Duara, *Rescuing History from the Nation: Questioning Narratives of Modern China* (Chicago: University of Chicago Press, 1996).

24. Susan L. Burns, "From 'Leper Villages' to Leprosaria: Public Health, Medicine, and the Culture of Exclusion in Japan," in *Isolation: Policies and Practices of Exclusion*, ed. Alison Bashford and Carolyn Stranger, 97–110 (London: Routledge, 2003).

25. Here I am paraphrasing Rose and Nova, "Biological Citizenship."
26. Adriana Petryna, *Life Exposed: Biological Citizenship after Chernobyl* (Princeton, NJ: Princeton University Press, 2002).
27. See Rose, *Politics of Life Itself.*
28. Arai Yūki, *Kakuri no bungaku: Hansenbyō ryōyōjo no jiko hyōgenshi* (Tokyo: Shoshiarusu, 2011), 80.
29. I am borrowing the concept of "testimony management" from my student Keyao (Kyle) Pan.
30. Giorgio Agamben, *Homo Sacer: Sovereign Power and Bare Life* (Palo Alto, CA: Stanford University Press, 1998), 181.
31. Susan Sontag, *Illness as Metaphor and AIDS and Its Metaphors* (New York: Anchor Books, 1990), 3.
32. Bruno Latour, *The Pasteurization of France*, trans. Allen Sheridan and John Law (Cambridge, MA: Harvard University Press, 1993).
33. F. Reibel et al., "Update on the Epidemiology, Diagnosis, and Treatment of Leprosy," *Médecine et maladies infectieuses* 45 (2015): 384, 387; Marc Monot et al., "On the Origin of Leprosy," *Science* 308, no. 5724 (2005): 1040–1042.
34. Verena J. Schuenemann et al., "Genome-Wide Comparison of Medieval and Modern *Mycobacterium leprae*," *Science* 341, no. 6142 (2013): 179–183.
35. Peter Richards, "Leprosy: Myth, Melodrama, and Mediaevalism," *Journal of the Royal College of Physicians* 24, no. 1 (1990): 55; B. Tabuteau, "Combien de lépreux au Moyen Âge? Essai d'étude quantitative appliquée à la lèpre. Les exemples de Rouen et de Bellencombre au XIIIᵉ siècle," *Sources: Travaux historiques* 13 (1988): 23.
36. Schuenemann et al., "Genome-Wide Comparison of Medieval and Modern *Mycobacterium leprae*," 183.
37. Lorentz M. Irgens and Tor Bjerkedal, "Epidemiology of Leprosy in Norway: The History of the National Leprosy Registry of Norway from 1856 until Today," *International Journal of Epidemiology* 2, no. 1 (1973): 82.
38. L. M. Bechelli and V. Martinez Domingues, "The Leprosy Problem in the World," *Bulletin of the World Health Organization* 34, no. 6 (1966): 811–826.
39. J. Fitness, K. Tosh, and A. V. Hill, "Genetics of Susceptibility to Leprosy," *Genes and Immunity* 3 (2002): 441–452; Elizabeth A. Misch et al., "Leprosy and the Human Genome," *Microbiology and Molecular Biology Review* 74, no. 4 (2010): 589–620; Andrea Alter et al., "Leprosy as a Genetic Disease," *Mammalian Genome* 22, no. 1 (2011): 19–31.

40. J. Parascandola, "Chaulmoogra Oil and the Treatment of Leprosy," *Pharmaceutical History* 45, no. 2 (2003): 47–57.

41. Robert H. Gelder and Jacques Grosset, "The Chemotherapy of Leprosy: An Interpretive History," *Leprosy Review*, no. 83 (2012): 221–240; Diana L. Williams and Thomas P. Gillis, "Drug-Resistant Leprosy: Monitoring and Current Status," *Leprosy Review* 83 (2012): 269–281; P. R. Saunderson, "Drug Resistant *M. leprae*," *Clinical Dermatology* 34, no. 1 (2016): 79–81.

42. See "Leprosy Elimination," World Health Organization, http://www.who .int/lep/en/, accessed July 12, 2016.

Chapter 1: The Geography of Exclusion

1. Marian Ury, trans., *Tales of Times Now Past: Sixty-Two Stories from a Medieval Japanese Collection* (Berkeley: University of California Press, 1979), 129.

2. Mabuchi Kazuo et al., eds., *Nihon koten bungaku zenshū*, vol. 37, *Konjaku monogatari shū*, vol. 3 (Tokyo: Shogakkan, 2001), 136–141.

3. Niunoya Tetsuichi, "Chūsei hinin to 'rai' sabetsu," in *Hansenbyō: Haijo, sabetsu, kakuri no rekishi*, ed. Okiura Kazuteru and Tokunaga Susumu, 85–86 (Tokyo: Iwanami Shoten, 2001).

4. Ōyama Kyōhei, *Nihon chūsei nōsonshi no kenkyū* (Tokyo: Iwanami Shoten, 390–392). Cited in Janet R. Goodwin, "Outcasts and Marginals in Medieval Japan," in *The Routledge Handbook of Premodern Japanese History*, ed. Karl F. Friday (London: Routledge, 2017), 399. Thomas Kierstead, "Outcasts before the Law: Pollution and Purification in Medieval Japan," in *Currents in Medieval Japanese History: Essays in Honor of Jeffrey P. Mass*, ed. Gordon M. Berger et al. (Los Angeles: Figueroa Press, 2009), 289.

5. For a lengthy list of those classified as *hinin*, see Kierstead, "Outcasts before the Law," 273.

6. Amino Yoshihiko, *Chūsei no hinin to yūjo* (Tokyo: Akashi Shoten, 1994), 25–63.

7. Kuroda Toshio, *Nihon chūsei kokka to shūkyō* (Tokyo: Iwanami Shoten, 1975), 351–398. See also Goodwin, "Outcasts and Marginals in Medieval Japan," 300. The phrase "freakish and aberrant" is from Kierstead, "Outcasts before the Law," 286.

8. Niunoya Tetsuichi, *Kebiishi: Chūsei no kegare to kenryoku* (Tokyo: Heibonsha, 1986), 20–66.

9. Kierstead, "Outcasts before the Law," 290. The text of this document is included in Buraku Mondai Kenkyūjo, ed., *Burakushi shiryō senshū*,

vol. 1, *Kodai chūsei hen* (Kyoto: Buraku Mondai Kenkyūjo Shuppanbu, 1988), 230–231.

10. Ibid.

11. Yokoi Kiyoshi, *Chūsei minshū no seikatsu bunka* (Tokyo: Tōkyō Daigaku Shuppankai, 1975), 295–334.

12. Yokoi Kiyoshi, "Raisha," in *Chūsei no minshū to geinō*, ed. Kyoto Burakushi Kenkyūjo (Kyoto: Aunsha, 1986), 130.

13. Duncan Ryūken Williams, *The Other Side of Zen: A Social History of Sōtō Zen Buddhism in Tokugawa Japan* (Princeton, NJ: Princeton University Press, 2009), 109.

14. Burton Watson, trans. *The Lotus Sutra* (New York: Columbia University Press, 1993), 324.

15. Yokoi, "Raisha," 311–312. Kuroda Hideo has analyzed the collection of forty-five *kishōmon* held by the Buddhist establishment at Kōyasan, which date from 1276 to 1333, and notes that thirty-one of them mention *rai*. Kuroda Hideo, *Kyōkai no chūsei shōchō no chūsei* (Tokyo: Tōkyō Daigaku Shuppankai, 1986), 256.

16. Aida Nirō, *Nihon no komonjo ge* (Tokyo: Iwanami Shoten, 1954), 517–518. On *kishōmon*, see also Chichiwa Itaru, "Kishōmon nōto: Keiyaku no sahō," *Jinmin no rekishigaku* 78 (1984): 1–7.

17. Digital text is available on the "Kishōmon Komonjo" section of the Ueda City Digital Archive http://museum.umic.jp/ikushima/kishomon/03-saigusa .html, accessed December 12, 2013.

18. Quoted in Satomichi Tokuo, "Suzuki Shosan 'Inga monogatari' ni miru bukkyō shinkō no kitei," in *Kinsei no seishin seikatsu*, ed. Ōkura Seishin Bunka Kenkyūjo (Tokyo: Zoku Gunsho Ruiju Kanseikai, 1996), 480.

19. Yoshida Eijirō, "Yakushiji saikō no shuku mura to kyūrai shisetsu Nishiyama Kōmyōin," *Regional* 4 (2006): 2; Niunoya, *Kebiishi*, 73.

20. Kobayashi Shigefumi, "Kodai-chūsei no 'raisha' to shūkyō," in *Reikishi no naka no raisha*, ed. Fujino Yutaka (Tokyo: Yumiru Shuppan, 1996), 24–26.

21. Ibid., 47–48.

22. Yoshida, "Yakushiji saikō no shuku mura to kyūrai shisetsu Nishiyama Kōmyōin," 13.

23. On the Empress Kōmyō legend, see ibid., 32–36.

24. Janet R. Goodwin, *Alms and Vagabonds: Buddhist Temples and Popular Patronage in Medieval Japan* (Honolulu: University of Hawai'i Press, 1994).

25. Niunoya, *Kebiishi*, 73.

26. On the founding of the Kitayama shelter, see Suzuki Motozo, "Nara, Kitayama Jūhachikenko," *Jinsen* 7 (1936): 105–136. On the Nishiyama hostel, see Yoshida Eijirō, "Yakushiji saikō no shuku mura to kyūrai shisetsu Nishiyama Kōmyōin," *Regional* 4 (2006): 1–13. On the shelter at Kamakura, see ibid., 58–60.

27. For a positive view of the medieval leprosy hostels, see Shinmura Taku, *Nihon iryō shakaishi no kenkyū* (Tokyo: Hōsei Daigaku Shuppan, 1985).

28. Fujiwara Yoshiaki, "Chūsei zenki no byōsha to kyūsai," *Rettō no bunkashi* 3 (1986): 79–114.

29. The story is related in Kobayashi, "Kodai-chūsei no 'raisha' to shūkyō," 38–39. For criticism of Ninshō's work, see Yoshida Fumio, "Ninshō no shaki jigyō ni tsuite," in *Nihon ni okeru shakai to shūkyō*, ed. Kasahara Kazuo, 114 (Tokyo: Yoshikawa Kōbunkan, 1969); and Hosokawa Ryōichi, *Chūsei mibunsei to hinin* (Tokyo: Nihon Editā Sukūru, 1994), 144.

30. On clothing and outcast status, see Kawata Mitsuo, "Chūsei hisabetsunin no yosoi," in *Kawata Mitsuo chosakushū*, vol. 2 (Tokyo: Akashi Shoten, 1995).

31. Kuroda, *Kyōkai no chūsei shōchō no chūsei*, 254–255.

32. Ibid., 238–239, 249–255.

33. Shimosaka Mamoru, "Chūsei hinin no sonzai keitai: Kiyomizu-zaka 'Chōtōdō' kō," *Geinōshi kenkyū* 110 (1990): 1–22.

34. Caroline Walker Bynum, *Fragmentation and Redemption: Essays on Gender and the Human Body in Medieval Religion* (New York: Zone Books, 1991), 183.

35. Chimoto Hideshi, "'Katai' kō: Setsuwa ni okeru raisha no mondai," *Ōsaka kyōiku daigaku kiyō*, ser. 1, 36, no. 1 (1987): 41.

36. David L. Howell, *Geographies of Identity in Nineteenth-Century Japan* (Berkeley: University of California Press, 2005), 26.

37. Kobayashi Keiichirō, "Raibyōnin no shiyaku chōshūken," *Nihon rekishi* 115 (1958): 49–50.

38. Kobayashi Keiichirō, "Zenkōji no raibyōnin buraku," *Nihon rekishi* 233 (1967): 64–72.

39. Kobayashi Keiichiro, *Nagano-shi shikō: Zenkōji machi no kenkyū* (Tokyo: Yoshikawa Kōbunkan, 1969).

40. On the controversy, see Higashi Eizō, "*Nagano-shi shikō* no mondai wo meguru shaken," *Shin Nihon bungaku* 36, no. 9 (1981): 84–97, and no. 10 (1981): 92–96; Aoki Takaju, "Buraku shi kenkyū no hoshō to dōwa gyōsei: *Nagano-shi shikō* wo megutte," *Buraku* 33, no. 8 (1981): 55–61;

Aoki Takaju, "*Nagano-shi shikō* mondai sono ato," *Buraku* 33, no. 14 (1981): 54–67. Members of the Buraku Liberation League published a pamphlet in defense of their position. See Buraku Kaihō Dōmei Nagano-ken Rengōkai, eds., *Nagano-shi shikō to buraku kaihō no kadai* (Nagano-shi: Buraku Kaihō Dōmei Nagano-ken Rengōkai, 1981).

41. Kobayashi, *Nagano-shi shikō*, 453.

42. Quoted in Aoki, "Buraku shi kenkyū no hoshō to dōwa gyōsei," 57. Kobayashi's recollection is included in his "Watakushi no tachiba wo kangae," *Buraku* 36, no. 9 (1984): 42.

43. Aoki, "Buraku shi kenkyū no hoshō to dōwa gyōsei," 57.

44. Kobayashi, "Watakushi no tachiba wo kangae," 46.

45. Yokota Noriko, "'Monoyoshi' kō: Kinsei Kyōto no raisha ni tsuite," *Nihonshi kenkyū* 352 (1991): 1–29.

46. Ibid., 1.

47. Ibid., 4–6.

48. Ibid., 9.

49. On the spatial demarcation of outcast villages, see Miyamae Chikako, "Zen-kindai ni okeru raisha no sonzai keitai ni tsuite, ge," *Buraku kaihō kenkyū* 167 (2005): 81.

50. Yoshida Eijirō, "Kyūrai shisetsu Kitayama Jūhachikenko itenron no airo wo megutte," *Regional* 3 (2006): 61–96.

51. Okamoto Takehiro, "Sono ato no Kitayama Jūhachikenko," *Nara kenritsu dōwa mondai kankei shiryō sentā kenkyū kiyō* 19 (2015): 44.

52. Nara Daigaku Sōgō Kenkyūjo, eds., *Nara Daibutsumae ezuya Tsutsui-ke kokusei ezu shūsei* (Nara: Nara Daigaku Sōgō Kenkyūjo, 2002), 25, 28.

53. Yoshida, "Yakushiji saikō no shuku mura to kyōrai shisetsu Nishiyama Kōmyōin," 1–3.

54. Miyamae Chikako, "'Raijin koya' no kanshin to chiiki shakai," *Buraku kaihō kenkyū* 197 (2013): 18.

55. Matsushita Shirō, *Kyūshū hisabestsu burakushi kenkyū* (Tokyo: Akashi shoten, 1985), 230.

56. Suzuki Noriko, "Kinsei raibyōkan no keisei to tenkai," in *Rekishi no naka no raisha*, ed. Fujino Yutaka, 124–128 (Tokyo: Yumiru shuppan, 1996). NB: Suzuki was the maiden name of Yokoto Noriko.

57. Yamashita Takaaki, "Kinsei Sanuki ni okeru hisabetsumin no kenkyū," *Buraku kaihō kenkyū* 124 (1998): 50.

58. Ibid.; Matsushita, *Kyūshū hisabetsu burakushi kenkyū*, 234; Ōuchi Hirotaka, "Kinsei Mutsu no kuni nanbu ni okeru hisabetsu mibun no jittai," *Bessatsu Tōhokugaku* 5 (2003): 220.

59. Howell, *Geographies of Identity in Nineteenth-Century Japan*, 27.

60. Ōuchi Hirotaka, "Kinsei ni okeru hisabestu mibun no jittai," in *Higashi Nihon no kinsei buraku no gutaizō*, ed. Higashi Nihon Buraku Kaihō Kenkyūjo, 391–393 (Tokyo: Akashi Shoten, 1992).

61. Ibid., 386–390.

62. Suzuki, "Kinsei raibyōkan no keisei to tenkai," 126.

63. Miyamae, "'Raijin koya' no kanshin to chiiki shakai," 21.

64. Kujirai Chisato, *Kyōkai no genba: Fōkuroa no rekishigaku* (Ibaragi: Henkyōsha, 2006), 142–154.

65. Yokota, "'Monoyoshi' kō: Kinsei Kyōto no raisha ni tsuite," 1–2.

66. Usami Hideki, "Kyō rakuchū rakugai bachō: Kinsei Kyōto raisha no kanshinba zu," pt. 1, *Buraku mondai kenkyū* 114 (1991): 64–77; pt. 2, *Buraku mondai kenkyū* 115 (1992): 100–114.

67. Buraku Mondai Kenkyūjo, ed., *Buraku no rekishi: Kinki hen* (Kyoto: Buraku Mondai Kenkyūjo Shuppanbu, 1982), 114–122.

68. Howell, *Geographies of Identity in Nineteenth-Century Japan*, 33–34.

69. Miyamae, "Zen kindai ni okeru raisha no sonzai keitai ni tsuite (ge)," 72–73.

70. Ōuchi, "Kinsei Mutsu no kuni nanbu ni okeru hisabetsu mibun no jittai," 224.

71. Matsushita, *Kyūshū hisabestsu burakushi kenkyū*, 230.

72. Ibid., 238.

73. Suzuki, "Kinsei raibyōkan no keisei to tenkai," 109.

74. See, for example, Miyagawa Ryō, "Kyūrai shiseki Nishiyama Kōmyōin ni tsuite," *Lepura* 6, no. 2 (1935): 93.

75. Miyamae, "'Raijin koya' no kanshin to chiiki shakai," 24–25.

76. Ibid.

77. Wakita Osamu, *Kawara makimono no sekai* (Tokyo: Tōkyō Daigaku Shuppankai, 1991), 304.

78. Miyamae, "'Raijin koya' no kanshin to chiiki shakai," 24–25.

79. Kobayashi, "Zenkōji no raibyōnin buraku," 72.

80. Kujirai, *Kyōkai no genba*, 141.

81. Miyamae, "'Raijin koya' no kanshin to chiiki shakai," 18.

82. Yamashita, "Kinsei Sanuki ni okeru hisabetsumin no kenkyū," 49–50; Teragi Nobuaki, "Kinsei ni okeru 'raisha' no shakaiteki ichi to seikatsu no shosokumen," in *Hansenbyō: Haijo, sabetsu, kakuri no rekishi*, ed. Okiura Kazuteru and Tokunaga Susumu, 102 (Tokyo: Iwanami Shoten, 2001).

83. Miyamae, "Zen kindai ni okeru raisha no sonzai keitai ni tsuite (ge)," 80.

84. Sawa Riichiro, "Nihon saisho no raibyōin ni tsuite," *Kyōto iji eisei shinbun* 100 (1902): 18.

85. On the involvement of the Buraku Liberation League, see Matsuda

Yoshinori, "Kitayama Jūhachikenko wo chūshin ni shita jinken no machizukuri," *Buraku kaihō* 542 (2003): 76.

86. Ibid.
87. Ibid.
88. "Kitayama Jūhachikenko no kengaku," Shiritsu Tsumizakakita Elementary School Homepage, 2012, http://www.naracity.ed.jp/ele04/index.cfm/20,2946,15,323,html, accessed July 22, 2016.

Chapter 2: From "Bad Karma" to "Bad Blood"

1. On Nakagami's background, see Kosoto Hiroshi, *Nihon kanpō tenseki jiten* (Tokyo: Taishūkan, 1999), 252.
2. Nakagami Kinkei, *Seiseidō idan* (Kyoto, 1795), in *KKIS*, vol. 17, 114. In identifying Edo-period medical texts on *rai*, I have benefited greatly from my reading of Harata Nobuo, "Tategaki de yonda rai," serialized in *Aisei*, nos. 387–415 (1972–1975).
3. Luke Demaitre, *Leprosy in Premodern Medicine: A Malady of the Whole Body* (Baltimore, MD: Johns Hopkins University Press, 2007), 19.
4. Angela Ki Che Leung, *Leprosy in China: A History* (New York: Columbia University Press, 2009), 19–20.
5. Tanba Yasunori, *Ishinpō*, vol. 3, ed. and trans. (modern Japanese) Maki Sachiko (Tokyo: Chikuma Shobō, 2002), 280.
6. Kosoto, *Nihon kanpō tenseki jiten*, 27.
7. Shinmura Taku, *Nihon iryō shakaishi no kenkyū* (Tokyo: Hōsei Daigaku Shuppankyoku, 1985), 209–210.
8. Koremune Tomotoshi, *Idansho*, ed. Minobe Shigekatsu (Tokyo: Miyai Shoten, 2006). *Rai* is discussed on 190–192. The quotation is from 191.
9. Andrew Edmund Goble, "Song Printed Medical Works and Medieval Japanese Medicine," in *Chinese Medicine and Healing: An Illustrated History*, ed. T. J. Hinrichs and Linda Barnes, 124 (Cambridge, MA: Belknap Press, 2013).
10. Kajiwara Seizen, *Ton'isho* (Tokyo: Kagaku Shoin, 1986), 534–545.
11. On the issue of medicalization, see Susan L. Burns, "Nanayama Jundō at Work: A Village Doctor and Medical Knowledge in Nineteenth-Century Japan," *East Asian Science, Technology, and Medicine* 29 (2008): 62–83.
12. Susan L. Burns, "The Body as Text: Confucianism, Reproduction, and Gender in Tokugawa Japan," in *Rethinking Confucianism: Past and Present in China, Japan, Korea and Vietnam*, ed. B. A. Elman, J. B. Duncan, and H. Ooms, 180–193 (Los Angeles: UCLA Asia Pacific Monograph Series, 2002).
13. Hartmut Rotermund, "Demonic Affliction or Contagious Disease?

Changing Perceptions of Smallpox in the Late Edo Period," *Japanese Journal of Religious Studies* 28, nos. 3–4 (2001): 373–398.

14. Daniel Trambaiolo, "Writing, Authority, and Practice in Tokugawa Medicine, 1650–1850" (PhD diss., Princeton University, 2014), chap. 4.

15. Satake Kūshaku, "Raibyō chiryō shinpō" (unpublished manuscript, n.d.), FYB-Kyoto.

16. "Sanbyō gorai wazurai no ken," Kobayashi Kyōichi Household Papers, no. H73-8-3 Kinsei, Archives of Gunma Prefecture.

17. Katsuki Gyūzan, *Kokuji isō*, vol. 5 (Kyoto: Ibaragi Tazaemon, 1737), National Diet Library, Rare Books and Old Materials Collection.

18. Minamisono Ishin, "Baisōchō" (manuscript, 1783), comp. Kuwabara Kenmei, n.p., FYB-Kyoto.

19. Okamura Wajun, *Iryōsatsu byōkō*, vol. 6 (Kyoto: Katsumura Jiuemon, 1831), 43–44, FYB-Kyoto.

20. Tatebe Seian, "Tenkei hiroku" (manuscript, 1785), n.p., Kyōu Shoya.

21. Katakura Kakuryō, *Bairai shinsho*, vol. 2 (Edo: Kyushokaku, 1786), 1–2, http://archive.wul.waseda.ac.jp/kosho/ya09/ya09_01176/, accessed February 2, 2018.

22. Hanaoka Seishū, "Tenkei hiroku" (manuscript, n.d.), n.p., FYB-Kyoto.

23. Ashikawa Keishū, *Byōmei ikai* (Kyoto, 1686), in *KKIS*, vol. 64, 329–331.

24. Tatebe Seian, "Tenkei hiroku," n.p.

25. Yamashita Yūhan (Genmon), *Iji sōdan* (Kyoto, 1850), FYB-Kyoto.

26. Katakura, *Bairai shinsho*, vol. 2, 1–2.

27. Kaibara Ekiken, *Yōjōkun*, ed. Matsuda Michio (Tokyo: Chūō Kōronsha, 1973), 59.

28. Ibid., 106–112.

29. Burns, "Body as Text," 178–219.

30. For examples of such work, see Yamamoto Masanori, ed., *Kakunshū* (Tokyo: Heibonsha, 2001).

31. Leung, *Leprosy in China*, 57.

32. Minamisono, "Baisōchō," n.p.

33. Tatebe Seian, "Tenkei hiroku," n.p.

34. Hans Martin Krämer, "'Not Befitting Our Divine Country': Eating Meat in Japanese Discourses of Self and Other from the Seventeenth Century to the Present," *Food and Foodways* 16 (2008): 33–62.

35. Arimochi Keiri, *Kōsei hōyogei* (pub. 1819), in *KKIS*, vol. 87, 483; Honma Sōken, *Ekika hiroku* (pub. 1847), in *KKIS*, vol. 114, 168.

36. Murai Kinzan, *Wahō ichimanpō*, in *Kinsei rekishi shiryō shūsei*, ed. Asami Megumi and Yasuda Kei, ser. 3, vol. 6, *Minkan chiryō* (Tokyo: Kasumigaseki Shuppan, 1995), 1941–1954.

37. Ibid., 1945–1948.
38. On Kitayama, see Tachibana Terumasa, *Nihon igaku senjin den: Kodai kara Bakumatsu made* (Tokyo: Ijiyakugyō Shinpōsha, 1969), 93–94.
39. On menstrual blood and leprosy, see, for example, Susan Zimmerman, "Leprosy in the Medieval Imagination," *Journal of Medieval and Early Modern Studies* 38 (2008): 559–587.
40. Kitayama Jūan, "Jishūroku" (manuscript, n.d.), n.p., FYB-Kyoto.
41. Charlotte Furth, *A Flourishing Yin: Gender in China's Medical History, 960–1665* (Berkeley: University of California Press, 1999), 58.
42. Katakura, *Bairai shinsho*, vol. 2, 2.
43. Arimochi, *Kōsei hōyogei*, 489–490.
44. For a discussion of the dangers posed by wet nurses, see Okamura Wajun, *Iryōsatsu byōkō*, 43–44.
45. Katakura, *Bairai shinsho*, vol. 2, 10–11.
46. Honma Sōken, *Ekika hiroku*, 164.
47. Ui Masatatsu, *Iryō sadan*, vol. 3 (Wakayama: Suharaya Mohē, 1830), 29–30, Tokyo University Library.
48. "Raifū ryōchi hiden" (manuscript, n.d.), personal collection of the author.
49. Murakami Ryōan, "Riraifū" (manuscript, 1785), n.p., FYB-Keiō.
50. Ibid.
51. Tatebe Seian, "Tenkei hiroku," n.p.
52. Timon Screech, *The Lens within the Heart: The Western Scientific Gaze and Popular Imagery in Later Edo Japan* (Cambridge: Cambridge University Press, 1996), esp. chap. 3.
53. Nakagami, *Seiseidō idan*, 112–113; Katakura, *Bairai shinsho*, vol. 2, 3–4.
54. Gotō Gonzan (Konzan), *Byōin kō* (manuscript, n.d.), n.p., FYB-Keio.
55. Hanaoka, "Tenkei hiroku"; Minamisono, "Baisōchō"; Honma, *Ekika hiroku*.
56. Leung, *Leprosy in China*, 55.
57. Hoashi Banri, "Raifūben" (manuscript, n.d.), n.p., FYB-Kyoto.
58. Yamazaki Teijirō, *Kinsei Nihon no iyaku bunka: miira, ahen, kōhī* (Tokyo: Heibonsha, 1995), 73.
59. On bloodletting, see Mieko Macé, "Dissection, Blood-Letting and Medicine as per Yamawaki Tōmon and Ogino Gengai," in *East Asian Science: Tradition and Beyond. Papers from the Seventh International Conference on the History of Science in East Asia, Kyoto, 2–7 August 1993*, ed. Hashimoto Keizō, Catherine Jami, and Lowell Skar, 353–357 (Osaka: Kansai University Press, 1995); Frederik Cryns, "Ranpō-i ga juyō shita jūhasseiki no seiyō iryō: chiryō no konkyo to riron tenkai," in *Jūhasseiki Nihon no bunka jōkyō to kokusai kankyō*, ed. Kasaya Kazuhiko, 103–119

(Kyoto: Shibunkaku Shuppan, 2011); Trambaiolo, "Writing, Authority, and Practice in Tokugawa Medicine," chap. 5.

60. Trambaiolo, "Writing, Authority, and Practice in Tokugawa Medicine," 189.

61. Katakura, *Bairai shinsho*, vol. 2, 3–6.

62. Nakagami, *Seiseidō idan*, 112–113.

63. Arimochi, *Kōsei hōyogei*, 490.

64. Katakura, *Bairai shinsho*, vol. 2, 10–11.

65. Arai Nobuaki, "Akago yōkun i-ro-ha uta," in *Nihon jinkōshi no kenkyū*, ed. Takahashi Bonsen, 851–855 (Tokyo: Sanyūsha, 1941).

66. Duncan Ryūken Williams, *The Other Side of Zen: A Social History of Sōtō Zen Buddhism in Tokugawa Japan* (Princeton, NJ: Princeton University Press, 2009), 108–110.

67. Sōda Hajime Collection, International Center for Japanese Studies Library, Kyoto.

68. Funagoshi Keiyū (Shin), *Ehon baisō gundan* (Osaka: Zorokutei, 1838), n.p. (advertisement inserted at the end of vol. 3), FYB-Kyoto.

69. Ibid., vol. 2; Funagoshi Keiyū, *Baisō chiken* (Osaka: Miyaji Kensuke, 1843), 45, http://libir.josai.ac.jp/contents/josai/kanpou/JOS-5201020061/index.html, accessed February 2, 2018.

70. Yanagiya Keiko, *Kinsei no josei sōzoku to kaigo* (Tokyo: Yoshikawa Kōbunkan, 2007), 202–203, 225.

Chapter 3: Rethinking Leprosy in Meiji Japan

1. Miyagawa Ryō, "Kyūrai shiseki Nishiyama Kōmyōin ni tsuite," *Lepura* 6, no. 2 (1935): 94–95.

2. Ibid., 98.

3. Yokota Noriko, "'Monoyoshi' kō: Kinsei Kyōto no raisha ni tsuite," *Nihonshi kenkyū* 352 (1991): 27.

4. Memorandum, May 18, 1874, document 606.B3.O3, TMA. A manuscript copy of "Repurabyō kō," dated 1874, is available in the FYB-Kyoto. Page numbers refer to this version of the text. I was alerted to the sources in the TMA by Yamaguchi Junko, "Gotō Masafumi Masanao fushi to Kihai Byōin no jiseki ni tsuite," *Hansenbyō shimin gakkai nenpō* (2005): 115–132.

5. Tsuda Kenpei, ed., *Meiji risshi hen* (Tokyo: Mochizuki Makoto, 1881), 81–90, NDL-Digital.

6. Tōfū Kyōkai, ed., *Mitsuda Kensuke to Nihon no rai yobō jigyō: Rai yobōhō gojūnen kinen* (Tokyo: Tōfū Kyōkai, 1958), 282–284.

7. Petition addressed to Iwakura Tomomi, 1880, document 265-0286, NAJ.

8. Shiomi Sen'ichirō, *Binmin no teito* (Tokyo: Bungei Shinsho, 2008), chap. 1.

9. *Nisshin shinjishi*, July 1, 1873. Quoted in Yamaguchi, "Gotō Masafumi Masanao fushi to Kihai Byōin no jiseki ni tsuite," 116.

10. For the provisions of the Medical Policy, see Kōseisho, ed., *Isei hachijūnenshi* (Tokyo: Insatsu Chōyōkai, 1955), 477–484.

11. Gotō, *Repurabyō kō*, 7–8.

12. Ibid., 1.

13. Ibid.

14. "Gotō Masafumi yori raibyō kanja kensa negai," document 608.A5.01, TMA.

15. Miyagi kenshi hensan iinkai, ed., *Miyagi kenshi*, vol. 18, *Iyaku taiiku* (Sendai: Miyagi Kenshi Kankōkai, 1959), 226–227, 231.

16. The report is reprinted in Naimusho, ed., *Meiji-ki eiseikyoku nenpō*, vol. 2, ed. Matsuda Takeshi (Tokyo: Tōyō Shorin, 1992), 262–267.

17. "Gotō Masafumi yori raibyō kanja kensa negai," document 608.A5.01, TMA.

18. "Gotō Masafumi yori raibyō kanja kensa sumi no todoke," document 608.C8.03, TMA.

19. *Yomiuri shinbun*, July 12, 1876, morning edition, 2.

20. *Yomiuri shinbun*, December 17, 1878, morning edition, 1.

21. *Tokyo nichi nichi shinbun*, July 6, 1873, 4.

22. See, for example, *Yomiuri shinbun*, April 14, 1875, 1; October 15, 1877, 3; February 17, 1878; March 21, 1878.

23. *Yomiuri shinbun*, February 17, 1878, 3.

24. *Chōya shinbun*, December 6, 1877.

25. Yamaguchi, "Gotō Masafumi Masanao fushi to Kihai Byōin no jiseki ni tsuite," 122; Kaneko Junji, *Nihon seishin igaku nenpyō* (Tokyo: Nihon Seishinbyōin Kyōkai, 1973), 150.

26. Attendance figures are cited in Tōfū Kyōkai, *Mitsuda Kensuke to Nihon no rai yobō jigyō*, 2–3. Gotō later published the text of his speech as a pamphlet. See Gotō Masafumi, *Gotō Masafumi Sensei Kōfu Mitsui-za enzetsu daiyō* (Tokyo: Aizensha, 1883), NDL-Digital. The quotation is from 3.

27. "Ryōbyōin ni tsuite no ikken," in "Kyōto-fu shiryō," document 59003-64, NAJ.

28. On the clinic in Ibaragi in Tochigi Prefecture, see *Yomiuri shinbun*, November 30, 1878, morning edition, 2. On Maebashi, see *Yomiuri shinbun*, February 22, 1879, morning edition, 1. On the Osaka hospital, see *Asahi shinbun*, April 24, 1881, morning edition, 3.

29. Petition to Iwakura Tomomi, 1880, document 265-0286, NAJ.

30. Akita-ken, ed., *Akita-ken shi*, vol. 5, *Meiji hen* (Akita: Akita-ken, 1979), 1179.

31. For statistics on average wages, see Japan Statistical Association, ed., *Historical Statistics of Japan*, vol. 4, *Labor, Wages, Housing, Prices* (Tokyo: Japan Statistical Association, 1987), 228–229.

32. Gotō Masafumi and Gotō Masanori, *Nanbyō jiryō* (Tokyo: Gotō Yakufu, 1882), pt. 1, 13–15, NDL-Digital. Similar metaphors are used in pt. 2, 13–14.

33. Ibid., pt. 2, 1–6.

34. Ibid.

35. The ad is reproduced in Hanejima Tomoyuki, ed., *Shinbun kōkoku bijutsu taikei Meiji hen*, vol. 1, *Iyaku keshō hen* (Tokyo: Ōzorasha, 1999), 45. Japan Statistical Association, *Historical Statistics of Japan*, vol. 4, 228–231.

36. *Asahi shinbun*, October 16, 1891, morning edition, 6.

37. Kaneko, *Nihon seishin igaku nenpyō*, 166.

38. Gotō and Gotō, *Nanbyō jiryō*, pt. 1, 38.

39. Ibid., pt. 1, 7.

40. Kobayashi Hiroshi, *Chirai shinron* (Tokyo: Shimamura Masanosuke, 1884), 30, NDL-Digital.

41. Ibid., 30.

42. Ibid., 25.

43. Ibid., 134.

44. Ibid.

45. Ibid., 140–150.

46. Murata Kentarō, "Raibyō no chiryō," *Tōkyō igakkai zasshi*, vol. 1, no. 4 (1887): 179–186.

47. Arai Saku, *Chirai keiken setsu* (Tokyo: Hashimoto Masashi, 1890), 8–13, NDL-Digital.

48. *Yomiuri shinbun*, March 9, 1883, morning edition, 1.

49. Kubo Takeo, director of the Kusuri no Doshōmachi Shiryōkan (Osaka), provided the biographical information on Mori.

50. Mori Kichibei, *Tsuzoku raibyō monogatari* (Osaka: Mori Kichibei, 1887), 2–3, NDL-Digital.

51. Douglas R. Howland, *Translating the West: Language and Political Reason in Nineteenth-Century Japan* (Honolulu: University of Hawai'i Press, 2001), 123–127.

52. Takayanagi Shinobu, "Nakamura Masanao to Yan Fu ni okeru J. S. Miru 'Jiyūron' honyaku no imi," Kyoto University, Institute for Research on

the Humanities, http://www.zinbun.kyoto-u.ac.jp/~rcmcc/h2-takayanagi. pdf, accessed November 15, 2017.

53. Yamaguchi, "Gotō Masafumi Masanao fushi to Kihai Byōin no jiseki ni tsuite," 121.

54. Arai Saku, *Chirai keikensetsu* (Tokyo: Hashimoto Masashi, 1890), 15–16, NDL-Digital.

55. Wei-ti Chen, "Cosmopolitan Medicine Nationalized: The Making of Japanese State-Empire and Migrant Physicians in a Global World" (PhD diss., University of Chicago, 2016), chap. 2.

56. Mitsuda Kensuke reportedly stated that Arai "had a bad reputation and was rumored to be a fraud," a view that contrasts with his favorable assessment of the Gotōs. Tōfū Kyōkai, *Mitsuda Kensuke to Nihon no rai yobō jigyō*, 3.

57. Kaji Jingo and Narita Ryūichi, eds., *Katō Tokijirō senshū* (Tokyo: Kōryūsha, 1981), 687–690.

58. Mori Shūichi and Ishii Norihisa, "Hansenbyō to igaku 1: Kakuri seisaku no teishō to sono haikei," *Japanese Journal of Leprosy* 75, no. 1 (2006): 8.

59. Ota Kōsaku, *Treatise on the Obstinate Herpes, as to Its Description, Pathology, Etiology, and Diagnosis* (Tokyo: Z. Maruya, 1888), NDL-Digital.

60. Ota Kōsaku, *Raibyō byōri benmō* (Tokyo: Moribe Kanshichi, 1891), NDL-Digital. For the discussion of smallpox vaccine and leprosy, see 23–27.

61. Quoted in Shimizu Kairyu, "Shūkyō Byōin DaiNihon Kyūsekan wo meguru jinbutsuzō: Ota Kōsaku," in *Indo bukkyōshi bukkyōgaku ronsō: Nakazawa Kōyū Hakushi koki kinen ronbunshū*, ed. Nakazawa Kōyū Hakushi koki kinen ronbunshū kankōkai, 364 (Tokyo: Sankibō Busshorin, 2011).

62. DaiNippon Kyūsekan, *Shūkyō Byōin DaiNippon Kyūsekan setsuritsu no shūi* (Tokyo: Saitō Shumin, 1892), n.p., NDL-Digital.

63. Miyagawa, "Kyūrai shiseki Nishiyama Kōmyōin ni tsuite,"100–101.

Chapter 4: Between the Global and the Local

1. "Sōkōshichō ni oite raibyō kanja wo Tōkyō Kihai Byōin ni sen to suru ken," October 14, 1893–January 23, 1894, document B12082195200, Diplomatic Archives of the Japanese Ministry of Foreign Affairs.

2. Henry Brown, "A Summary of Leprosy Cases," in *San Francisco Municipal Reports, 1893–1894*, 1026–1034 (San Francisco: Jas. H. Barry, 1894).

3. On US immigration policy towards leprosy, see Walter Wyman, "National Control of Leprosy," *Transactions of the Congress of American*

Physicians and Surgeons (New Haven, CT: Congress of American Physicians and Surgeons, 1894), 10.

4. Zachary Gussow, *Leprosy, Racism, and Public Health: Social Policy in Chronic Disease Control* (Boulder, CO: Westview Press, 1989).

5. Sawano Masaki, *Raisha no sei: Bunmei kaika no jōken toshite no* (Tokyo: Seikyūsha, 1994), 166.

6. On nineteenth-century medical internationalism, see W. F. Bynum, "Policing Hearts of Darkness: Aspects of the International Sanitary Conferences," *History and Philosophy of the Life Sciences* 15, no. 3 (1993): 421–434.

7. Letter to J. O. Carter, October 3, 1879, Board of Health Records, Box 334-34, HSA.

8. D. B. Simmons, letter to Colonel Judd, March 13, 1881, Board of Health Records, Box 334-34, HSA.

9. "Hawaiikokujin Giruberuto fufu Kihai Byōin shutsuin no ken," document 613.D5.O5, TMA; "Kihai Byōin he Amerikajin Furansesu hoka ichimei nyūin," document 604.D7.04, TMA. See also *Yomiuri shinbun*, February 14, 1886, morning edition, 2.

10. Quoted in Anwei Skinsnes Law, *Kalaupapa: A Collective Memory* (Honolulu: University of Hawai'i Press, 2012), 185.

11. Correspondence, Gotō Masanao to the Board of Health, Board of Health Records, Box 334-24, HSA.

12. Law, *Kalaupapa*, 333.

13. "Kihai Byōin Amerikajin Jōji Gire tsuma narabi ni musume Sorē taiin no ken," document 619.D5.09, TMA.

14. Hajima Tomoyuki, ed., *Shinbun kōkoku bijutsu taikei, Meiji hen*, vol. 1 (Tokyo: Ōzorasha, 1999), 45.

15. S. Arai, "The Treatment of Leprosy: A Lecture," medical pamphlet collection, box 67, no. 102706, library of the New York Academy of Medicine.

16. Suzuki Noriko, "Kinsei raibyōkan no keisei to tenkai," in *Rekishi no naka no raisha*, ed. Fujino Yutaka, 133 (Tokyo: Yumiru Shuppan, 1996).

17. Kuryū Rakusen'en Kanja Jichikai, ed., *Fūsetsu no mon: Kuryū Rakusen'en kanja gojūnenshi* (Gumma: Kuryū Rakusen'en Kanja Jichikai, 1982), 10–11.

18. Eric T. Jennings, *Curing the Colonizers: Hydrotherapy, Climatology, and French Colonial Spas* (Durham, NC: Duke University Press, 2006), 8–9.

19. Narusawa Hiroyuki, "Kankō bunka to kindai onsen ryōyō: Kusatsu onsen to Eruvuin Berutsu," *Keizaigaku ronsō* 13, no. 1 (2004): 85–112.

20. Lewis Strange Wingfield, *Wanderings of a Globe-Trotter in the Far East* (London: R. Bentley and Sons, 1889), 123.

21. Basil Hill Chamberlain, *A Handbook for Travellers in Japan* (London: John Murray, 1891), 186–187.

22. Kuryū Rakusen'en Kanja Jichikai, 14–15; Furumi Kiichi, ed., "Yuno-sawa buraku rokujunen shikō" (1941), in *Kindai shomin seikatsushi*, vol. 20, *Byōki eisei*, ed. Minami Hiroshi (Tokyo: San'ichi Shobō, 1995), 426–427.

23. W. K. Burton, "Hot Bathing in Japan, the Kusatsu Baths, Cure of Leprosy," *Annals of Hygiene* 11, no 10 (October 1, 1891): 473–475. See also *Boston Medical and Surgical Journal* 129, no. 9 (December 21, 1893): 630–631; *New England Journal of Medicine* 129 (1893): 630.

24. Erwin von Bälz, "Das heisse Bad in physiologischer und therapischer Hinsicht," *Münchener Medizinische Wochenschrift* 40 (1893); 351–352. For reprints, see *Medical World* 11 (1893): 287; *Western Medical Reporter* 15 (1893): 156; *Canadian Lancet and Practitioner* 1 (1893): 21–22.

25. "Wonderful Japanese Baths, Where the Leprous Are Made Clean," *San Francisco Chronicle*, June 3, 1900, 23. See also "Kusatsu: The Painful Cure of Japan," *San Francisco Chronicle*, May 18, 1902, and the account of Kusatsu in J. H. Deforest, "Why Nik-ko Is Beautiful," *National Geographic* 19, nos. 1–6 (January–June 1908): 305–308.

26. J. M. Comelles, "The Role of Local Knowledge in Medical Practice: A Trans-historical Perspective," *Culture, Medicine, Psychiatry* 24, no. 1 (2000): 41–75.

27. Hoi-eun Kim, *Doctors of Empire: Medical and Cultural Encounters between Imperial Germany and Meiji Japan* (Toronto: University of Toronto Press, 2014), chap. 5.

28. Erwin von Bälz, "Beiträge zur Lehr von der Lepra," in *Lepra Studien*, ed. Gregor N. München, 22–32 (Hamburg: Verlag von Leopold Voss, 1885).

29. Jo Robertson, "Leprosy and the Elusive *M. leprae*: Colonial and Imperial Medical Exchanges in the Nineteenth Century," *História, Ciências, Saúde-Manguinhos* 10, supp. 1 (2003): 13–40.

30. Bälz, "Beiträge zur Lehr von der Lepra," 23.

31. Ibid., 27.

32. E. H. Ackernecht, "Anti-Contagionism between 1821–1867," *Bulletin of the History of Medicine* 22 (1948): 562–593.

33. Bälz, "Beiträge zur Lehr von der Lepra," 27–28.

34. R. Koch, *Die Lepra-Erkrankungen in Kreise Memel* (Jena: Verlag von Gustav Fischer, 1897). See also M. Hundeiker and H. Brömmelhaus, "Leprakranke in Deutchland und Einführung industriell hergestellter Lepramedikamente von 100 Jahnen," *Dermatologie in Kunst und Geschichte* 58 (2007): 899–903.

35. Erwin von Bälz, "Zur Lehre von der Lepra und ihrer Behandlung," *Berliner Klinische Wochenshrift* 34, no. 46 (November 15, 1897): 998.

36. Erwin von Bälz, "Zur Lehre von der Lepra und ihrer Behandlung," *Berliner Klinische Wochenshrift* 34, no. 47 (November 22, 1897): 1031–1034.

37. "Correspondence," *Philadelphia Medical Times*, January 16, 1875, 5.

38. Albert S. Ashmead, "Leprosy in Japan—Intermediary-Host Function in Its Propagation," *Journal of Cutaneous and Genito-Urinary Diseases* 8, no. 93 (June 1890): 220–227.

39. Albert S. Ashmead, "The Propagation of Leprosy," *New York Times*, September 19, 1901, 19.

40. See, for example, Hansen's remarks on Ashmead in International Congress of Leprosy, ed., *Mittheilungen und Verhandlungen der Internationalen Wissenschaftlichen Lepra-Conferenz zu Berlin im October 1897*, vol. 1 (Berlin: A. Hirschwald, 1897), 165.

41. See, for example, "Plan for National Colony of Lepers," *New York Times*, December 16, 1901, 2.

42. Albert S. Ashmead, "Opinions of a Noted Japanese Specialist in Matters of Leprosy," *Journal of Cutaneous Diseases and Genito-Urinary Diseases* 12 (January 1894): 107–117.

43. *San Francisco Chronicle*, July 4, 1896, 16; October 15–16, 1896, 8. Los Angeles, too, was importing the Gotōs' medicines in this year. See "Hope for the Lepers: Dr. Barber Will Import the Goto Remedy," *Los Angeles Times*, March 16, 1896, 7. Barber was a staff member at the Los Angeles County Hospital.

44. "Two Lepers Leave the Pesthouse," *San Francisco Chronicle*, October 24, 1896, 14.

45. Rod Edmond, *Leprosy and Empire: A Medical and Cultural History* (Cambridge: Cambridge University Press, 2006) 155.

46. Shubhada S. Pandya, "The First International Leprosy Conference, Berlin, 1897: The Politics of Segregation," *História, Ciências, Saúde-Manguinhos* 10, supp. 1 (2003): 161–177.

47. International Congress of Leprosy, *Mittheilungen und Verhandlungen der Internationalen Wissenschaftlichen Lepra-Conferenz*, vol. 1, v–x.

48. Sanjiv Kakar, "Leprosy in British India, 1860–1940: Colonial Politics and Missionary Medicine," *Medical History* 40 (1996): 215–230. On British unwillingness to engage with segregationists, see Pandya, "First International Leprosy Conference, Berlin, 1897," 171.

49. A. Nakagawa, "Progress of Kitasato's Institute for Infectious Disease at Tokio," *Science* 6, no. 39 (August 27, 1897): 314. For a skeptical report, see "Has Kitasato Found It?" *New York Times*, January 29, 1896, 4.

50. "Raibyō ni kansuru bankoku iji kaigi," *Yomiuri shinbun*, August 1, 1897, morning edition, 2.

51. Kitasato, "Statistik der Leprakrankheiten in Japan," in International Congress of Leprosy, *Mittheilungen und Verhandlungen der Internationalen Wissenschaftlichen Lepra-Conferenz*, vol. 3, 269.

52. K. Dohi, "Ueber die Lepa in Japan," in International Congress of Leprosy, *Mittheilungen und Verhandlungen der Internationalen Wissenschaftlichen Lepra-Conferenz*, vol. 1, 141–145.

53. Koyama Fūkusei Byōin Hyakunen Henshū Iinkai, ed., *Koyama Fūkusei Byōin Hyakunen shi* (Tokyo: Shunjusha, 1989), 12–42.

54. Kōzensha, ed., *Aru gunzō: Kōzensha no hyakunen no ayumi* (Tokyo: Nihon Kirisutokyōdan Shuppankyoku, 1978).

55. On Hannah Riddell, see Jingo Tobimatsu, *Hannah Riddell: Known in Japan as "The Mother of Lepers"* (Kumamoto: Kaishun Byōin Jimusho, 1937); and Julia Boyd's *Hannah Riddell: An Englishwoman in Japan* (Rutland, VT: Charles E. Tuttle, 1996).

56. Kakar, "Leprosy in British India, 1860–1940," 218.

57. D. George Joseph, "'Essentially Christian, Eminently Philanthropic': The Mission to Lepers in India," *História, Ciências, Saúde-Manguinhos* 10, supp. 1 (2003): 250.

58. See, for example, Lila Watt, "Life among the Lepers," *Missionary Review of the World* 8 (1897): 346, 348.

59. On the discussion of the colony model, see Susan L. Burns, "Reinvented Places: Tradition, Family Care, and Psychiatric Institutions in Japan," *Social History of Medicine*, September 25, 2017, https://doi.org/10.1093/shm/hkx066.

60. Lorentz M. Irgens and Tor Bjerkedal, "Epidemiology of Leprosy in Norway: The History of the National Leprosy Registry of Norway from 1856 until Today," *International Journal of Epidemiology* 2, no. 1 (1973): 85.

61. Pandya, "First International Leprosy Conference, Berlin, 1897," 171–172.

62. Joseph, "'Essentially Christian, Eminently Philanthropic,'" 252–253.

63. On leprosy policy in Iceland and Scandinavia, see Peter Richards, *The Medieval Leper and His Northern Heirs* (Totowa, NJ: Rowman and Littlefield, 1977), 93–94; on German policy, see Hundeiker and Brömmelhaus, "Leprakranke in Deutschland"; on Culion, see Warwick Anderson, *Colonial Pathologies: American Tropical Medicine, Race, and Hygiene in the Philippines* (Durham, NC: Duke University Press, 2006), chap. 6; on Colombia, see Diana Obregón, "The State, Physicians, and Leprosy in

Modern Colombia, in *Disease in the History of Modern Latin America*, ed. Diego Armus and Nancy Lews Stepan, 130–157 (Durham, NC: Duke University Press, 2003); on Penikese Island, see I. Thomas Buckley and Meg B. Springer, *Penikese: Island of Hope* (Brewster, MA: Stoney Brook Publishing, 1997); on leprosy policy in Australia, see Alison Bashford, *Imperial Hygiene: A Critical Study of Colonialism, Nationalism, and Public Health* (Basingstoke: Palgrave MacMillan, 2004), esp. chap. 4.

64. Inoue Ken, "Rai yobō hōsaku no hensen," *Aisei* (September 1955): 2–12.

65. D. N. Durrheim and R. Speare, "Global Leprosy Elimination: Time to Change More than the Elimination Date," *Journal of Epidemiology and Community Health* 57, no. 5 (2003): 316–317.

66. See, for example, the remarks of Saitō Hisao during the 1902 Diet session, "Raibyōsha torishimari ni kansuru kengian," *Shūgiin giji sokkiroku* no. 25 (March 6, 1902), in *KNHMSS, Senzenhen*, vol. 8, 3.

67. "Rai yobō ni kansuru hōritsuan," *Kizokuin giji sokkiroku*, no. 9 (February 26, 1907), in *KNHMSS, Senzenhen*, vol. 8, 58.

68. See, for example, "Raibyō no chiriteki bunbu oyobi meisho ni tsuite," *Dai Nihon shiritsu eiseikai zasshi*, no. 273 (February 26, 1906): 42.

69. Quoted in Fujino Yutaka, *Nihon fashizumu to iryō: Hansenbyō wo meguru jisshōteki kenkyū* (Tokyo: Iwanami Shoten, 1993), 12.

70. Nakayama Yasumasa, ed., *Shinbun shūsei: Meiji-hennenshi*, vol. 11 (Tokyo: Honpō Shoseki, 1982), 414.

71. Mitsuda Kensuke, "Raibyō kakurijo setsuritsu no hitsuyō ni tsuite," in *Mitsuda Kensuke to Nihon no rai yobō jigyō: Rai yobōhō gojūnen kinen*, ed. Tōfū Kyōkai, 3–7 (Tokyo: Tōfū Kyōkai, 1958).

72. Ibid., 6.

73. Ibid., 7.

74. Sawa Riichirō, "Nihon saisho no raibyōin ni tsuite, jō," *Kyōto iji eisei shi*, no. 101 (1902): 3.

75. Sawa Riichirō, "Nihon saisho no raibyōin ni tsuite, ge," *Kyōto iji eisei shi*, no. 100 (1902): 18.

76. Takahashi Seii, "Kyōto no raibyōin ni tsuite," *Kyōto iji eisei shi*, nos. 101–121 (1902–1904).

77. "Raibyōsha torishimari ni kansuru kengian," 3.

78. Quoted in Yamamoto Shun'ichi, *Nihon raishi* (Tokyo: Tokyo Daigaku Shuppankai, 1993), 56–57.

79. Kōseishō Imukyoku, ed., *Isei hyakunenshi* (Tokyo: Gyōsei, 1976): 264–266.

80. Komatsu Yoshio, *Kekkaku: Nihon kindaishi no uragawa* (Osaka: Seifūdō, 2000), 404.

81. William Johnston, *The Modern Epidemic: A History of Tuberculosis in Japan* (Cambridge, MA: Harvard East Asian Monographs, 1995), 220–228; the quotation is from 227–228.

82. Kōzensha, *Aru gunzō*, 77–80; Hirai Yuichirō, "Yōikuen kara Ihaien he: Hansenbyō seisaku zenya no issōwa," *Shibusawa kenkyū* 13 (2000): 65–82.

83. Tanaka Sukeichi, *Hagi no unda kindai Nihon no iseika Yamane Masatsugu* (Hagi: Daiaikai, 1967).

84. "Mansei oyobi kyū densenbyō yobō ni kansuru shitsumonsho," *Shūgiin giji sokkiroku*, no. 5 (May 28, 1903), in *KNHMSS, Senzenhen*, vol. 8, 7.

85. Ibid., 8.

86. Ikai Takaaki, *Hanna Rideru to Kaishun Byōin* (Tokyo: Sōryū Shuppan, 2005), 201.

87. *Densenbyō yobō hō kaisei hōritsuan iinkai kaigiroku dainikai* (February 6, 1905), in *KNHMSS, Senzenhen*, vol. 8, 23–24.

88. Kubota Seitarō, "Rai yobō seido sōsetsu tōji wo kaigan su," in *Kubota Seitarō ronshū*, ed. Nihon Shakai Jigyō Daigaku, 305–310 (Tokyo: Nihon Shakai Jigyō Daigaku, 1980).

89. Ibid., 306.

90. David R. Ambaras, *Bad Youth: Juvenile Delinquency and the Politics of Everyday Life in Japan* (Berkeley: University of California Press, 2005), 34.

91. Yoshida Hisaichi, "Kubota Seitarō to shakai jigyō," in Nihon Shakai Jigyō Daigaku, *Kubota Seitarō ronshū*, 536–542.

92. "Raiyobō hōan," *Shūgiin giji sokkiroku*, no. 21 (March 25, 1906), in *KNHMSS, Senzenhen*, vol. 8, 37–38.

93. Yamamoto, *Nihon raishi*, 65.

94. "Raiyobō ni kansuru hōritsuan," *Shūgiin giji sokkiroku*, no. 21 (February 17, 1907), in *KNHMSS, Senzenhen*, vol. 8, 51–52.

95. *Raiyobō hō ni kansuru hōritsuan tokubetsu iinkai giji sokkiroku*, no. 1 (March 5, 1907), in *KNHMSS, Senzenhen*, vol. 8, 67.

96. Ibid., 3.

97. Ibid., 2, 4, 5.

98. Ibid., 5.

99. Ibid., 7–8.

100. Ibid., 3, 5, 7.

101. Kubota, "Rai yobō seido sōsetsu tōji wo kaigan su," 307–309.

102. Ibid., 309.

Chapter 5: Not Quite Total Institutions

1. "The Christ-Treatment in Japan," *Without the Camp*, no. 64 (October 1912): 201.

2. Naimusho Eiseikyoku, ed., *Raikanja no kokuhaku* (Tokyo: Naimusho Eiseikyoku, 1923), 55–59.

3. Koyama Fūkusei Byōin Hyakunen Henshū Iinkai, ed., *Koyama Fūkusei byōin 100-nen shi* (Tokyo: Shunjusha, 1989), 40–42.

4. See, for example, Kokuritsu Hansenbyō Shiryōkan, ed., *Zensei Byōin wo aruku—Utsusareta 20-seiki zenhan no ryōyōjo* (Higashimurayama: Kokuritsu Hansenbyō Shiryōkan, 2010), 7.

5. Erving Goffman, *Asylums: Essays on the Social Situation of Mental Patients and Other Inmates* (Garden City, NY: Anchor Books, 1961).

6. Yamamoto Shun'ichi, *Zōho Nihon raishi* (Tokyo: Tōkyō Daigaku Shuppankai, 1993), 73.

7. Mitsuda Kensuke, *Kaishun byōshitsu: Kyūrai Gojūnen no kiroku* (Tokyo: Asahi Shinbun, 1950), 39.

8. "Fuka no raibyō ryōyōjo," *Asahi shinbun*, July 23, 1908, 3.

9. Katō Naoko, *Moto Minobu Jinkyōenchō Tsunawaki Michi-san ni kiku: Yama no naka no chiisana en ni te: Mōhitotsu no Hansenbyō shi* (Tokyo: Iryō Bunkashi, 2005).

10. "Meguro no hantai," *Asahi shinbun*, September 1, 1908, 6.

11. Meguro-ku Kyōdo Kenkyūkai, ed., *Meguro-ku no rekishi* (Tokyo: Meicho Shuppan, 1978), 110–111.

12. Kōzensha, ed., *Aru gunzō: Kōzensha no hyakunen no ayumi* (Tokyo: Nihon Kirisutokyōdan Shuppankyoku, 1978), 76.

13. "Meguro sonmin fuchō ni semaranto su," *Asahi shinbun*, October 20, 1908, 3; "Meguro sonmin mata sōshō," *Asahi shinbun*, October 28, 1908, 6.

14. Tōkyō Toritsu Daigaku Gakujutsu Kenkyūkai, ed., *Meguro-ku shi*, vol. 1 (Tokyo: Meguro-ku, 1961), 624–625.

15. Ibid., 627–628.

16. Ibid., 640.

17. "Meguro sonmin no ensei," *Asahi shinbun*, September 2, 1908, 6.

18. "Meguro sonmin mata sōshō," 6.

19. "Meguro sonmin daikyo," *Asahi shinbun*, September 7, 1908, 6.

20. Kōzensha, *Aru gunzō*, 86–87.

21. "Mata mata Meguro sonmin oshiyosu," *Asahi shinbun*, November 26, 1908, 4.

22. Higashimurayama-shi hensan iinkai, *Higashimurayama-shi shi*, vol. 2 (Tokyo: Higashimurayama, 1981), 253.

23. "Rai ryōyōjo kettei," *Asahi shinbun*, February 20, 1909, 2. Land values are discussed in Higashimurayama-shi hensan iinkai, *Higashimurayama-shi shi*, 253.

24. "Rai ryōyōjo kangei," *Asahi shinbun*, February 21, 1909, 5.

25. See "Raibyō sōdō kōban," *Asahi shinbun*, June 2, 1909, 2; "Rai ryōyōjo jiken no gimon," *Asahi shinbun*, June 13, 1909, 4; "Raibyō sōdō no benrin," *Asahi shinbun*, June 23,1909, 5.

26. Higashimurayama-shi hensan iinkai, *Higashimurayama-shi shi*, 253.

27. Ibid.

28. Itakura Kazuko, "Shiritsu rai ryōyōjo Biwasaki Tairōin no rekishi," *Nihon Hansenbyō gakkai zasshi* 61, no. 2 (1992): 112–116.

29. Kokuritsu Hansenbyō Shiryōkan, *Hyakunen no kakuri: Kōritsu rai ryōyōjo no tanjō* (Higashimurayama: Kokuritsu Hansenbyō Shiryōkan, 2009), 50.

30. Ibid., 36.

31. Ibid., 44.

32. Ibid., 28.

33. Mitsuda, *Kaishun byōshitsu*, 43–46.

34. Kokuritsu Hansenbyō Shiryōkan, *Hyakunen no kakuri*, 51.

35. Daniel Botsman, *Punishment and Power in the Making of Modern Japan* (Princeton, NJ: Princeton University Press, 2005), 198.

36. The plans for the institutions are reproduced in Kokuritsu Hansenbyō Shiryōkan, *Hyakunen no kakuri*, 20, 30, 38, 46, 54.

37. See, for example, the photographs in ibid., 21, 31.

38. Diagrams of the prefectural psychiatric hospital can be found in Okada Yasuo, *Shisetsu Matsuzawa Byōin shi, 1879–1980* (Tokyo: Iwasaki Gakujutsu Shuppankai, 1981), 58–59, 132–133.

39. Mitsuda, *Kaishun byōshitsu*, 41.

40. Yamamoto, *Zōho Nihon raishi*, 79.

41. Naimusho Eiseikyoku, *Raikanja no kokuhaku*, 157.

42. Ibid., 252–253.

43. Ibid., 28, 44, 166, 219.

44. Ibid., 162.

45. Ibid., 129, 241, 331.

46. On the Aomori sanitarium, see "Hokubu hoyōin wo tazuneru," *Tōoku nippō*, June 18, 1909, quoted in Kokuritsu Hansenbyō Shiryōkan, *Hyakunen no kakuri*, 33. On the Kyūshū Sanitarium, see Kokuritsu Ryōyōjo Kikuchi Keifūen, ed., *Kikuchi Keifūen 50-nen shi* (Kumamoto: Kokuritsu Ryōyōjo Kikuchi Keifūen, 1960), 135.

47. "Meiji 45-nen hōritsu daijūichigō chū kaisei hōritsuan iinkaigi roku, dai ikkai," March 2, 1916, in *KNHMSS, Senzenhen*, vol. 8, 2.

48. Mitsuda, *Kaishun byōshitsu*, 55.

49. "Rai kanja dashutsu ni kansuri ken," document 603.B2.18, TMA; "Zensei Byōin nai chitsujo ni kansuru ken," document 603.A5.13, TMA.

50. Mitsuda, *Kaishun byōshitsu*, 55–64.

51. Kokuritsu Ryōyōjo Kikuchi Keifūen, *Kikuchi Keifūen 50-nen shi*, 132–135.

52. Naimusho Eiseikyoku, ed., *Rai ryōyōjo shūyū kanja tōkei* (Tokyo: Naimusho Eiseikyoku, 1917), 2, 22–23.

53. Sakurazawa Fusayoshi, *Zensei konjaku* (Tokyo: Miwa Shōhō, 1991), 36.

54. Ibid., 34.

55. Kokuritsu Ryōyōjo Kikuchi Keifūen, *Kikuchi Keifūen 50-nen shi*, 47.

56. Kokuritsu Hansenbyō Shiryōkan, ed., *Kimono ni miru ryōyōjo no kurashi* (Tokyo: Kokuritsu Hansenbyō Shiryōkan, 1910).

57. On Zensei Hospital's responses to the runaway problem, see Sakurazawa, *Zensei konjaku*, 36–39; Mitsuda, *Kaishun byōshitsu*, 55–59; Mitsuda Kensuke, "Hori wo uzumuru made," in *Mitsuda Kensuke to Nihon no rai yobō jigyō: Rai yobōhō gojūnen kinen*, ed. Tōfū Kyōkai, 103–106 (Tokyo: Tōfū Kyōkai, 1958).

58. Mitsuda, *Kaishun byōshitsu*, 45–46; Sakurazawa, *Zensei konjaku*, 101.

59. Sakurazawa, *Zensei konjaku*, 46.

60. Kokuritsu Ryōyōjo Kikuchi Keifūen, *Kikuchi Keifūen 50-nen shi*, 46.

61. Kōzensha, *Aru gunzō*, 97–99.

62. Mitsuda, *Kaishun byōshitsu*, 77–78.

63. Sakurazawa, *Zensei konjaku*, 62–63; Mitsuda, *Kaishun byōshitsu*, 75–77.

64. Sakurazawa, *Zensei konjaku*, 49–51.

65. Kokuritsu Ryōyōjo Kikuchi Keifūen, *Kikuchi Keifūen 50-nen shi*, 143.

66. Yamamoto, *Zōho Nihon raishi*, 75. Mitsuda compared the funding of Zensei and the Northern Area Rest Home in *Kaishun byōshitsu*, 91.

67. Naimusho Eiseikyoku, *Raikanja no kokuhaku*, 247.

68. Mitsuda, *Kaishun byōshitsu*, 42; Sakurazawa, *Zensei konjaku*, 32, 43.

69. Mitsuda, *Kaishun byōshitsu*, 75.

70. Sakurazawa, *Zensei konjaku*, 57–59.

71. Naimusho Eiseikyoku, *Raikanja no kokuhaku*, 55–59.

72. Sakurazawa discusses wages in *Zensei konjaku*, 32–33. For information on wages outside the sanitaria, see Japan Statistical Association, ed., *Historical Statistics of Japan*, vol. 4, *Labor, Wages, Housing, Prices* (Tokyo: Japan Statistical Association, 1987), 230–231.

73. Sakurazawa, *Zensei konjaku*, 42, 143–144.

74. Ibid., 38–39.

75. Mitsuda, *Kaishun byōshitsu*, 40.

76. Ibid., 91.

77. Sakurazawa, *Zensei konjaku*, 105–106, 144–145, 149–158.

78. Mitsuda Kensuke, "Raibyō ni taisuru daifūshiyu no kachi," *Hifuka*

hinyōkika zasshi 12 (December 1912); J. Parascandola, "Chaulmoogra Oil and the Treatment of Leprosy," *Pharmaceutical History* 45, no. 2 (2003): 47–57.

79. Sakurazawa, *Zensei konjaku*, 74–76, 79.

80. "Meiji 40-nen hōritsu dai-jūichigō chū kaisei hōritsuan iin kaigiroku dai-ikkai," March 2, 1916, 78, in *KNHMSS, Senzenhen*, vol. 8, 78.

81. Ibid., 79.

82. Mitsuda, *Kaishun byōshitsu*, 46–47.

83. Mitsuda Kensuke, "Raibyō kanja danjo kyōdō shūyō wo ka suru iken," in Tōfū Kyōkai, *Mitsuda Kensuke to Nihon no rai yobō jigyō*, 55.

84. Naimusho Eiseikyoku, *Rai ryōyōjo shūyū kanja tōkei*, 5–8.

85. Mitsuda Kensuke, "Wazekutomī nijū shūnen," in Tōfū Kyōkai, *Mitsuda Kensuke to Nihon no rai yobō jigyō*, 233–234.

86. M. E. Duncan, "An Historical and Clinical Review of Leprosy and Pregnancy: A Cycle to Be Broken," *Social Science Medicine* 37, no. 4 (1993): 457–472.

87. Nakajō Suketoshi, "Shoseiji no shohatsu rai ni tsuite," *Hifuka hinyōkika zasshi* 14, no. 11 (1914): 1026, and "Sentenrai no kinketsusho narabini taiban rai ni tsuite," *Hifuka hinyōkika zasshi* 15, no. 6 (1915): 446. In 1938, a Japanese researcher would succeed in identifying *M. leprae* in placental tissue and cord blood. See M. L. Brubaker, "Leprosy in Children One Year of Age and Under," *International Journal of Leprosy and Other Mycobacterium Diseases* 53, no. 4 (1985): 517–523.

88. Sugai Takekichi and Monobe Kazuji, "Rai kanja shoseiji no keneki kensa to ketsueki no kensa," *Ōsaka igakkai zasshi* (1911); Sugai Takekichi and Kumatani Kensaburō, "Rai kanja no nūjūchū no kin," *Tōkyō iji zasshi* (1915); Sugai Takekichi and Miyahara Jun, "Rai kanja yōsuichū no ken," *Igaku chūō zasshi* (1915); Sugai Takekichi and Monobe Kazuji, "Kiō jūnenkan honkoku ryōyojo shūyō kanja benji no tōkei," *Hifuka hinyōkika zasshi* 21, no. 2 (1921).

89. Nichibenren Hōmu Kenkyū Zaidan, *Hansenbyō mondai ni kansuru kenshō kaigi saishū hōkokusho*, vol. 2 (Tokyo: Akashi Shoten, 2007), 1.

90. On the Declaration of Helsinki and its aftermath, see Charo Ra, "Body of Research: Ownership and Use of Human Tissue," *New England Journal of Medicine* 355 (2005): 1517–1519.

91. Duncan, "Historical and Clinical Review of Leprosy and Pregnancy," 457–472.

92. Mitsuda, *Kaishun byōshitsu*, 49.

93. Philip R. Reilly, *The Surgical Solution: A History of Involuntary Sterilization in the United States* (Baltimore, MD: Johns Hopkins University Press, 1991), 30–31.

94. Mitsuda, *Kaishun byōshitsu*, 53.

95. Ujihara Sukezo, annotated by Kitashima Ta'ichi, *Minzoku eiseigaku* (To-kyo: Naneidō Shoten, 1914), in Ogino Miho et al., eds., *Sei to seishoku no jinken mondai shiryō shūsei*, vol. 16 (Tokyo: Fuji Shuppan, 2000), 1–23.

96. Sheldon Garon, *Molding Japanese Minds: The State in Everyday Life* (Princeton, NJ: Princeton University Press, 1997), 103.

97. Mitsuda, *Kaishun byōshitsu*, 53–55.

98. Naimusho Eiseikyoku, ed., *Hoken eisei chōsakai dai-4 bu (rai) giji sokki roku* (Tokyo: Naimusho Eiseikyoku, 1920), 79.

99. Ibid., 6.

100. H. Riddel [*sic*], "Rai no kyūsai oyobi yobō mondai," *Nihon no ikai*, no. 124 (February 1914): 4–5.

101. Naimusho Eiseikyoku, *Hoken eisei chōsakai dai-4 bu (rai) giji sokki roku*, 7–9.

102. Ibid., 113–118.

103. Ibid., 21–24.

104. Ibid., 26–27.

105. Warwick Anderson, "States of Hygiene: Race 'Improvement' and Bio-medical Citizenship in Australia and the Colonial Philippines," in *Haunted by Intimacy: Geographies of Intimacy in North American History*, ed. Ann Laura Stoler, 94 (Durham, NC: Duke University Press, 2006).

106. C. B. Lara and C. A. Palafox, "The Care of Culion-Born Children," in *Culion: A Record of Fifty Years Work with the Victims of Leprosy at the Culion Sanitarium, Prepared by Members of the Staff and Patient Body* (Manila: Bureau of Printing, 1956), 28. My thanks to Jo Robertson for pointing me towards this source.

107. Naimusho Eiseikyoku, *Hoken eisei chōsakai dai-4 bu (rai) giji sokki roku*, 28–29.

108. Ibid., 51.

109. Ibid., 62–63.

110. Ibid., 68–69.

111. Ibid., 33–37.

112. Naimusho Eiseikyoku, *Raikanja no kokuhaku*, 1–2.

113. Ibid., 2.

114. Ibid., 144

115. Ibid., 101.

116. Ibid., 408.

117. Murakami Kimiko, "Kekkaku yobohō no seiritsu yōin ni kansuru kōsatsu," *Kansai Fukushi Daigaku shakai fukushi gakubu kiyō* 17, no. 1 (2013): 31–32.

118. Komatsu Yoshio, *Kekkaku: Nihon kindaishi no uragawa* (Osaka: Seifūdō, 2000), 268–271.

119. William Johnston, *The Modern Epidemic: A History of Tuberculosis in Japan* (Cambridge, MA: Harvard East Asian Monographs, 1995), 248.

120. Utsunomiya Minori, "Taisho 8-nen Seishin Byōinhō no rippō teian to sono giron," *Kinjō Gakuin Daigaku ronshū shakaigakuhen* 8, no. 1 (2011): 6.

121. Kure Shūzō, *Seishinbyō no shitaku kanchi no jikkyō* (Tokyo: Naimusho Eiseikyoku, 1918).

122. Utsunomiya, "Taisho 8-nen Seishin Byōinhō no rippō teian to sono giron," 11.

123. Kan Osamu, "Honpō ni okeru seishinbyōsha narabi ni kore ni kensetsu suru seishin ijōsha ni kansuru chōsetsu," *Shinkeigaku zasshi* 41, no. 10 (1937): 52.

124. Kōseishō Imukyoku, ed., *Isei hachijūnenshi* (Tokyo: Gyōsei, 1976), 747.

Chapter 6: The National Culture of Leprosy Prevention

1. From a Leprosy Prevention Day poster in *KNHMSS, Senzenhen*, Hokan 9, 177.

2. Rai Yobō Kyōkai, ed., *Raisha sakuhin eiga sosaishū* (n.p.: Rai Yobō Kyōkai, 1933), 119.

3. Naimushō Eiseikyoku, ed., "Rai yobō ni kansuru ken," in *KNHMSS, Senzenhen*, vol. 2, 131.

4. Quoted in Yamamoto Shun'ichi, *Zōho Nihon raishi* (Tokyo: Tokyo Daigaku Shuppankai, 1997), 164.

5. Naimusho Eiseikyoku, *Rai ryōyōjo shūyū kanja tōkei* (Tokyo: Naimusho Eiseikyoku, 1917), 10.

6. Naimushō Eiseikyoku, "Rai yobō ni kansuru ken," 131.

7. For an account of Yunosawa that relies heavily on oral history, see Kuryū Rakusen'en Kanja Jichikai, ed., *Fūsetsu no mon: Kuryū Rakusen'en kanja gojūnenshi* (Gumma: Kuryū Rakusen'en Kanja Jichikai, 1982). For a work based on documentary evidence, see Hirokawa Waka, *Kindai Nihon no Hansenbyō mondai to chiiki shakai* (Osaka: Osaka Daigaku Shuppankai, 2011), chaps. 2–3.

8. Kuryū Rakusen'en Kanja Jichikai, *Fūsetsu no mon*, 38–39.

9. Mitsuda Kensuke, "Meiji yonjūninen igo ni ha Kusatsu ni okeru raikanja wa ikan ni shochi serarubeki ya" (1910), in *Mitsuda Kensuke to Nihon no rai yobō jigyō: Rai yobōhō gojūnen kinen*, ed. Tōfū Kyōkai, 33 (Tokyo: Tōfū Kyōkai, 1958).

10. Kuryū Rakusen'en Kanja Jichikai, *Fūsetsu no mon*, 30–36.

11. Ibid., 33.

12. For criticism of Kusatsu, see Naimusho Eiseikyoku, ed., *Raikanja no kokuhaku* (Tokyo: Naimusho Eiseikyoku, 1923), 224–225, 232–233.
13. Mary Cornwallis-Legh, *Church Work for Lepers in Japan* (New York: National Council, Protestant Episcopal Church, Department of Missions, n.d.), 16, pamphlet collection, Archives of the Episcopal Church, Austin, Texas.
14. "Rai yobō kankei hōki kaisei ni kansuru kengian," Dai 44-kai teikoku gikai shūgiin giji sokki kiroku, quoted in Yamamoto Shun'ichi, *Zōhō Nihon raishi* (Tokyo: Tokyo Daigaku Shuppankai, 1997), 165.
15. Ibid., 13.
16. Hirokawa, *Kindai Nihon no Hansenbyō mondai to chiiki shakai*, 152–153.
17. Ibid., 117–122.
18. Mitsuda Kensuke, *Kaishun byōshitsu: Kyūrai Gojūnen no kiroku* (Tokyo: Asahi Shinbun, 1950), 92.
19. Eiseikyoku Chōsabu, *Kaku chihō ni okeru rai buraku rai shūgōchi ni kansuru gaikyō* (Tokyo: Naimusho Eiseikyoku, 1920), in *KNHMSS, Senzenhen*, vol. 2, 97–113.
20. Lois Danner, "Cleansing Lepers Today in Kusatsu, Japan: An Account of a Visit to an Appealing Missionary Center Where Bishop McKim Ministers," *Spirit of Missions* (May 1926): 292.
21. J. B. Teusler, letter to Rev. John McKim, November 15, 1926, Archives of the Episcopal Church, Austin, Texas.
22. Hirokawa, *Kindai Nihon no Hansenbyō mondai to chiiki shakai*, 146–147.
23. Ellen J. Amster, *Medicine and the Saints: Science, Islam, and the Colonial Encounter in Morocco, 1877–1956* (Austin: University of Texas Press, 2013), 76–77.
24. Émile Marchoux, ed., *IIIe conférence international de la lepre: Strasbourg, 28 au 31 juillet 1923: communications et débats* (Paris: J. B. Baillière et Fils, 1924), 8–15.
25. Ibid., 493–502.
26. Donald H. Currie, "The Second International Conference on Leprosy, Held in Bergen, Norway," *Public Health Reports* 24, no. 38 (September 17, 1909): 1537–1561.
27. Marchoux, *IIIe conférence international de la lepre*, 507–508.
28. Ibid., 181.
29. Ibid.,186–187.
30. Mitsuda Kensuke, *Apercu général sur le traitement de la lèpre au Japon, présenté à la troisième Conférence international scientifique de la lèpre réunie à Strasbourg, le 28 juillet 1923* (Paris: Presses Universitaires, 1923).

31. Mitsuda, *Kaishun byōshitsu*, 96–97.

32. Ibid., 97.

33. Mitsuda Kensuke, "Hoken eisei chōsakai iin Mitsuda Kensuke Okinawa-ken Okayama-ken oyobi Taiwan shutchō fukumeisho," in *KNHMSS, Senzenhen*, vol. 2, 28.

34. Mitsuda, *Kaishun byōshitsu*, 123.

35. Mitsuda, "Nagashima no sentaku," *Aisei*, no. 1 (1931).

36. Mitsuda, *Kaishun byōshitsu*, 123.

37. Nagashima Aiseien Iankai, ed., *Nagashima kaitaku* (Tokyo: Nasasaki Shoten, 1932), in *KNHMSS, Senzenhen*, vol. 3, 57.

38. Ibid., 130.

39. Hirokawa, *Kindai Nihon no Hansenbyō mondai to chiiki shakai*, 312–314.

40. Fujino Yutaka, *Nihon fashizumu to iryō: Hansenbyō wo meguru jisshōteki kenkyū* (Tokyo: Iwanami Shoten, 1993), 90.

41. Hirokawa, *Kindai Nihon no Hansenbyō mondai to chiiki shakai*, 71–73.

42. Dai 59-kai Teikoku Gikai Kizokuin, *Eisei kumiai hōan tokubetsu iinkaigiji sokkiroku*, daisangō, February 14, 1931, in *KNHMSS, Senzenhen*, vol. 8, 28.

43. Dai 59-kai Teikoku Gikai Shūgiin, *Kisei chūbyō yobōhō annai hoka ikken iinkaigiroku (sokki)*, daiyonkai, February 28, 1931, in *KNHMSS, Senzenhen*, vol. 8, 133.

44. Ibid., 135–136.

45. Ibid., 139–140.

46. Ibid., 140.

47. "Kanja shūyōbō" (1931), in *NHK*, vol. 1, 75–78.

48. "Nyūtaien jōkyō ni tsuki chōsa tōkei," in *NHK*, vol. 1, 197.

49. Nagashima Aiseien Nyūensha Jichikai, ed., *Kakuzetsu no ritei: Nagashima Aiseien nyūensha 50-nenshi* (Okayama: Nagashima Aiseien Nyūensha Jichikai, 1982), 126.

50. Information on the finances and membership of the organization can be found in Zaidan Hōjin Rai Yobō Kyōkai, ed., *Showa roku nendo jigyō seiseki hōkokusho* (Tokyo: Zaidan Hōjin Rai Yobō Kyōkai, 1933), in *KNHMSS, Senzenhen*, vol. 3, 133–185.

51. Ibid., 72. On outpatient care, see Kokuritsu Ryōyōjo Kikuchi Keifūen, ed., *Kikuchi Keifūen 50-nen shi* (Kumamoto: Kokuritsu Ryōyōjo Kikuchi Keifūen, 1960), 66.

52. Kuryū Rakusen'en, *Rakusen'en nenpō Showa 9-nen* (Kusatsu: Rakusen'en, 1935), 49.

53. An example of an intake form can be found in *KNHMSS, Senzenhen*, Hokan 9, 161.

54. Calculated from information in the chart in Kokuritsu Ryōyōjo Kikuchi Keifūen, *Kikuchi Keifūen 50-nen shi*, 66.
55. Zaidan Hōjin Rai Yobō Kyōkai, *Rai no hanashi* (Tokyo: Zaidan Hōjin Rai Yobō Kyōkai, 1931), in *KNHMSS, Senzenhen*, vol. 2, 356.
56. Ibid., 357.
57. Nagashima Aiseien Iankai, *Toppō jūtaku* (Okayama: Sanyō Shinbunsha, 1934), in *KNHMSS, Senzenhen*, vol. 3, 288.
58. Ibid., 287.
59. Ibid., 294.
60. On the leprosy-free prefecture movement, see Satō Tsutomu's "Hansenbyō 'muraiken undō' no hatten ni tsuite," *Hansenbyō shimin gakkai nenpō*, no. 3 (2007): 44–53.
61. Naimusho Eiseikyoku, *Raikanja tōkei* (1922), in *KNHMSS, Senzenhen*, vol. 2, 141–142; Tottori-ken Sōmubu Sōmuka Kenshi Hensanshitsu, *Tottori-ken no muraiken undō: Hansenbyō no kindaishi* (Tottori-shi: Tottori Heibonsha, 2008), 37–38.
62. Tottori-ken Sōmubu Sōmuka Kenshi Hensanshitsu, *Tottori-ken no muraiken undō*, 56.
63. Sugiyama Hiroaki, "Yamaguchi-ken ni okeru Hansenbyō taisaku no tenkai: Muraiken undōki wo chūshin ni," *Yamaguchi kenshi kenkyū* 14 (2006), http://takaamami.fc2web.com/sugiyama_yamaguchiken.html, accessed November 9, 2017.
64. Mitsuda Kensuke, *Aiseien nikki* (Tokyo: Mainichi Shinbunsha, 1958), 180–181.
65. "Kaisetsu," *NHK*, vol. 1, 60
66. Fukumoto Ichirō, *Haiku no hakken: Masaoka Shiki to sono jidai* (Tokyo: Nihon Hōsoku Shuppan Kyōkai, 2007).
67. Sakurazawa Fusayoshi, *Zensei konjaku* (Tokyo: Miwa Shōhō, 1991), 85–86.
68. Tama Zenshōen Kanja Jichikai, ed., *Kue issho: Kanja ga tsuzuru Zenshōen no nanajūnen* (Tokyo: Ikkōsha, 1979), 62–63.
69. Ibid.
70. Uchida Mamoru, *Hinoki no kage* (Kumamoto: Kyūshū ryōyōjo hinoki no kage kai, 1926), 4.
71. Matsuoka Hōyōen 70-nen Kinenshi Kankō Iinkai, *Hikkyō wo hiraku* (Aomori: Aomori Kyūrai Kyōkai, 1979), 62–64.
72. Ōshima Seishōen Nyūensha Jichikai, ed., *Tōzasareta shima no Shōwashi* (Ajichō, Kagawa-ken: Ōshima Seishōen Nyūensha Jichikai, 1981): 57.
73. Uchida Mamoru, "Rai kanja to bungei seikatsu," *Shakai jigyō no tomo* 27 (February 1931): 151.

74. Ibid.,153.
75. Tsubota Kimiko, "Hikari wo motomete," *Yamazakura* (December 1934): 59–66.
76. Ibid., 62.
77. Ibid., 64.
78. Shiba Tomotsu, "Ichiji kisei," *Yamazakura* (December 1934): 72.
79. Yokoyama Ishitori, "Tenkanki no kanja undō ni riron no urazuke wo," *Takahara* 15, no. 4 (April 1960): 5.
80. Yamashita Michisuki and Arai Yūki, *Hansenbyō bungaku shiryō shūi*, vol. 1 (Higashimurayama: Kokuritsu Ryōyōjo Tama Zenshōen Jichikai Hansenbyō Toshokan, 2004), 4–5.
81. Rai Yōbō Kyōkai, ed., *Kanja sakuhin: Eiga sosaishū* (Tokyo: Rai Yōbō Kyōkai, 1933), 29–33.
82. Yamashita and Arai, *Hansenbyō bungaku shiryō shūi*, vol. 1, 47–51.
83. Konami Yokobue, "Kawa no men," in Yamashita and Arai, *Hansenbyō bungaku shiryō shūi*, vol. 1, 20–23; Kubota Meisei, "Haha ni dakareru made," in Yamashita and Arai, *Hansenbyō bungaku shiryō shūi*, vol. 1, 34–37.
84. Kubota, "Haha ni dakareru made," 37–42.
85. Ōni Tomozō, "Odori no yoru," in Rai Yōbō Kyōkai, *Kanja sakuhin*, 29–33.
86. Arai Yūki, "Kakuri suru bungaku: Rai Yōbo Kyōkai no bungaku senryaku," *Shōwa bungaku kenkyū* 50 (March 2005): 26.
87. See, for example, Katherine Tanaka, "Through the Hospital Gates: Hansen's Disease and Modern Japanese Literature" (PhD diss., University of Chicago, 2012).
88. Nishio Tadashi, "Dozō," *Purufuiru* (January 1935): 72–82.
89. Yokomitsu Riichi, "Basha," *Kaizō* (January 1932): 1–32. Quotations are from Dennis Keene, trans., *Love and Other Stories of Yokomitsu Riichi* (Tokyo: Tokyo University Press, 1979), 181–226. William Johnston, *The Modern Epidemic: A History of Tuberculosis in Japan* (Cambridge, MA: Harvard East Asian Monographs, 1995), 144–148.

Chapter 7: The Sanitaria in the Time of National Emergency

1. Nagashima Aiseien Nyūensha Jichikai, ed., *Kakuzetsu no ritei: Nagashima Aiseien nyūensha 50-nenshi* (Okayama: Nagashima Aiseien Nyūensha Jichikai, 1982), 14–15.
2. Andrew Gordon, *Labor and Imperial Democracy in Prewar Japan* (Berkeley: University of California Press, 1991).

3.　Tama Zenshōen Kanja Jichikai, ed., "Nenpyō," in *Kue issho: Kanja ga tsuzuru Zenshōen no nanajūnen* (Tokyo: Ikkōsha, 1979), 28.

4.　Mitsuda Kensuke, *Aiseien nikki* (Tokyo: Mainichi Shinbunsha, 1958), 156.

5.　Nagashima Aiseien Iankai, *Nagashima annai* (Okayama: Sanyō Shinbunsha, 1934), in *KNHMSS, Senzenhen*, Hokan 9, 184.

6.　Ogawa Masako, *Kojima no haru* (Tokyo: Nagasaki Shoten, 1938).

7.　"Showa 11-nen Shochō kaigi jiroku," in *NHK*, vol. 1, 499.

8.　Kokuritsu Ryōyōjo Kikuchi Keifūen, ed., *Kikuchi Keifūen 50-nen shi* (Kumamoto: Kokuritsu Ryōyōjo Kikuchi Keifūen, 1960), 50.

9.　*Nyūen no susume* (Kusatsu: Kuryū Rakusen'en, 1935).

10.　Kuryū Rakusen'en Kanja Jichikai, ed., *Fūsetsu no mon: Kuryū Rakusen'en kanja gojūnenshi* (Gumma: Kuryū Rakusen'en Kanja Jichikai, 1982), 109–111.

11.　Kuryū Rakusen'en, *Rakusen'en nenpō Showa 8-nen* (Kusatsu: Rakusen'en, 1935), 11; Kuryū Rakusen'en, *Rakusen'en nenpō Showa 9-nen* (Kusatsu: Rakusen'en, 1935), 11.

12.　Matsuoka Hiroyuki, *Kakuri no shima ni ikiru: Okayama Hansenbyō mondai kiroku* (Okayama: Fukuro Shuppan, 2011), 112, 129.

13.　Nagashima Aiseien Nyūensha Jichikai, *Kakuzetsu no ritei*, 11–12.

14.　Ibid., 4.

15.　Ibid., 42–43.

16.　Ibid., 75.

17.　Mitsuda, *Aiseien nikki*, 144–148.

18.　Ibid., 146.

19.　Matsuoka, *Kakuri no shima ni ikiru*, 67.

20.　Ibid., 31.

21.　Ibid., 121.

22.　Matsuoka Hiroyuki, "Hansenbyō ryōyōjo ni okeru kanja jichi no mosaku: Daisan fukenritsu no ryōyōjo Sotojima Hoyōin ni tsuite," *Buraku mondai kenkyū*, no. 173 (2005): 2–21.

23.　For a patient's account of Murata's work at Sotojima, see Abe Reiji, "Sotojima Hoyōin shoshi," in *Kindai shomin seikatsushi*, vol. 20, *Byōki eisei*, ed. Minami Hiroshi, 457–482 (Tokyo: San'ichi Shobō, 1984).

24.　Ibid., 472–473.

25.　"Sayoku kanja 20-mei yain hoyōin wo dassō su," *Ōsaka mainichi shinbun*, September 3, 1933.

26.　See, for example, "Repura kanja ni akaibiyaku," *Ōsaka mainichi shinbun*, August 27, 1933.

27. "Senei raikanja dasshutsu mokunin no kamon," *Ōsaka mainichi shinbun*, September 3, 1933.
28. "Hayashi Yoshinobu ate nyūjosha shojō," in *NHK*, vol. 1, 475.
29. "Shōdokuba Nakajima Hideo kinmu nisshi," in *NHK*, vol. 1, 422.
30. "Mamoru shojō ni miru jiken," in *NHK*, vol. 1, 427.
31. Nagashima Aiseien Nyūensha Jichikai, *Kakuzetsu no ritei*, 18–19.
32. "Miyagawa Hakaru ate Imatani Itsunosuke shojō," in *NHK*, vol. 1, 493.
33. "Sasaki Mamoru shojō ni miru jiken," in *NHK*, vol. 1, 429–430.
34. "Mitsuda no saibanjo ate kokuhatsujo," in *NHK*, vol. 1, 463–466. The term "pathetic cripple" was used in the petition submitted to Home Minister Ushio on August 15. See Nagashima Aiseien Nyūensha Jichikai, *Kakuzetsu no ritei*, 24. On Mitsuda's motives, see 23–24.
35. "Aiseien wo tsutsumu: hi no te tsui ni ikiyu," *Ōsaka asahi shinbun*, August 24, 1936; "Jichi ka kazokushūgi? Kyūrai jigyō no jūjiro," *Ōsaka asahi shinbun*, August 23, 1936; "Kyūrai jigyō keieini kenkyū mondai wo nagekaku," n.d., all from a scrapbook of newspapers clippings compiled by Aiseien staff and now on display at the Aiseien Historical Museum.
36. On the patients' view of the Home Ministry, see "Sasaki Mamoru shojō ni miru jiken," 430. On Ushio's response, see Nagashima Aiseien Nyūensha Jichikai, *Kakuzetsu no ritei*, 25.
37. "Totsujo raikanja senyomei hansuto wo kekkō," *Asahi shinbun*, August 19, 1936.
38. Nagashima Aiseien Nyūensha Jichikai, *Kakuzetsu no ritei*, 26.
39. "Nijūgokai Kansai MTL shusai kyūrai zadankai kiroku," in *NHK*, vol. 1, 479–480.
40. "Kyō saigo no kaiken," *Chūgoku minpō*, August 23, 1936.
41. "Raikyūryō jigyō no konpon shisetsu," *Ōsaka asahi shinbun*, August 24, 1936.
42. See, for example, the remarks by Shimomura Hiroshi, longtime bureaucrat and former colonial official, and Tsukada Kitarō in *NHK*, vol. 1, 481–482.
43. Ibid.
44. Ibid., 485–486.
45. "Nagashima Aiseien jiken kara manabitorubeki mono," *Chūgai nippō*, September 2–3, 1936.
46. "Showa 11-nen Shochō kaigi jiroku," in *NHK*, vol. 1, 494–508.
47. "Ryōyōjo kankinjo shirabe," in *NHK*, vol. 1, 715.
48. "Chōkei kensoku shirabe," in *NHK*, vol. 1, 718.
49. On the history of Japanese leprosy policy in colonial Korea and the Sorokdo institutions, see Takio Eiji, *Chōsen Hansenbyō shi: Nihon*

shokuminchika no Sorokuto (Tokyo: Miraisha, 2001). On policy in Taiwan, see Serizawa Ryōko, "Hansenbyō iryō wo meguru seisaku to dendō: Nihon tōchiki Taiwan ni okeru jirei kara," *Rekishigaku kenkyū*, no. 834 (2007): 27–36.

50. "Showa 11-nen Shochō kaigi jiroku," in *NHK*, vol. 1, 494–508.
51. "Chōkei kensoku shirabe," in *NHK*, vol. 1, 718.
52. Information on confinees is from an exhibit at Jyu-kanbo National Museum.
53. Nagashima Aiseien Nyūensha Jichikai, *Kakuzetsu no ritei*, 32.
54. Kokuritsu Ryōyōjo Kikuchi Keifūen, *Kikuchi Keifūen 50-nen shi*, 52.
55. Kuryū Rakusen'en Kanja Jichikai, ed., *Fūsetsu no mon: Kuryū Rakusen'en kanja gojūnenshi* (Gumma: Kuryū Rakusen'en Kanja Jichikai, 1982), 91–100.
56. Julia Boyd, *Hannah Riddell: An Englishwoman in Japan* (Rutland, VT: Charles E. Tuttle, 1996), 192–193.
57. Kokuritsu Hansenbyō Shiryōkan, ed., *Shiritsu Hansenbyō ryōyōjo Tairōin no arumi: Sōritsu kara heiin made no 115-nen* (Higashimurayama: Kokuritsu Hansenbyō Shiryōkan, 2015).
58. William Johnston, *The Modern Epidemic: A History of Tuberculosis in Japan* (Cambridge, MA: Harvard East Asian Monographs, 1995), 277–285.
59. Nagashima Aiseien Nyūjosha Jichikai, ed., *Akebono no shiokaze* (Okayama: Nihon Bunkyō Shuppan, 1998), 196–197.
60. Ibid., 335.
61. Matsubara Yōko, "Minzoku yūseihogohō to Nihon no yūseihō no keifu," *Nihon kagakushi gakkai zasshi* 36, no. 201 (1997): 42–50; and Yokoyama Takashi, *Nihon ga yūsei shakai ni naru made: Kagaku keimō, media, seishoku no seiji* (Tokyo: Keisō Shobō, 2015), chap. 2.
62. Mitsuda Kensuke, "Wasekutomī nijū shūnen," in *Mitsuda Kensuke to Nihon no rai yobō jigyō: Rai yobōhō gojūnen kinen*, ed. Tōfū Kyōkai, 233–234 (Tokyo: Tōfū Kyōkai, 1958).
63. Tamamura Kōzō and Yajima Ryōichi, "Rai kanja ni taisuru danshu shujutsu ni tsuite," *Kōshū eisei hoken kyōkai zasshi* 16, no. 2 (1942).
64. Fujino Yutaka, *"Inochi" no kindaishi: "Minzoku jōka" no na no motoni hakugai sareta Hansenbyō kanja* (Kyoto: Kamogawa Shuppan, 2001), pt. 4, chap. 2.
65. "Rai yobōhō chū kaisei hōritsu an, Dai-ikkaigi," *Shūgiin giji sokki roku*, no. 26 (March 15, 1940), in *KNHMSS, Senzenhen*, vol. 8, 210.
66. Mitsuda, "Wasekutomī nijū shūnen," 235.
67. Fujino Yutaka, "Eugenics and Hansen's Disease Patients," in *Eugenics*

in Japan, ed. Karen J. Schafner, 123–125 (Fukuoka: Kyushu University Press, 2014).

68. "Rai yobōhō chū kaisei hōritsu an, Dai-ikkaigi," 211–218.

69. Yamamoto Sumiko and Katō Naoko, *Hansenbyō ryōyōjo no esunogurafi: Kakuri no naka no kekkon to kodomo* (Tokyo: Iryō Bunkasha, 2008), 226–228.

70. "Nyūjosha toshite o seikatsu: Kaisetsu," in *NHK*, vol. 1, 610.

71. Nichibenren Hōmu Kenkyū Zaidan, *Hansenbyō mondai ni kansuru kenshō kaigi saishū hōkokusho*, vol. 2 (Tokyo: Akashi Shoten, 2007). For information on participants in the survey, see 15–16; on its design, see 10–14. The narrative responses to questions on "eugenics" are found on 583–584.

72. Ibid., 110–113.

73. Yamamoto and Katō, *Hansenbyō ryōyōjo no esunogurafi*, 234.

74. Ibid., 215.

75. Hōjō Tamio, "Rai kazoku," in *HBZ*, vol. 1, 107–128.

76. Hōjō Tamio "Raiin jutai," in *HBZ*, vol. 1, 49–86.

Chapter 8: Leprosy in Postwar Japan

1. For some of the press coverage of the protests, see "Raibyōsha suwarikomu," *Asahi shinbun*, July 4, 1953, evening edition, 3; "Raikanji hikiageru," *Asahi shinbun*, July 9, 1953, evening edition, 7; "Raikanja keitsatsu to momu," *Asahi shinbun*, July 31, 1953, evening edition, 3; "Mata suwari komi," *Asahi shinbun*, August 1, 1953, evening edition, 7. See also the account of the events offered to the members of the Health and Welfare Committee of the lower house. Shūgiin Kōsei Iinkai Kaigiroku, no. 9 (July 6, 1953), in *KNHMSS, Sengohen*, vol. 10, 242–243.

2. Zenkoku Hansenshibyō Kanja Kyōgikai, ed., *Zenkankyō undōshi* (Tokyo: Ikkōsha, 1977), 31–32.

3. Kikuchi Keifūen Jichikai, ed., *Jichikai Gojūnenshi* (Kumamoto: Kokuritsu Ryōyōjo Kikuchi Keifūen, 1977), 29. For reports of damage, see letters addressed to MacArthur by patients and the sanitarium's director, Records of SCAP, Public Health and Welfare Administrative Bureau, 775024, 331-9439, folder 1, USNA.

4. Both in Records of SCAP, Public Health and Welfare Administrative Bureau, 770524, 331-9431, folder 8, USNA.

5. Brigadier General Crawford F. Sams, letter to Colonel J. H. McNinch, June 6, 1950, Records of SCAP, Public Health and Welfare Administrative Bureau, 770524, 331-9431, folder 8, USNA.

6. Kikuchi Keifūen Jichikai, *Jichiikai Gojūnenshi*, 32.

7. Kōseisho Imukyoku, ed., *Isei hyakunenshi* (Tokyo: Gyōsei, 1976), 294.

8. Zenkoku Hansenshibyō Kanja Kyōgikai, *Zenkankyō undōshi*, 193.

9. Nagashima Aiseien Nyūensha Jichikai, ed., *Kakuzetsu no ritei: Nagashima Aiseien nyūensha 50-nenshi* (Okayama: Nagashima Aiseien Nyūensha Jichikai, 1982), 34.

10. Ibid., 34–35.

11. Tama Zenshōen Kanja Jichikai, ed., *Kue issho: Kanja ga tsuzuru Zenshōen no nanajūnen* (Tokyo: Ikkōsha, 1979), 167–168.

12. Kuryū Rakusen'en Kanja Jichikai, ed., *Fūsetsu no mon: Kuryū Rakusen'en kanja gojūnenshi* (Gumma: Kuryū Rakusen'en Kanja Jichikai, 1982), 224–225.

13. "Shimei, Kokuritsu Ryōyōjo Hoshizuka Keiaien kanja ichidō," in *KNHMSS, Sengohen*, vol. 1, 74.

14. "Shimeisho, Zenkoku Raikanja Seikatsu Yōgo Renmei ni kanyū shinai riyū," in *KNHMSS, Sengohen*, vol. 1, 75.

15. Zenkoku Hansenshibyō Kanja Kyōgikai, *Zenkankyō undōshi*, 193–195.

16. Christina Norgen, *Abortion before Contraception: The Politics of Reproduction in Postwar Japan* (Princeton, NJ: Princeton University Press, 2001), 37–38.

17. Ogino Miho et al., *Sei to seishoku no jinken mondai shiryō shūsei*, vol. 15, *Yūsei mondai jinkō seisaku* (Tokyo: Fuji Shuppan, 2002), 212–217.

18. Matsubara Yōko, "Nihon no yūseihō no rekishi," in *Yūsei hogohō ga okashita tsumi*, ed. Yūsei shujutsu ni taisuru shazai wo motomeru kai, 104–115 (Tokyo: Gendai Shokan, 2003).

19. Toyota Kazuo, "Anatatachi ni iitai," *Aisei* 7, no. 11 (1953): 4–5.

20. Toyota Kazuo, "Shakai fukkisha zōka no mondai ni tsuite: 'Anatatachi ni iitai' ni taisuru bakuron ni kotaete," *Aisei* 8, no. 12 (1954): 3.

21. Ibid., 4.

22. Hoshi Seiji, "'Anatatachi ni iitai' to iu ronbun wo yomite," *Kōda no suso* 25, no. 4 (1954): 20.

23. Kai Hachirō, "Enpō kara no tegami: Arui ha 'Anatatachi ni iitai' hihan," *Takahara* 9, no. 1 (1954): 17.

24. "Summary of vital statistics," Ministry of Health, Labour and Welfare website, http://www.mhlw.go.jp/english/database/db-hw/populate/xls/inter2.xls, accessed November 14, 2017.

25. Fujino Yutaka, "'Sengo minshū shūgi' no naka no Hansenbyō kanja," in *Rekishi no naka no raisha*, ed. Fujino Yutaka, 203 (Tokyo: Yumiru Shuppan, 1996).

26. Ibid.

27. Toyota, "Shakai fukkisha zōka no mondai ni tsuite," 3.

28. Guy Henry Faget et al., "The Promin Treatment of Leprosy: A Progress Report," *Public Health Reports* 58, no. 48 (1943): 1729–1741. On the development and testing of Promin, see John Parascandola, "Miracle at Carville: The Introduction of the Sulfones for the Treatment of Leprosy," *Pharmacy in History* 40, nos. 2–3 (1998): 59–66. Yuasa Yō, "Nihon de puromin no gassei to sekai no Hansenbyō seiatsu," *Yakugaku zasshi*, no. 117 (1997): 957–962.

29. Tama Zenshōen Kanja Jichikai, *Kue issho*, 174; Ōshima Seishōen Nyūensha Jichikai, ed., *Tozasareta shima no Shōwashi* (Ajicho, Kagawa-ken: Ōshima Seishōen Nyūensha Jichikai, 1981), 128.

30. Tama Zenshōen Kanja Jichikai, *Kue issho*, 174.

31. "Ware ni mo puromin wo, Puromin kakutoku sokushin undō ni tsuite zenkoku ryōyōjo kanja no minasama he," in *KNHMSS, Sengohen*, vol. 1, 114.

32. "Rai no shinyaku puromin," in *KNHMSS, Sengohen*, vol. 1, 125–132.

33. "Kanpō gogai, Shūgiin kaigiroku," no. 28 (May 17, 1947), in *KNHMSS, Sengohen*, vol. 1, 50.

34. "Memorandum for Record: Hunger Strike in Leprosarium," March 7, 1949, Records of SCAP, Public Health and Welfare Administrative Bureau, 770524, 331-9372, folder 10, USNA.

35. Crawford Sams, letter to Charles L. Wilbur, October 12, 1949, Records of SCAP, Public Health and Welfare Administrative Bureau, 775024, 331-9431, folder 8, USNA.

36. Hajime Sato and Janet E. Frantz, "Termination of the Leprosy Isolation Policy in the US and Japan: Science, Policy Changes, and the Garbage Can Model," *BMC International Health and Human Rights* 5 (2005): 5.

37. Michelle Moran, *Colonizing Leprosy: Imperialism and Public Health in the United States* (Chapel Hill: University of North Carolina Press, 2007), 178.

38. Ibid., 178–179.

39. Sato and Frantz, "Termination of the Leprosy Isolation Policy in the US and Japan," 5.

40. Moran, *Colonizing Leprosy*, 169.

41. Ibid., 184–185.

42. Yamamoto Shun'ichi, *Zōhō Nihon raishi* (Tokyo: Tokyo Daigaku Shuppankai, 1997), 268–269.

43. Ibid., 274.

44. "Wareware wa kyū kenpōka ni ikasarete iru rai yobō hō wo kaku uttaeru, *Zenrai kankyō nyūzu*, no. 21 (September 30, 1952): 2.

45. "Omura Kokuritsu Ryōyōjo kachō rai yobōhō kaisei mondai ni tsuite sokushin iinkai to nendan," *Zenrai kankyō nyūzu*, no. 23 (November 30, 1952): 1.

46. For the text of the draft law, see "Rai yobō hōan, *Dai 16-kai Kokkai Shūgiin Kōsei Iinkai kaigiroku*, no. 11 (July 2, 1953), in *KNHMSS, Sengohen*, vol. 10, 213–216.

47. Letter to Eleanor Roosevelt, in *KNHMSS*, Hokan 12, 205.

48. For evidence of the NCSP's evolving position, see the various petitions and declarations collected in *KNHMSS*, Hokan 12, such as 228–229, 243, as well as essays published in the sanitarium journals, such as Yokohama Ishitori, "'Rai yobō hōan' ha naniyue warui ka," *Takahara* 8, no. 5 (May 1953): 4–9.

49. Aoki Jun'ichi, "Nihon ni okeru kekkaku ryōyōjo no rekishi to jiki kubun ni kansuru kōsatsu," *Senshū Daigaku shakai kagaku nenpō*, no. 50 (2016): 8–9.

50. "Kekkaku Yobōhō" is available on www.houko.com, a digital archive of Japanese laws. See http://www.houko.com/00/01/S26/096.HTM, accessed July 23, 2018. See also Johnston, *The Modern Epidemic: A History of Tuberculosis in Japan*, 286–289.

51. P. T. Erickson, "Relapse Following Apparent Arrest of Leprosy by Sulfone Therapy," *Public Health Report* 65 (1950): 1147–1157.

52. See, for example, the discussion within the Committee on Health and Welfare of the upper house, in *Dai 16-kai Kokkai Sangiin Kōsei Iinkai kaigiroku*, no. 7 (July 2–3, 1953), in *KNHMSS, Sengohen*, vol. 10, 217–224.

53. Lee Pennington, *Casualties of History: Wounded Japanese Servicemen and the Second World War* (Ithaca, NY: Cornell University Press, 2015), 198–199.

54. Shima Hiroshi (Ishimura Michiaki), "Raiyobō hō kaisei undō ni tsuite warera no hansei," in *HBZ*, vol. 5, 125–128.

55. The critic was Tsukida Masashi. See Tsukida Masashi, "'Raiyobō hō kaisei undō ni tsuite warera no hansei' no sakusha ni hitokoto," in *HBZ*, vol. 5, 120.

56. Aoki, "Nihon ni okeru kekkaku ryōyōjo no rekishi to jiki kubun ni kansuru kōsatsu," 9.

57. Mori Mikio, "Atarashiki jidai no atarashiki ryōyōjo," *Kaede* (September 1956).

58. Kokuritsu Hansenbyō Shiryōkan, ed., *Seinentachi no "shakai fukki"* (Higashimurayama: Kokuritsu Hansenbyō Shiryōkan, 2011), 8.

59. Ibid., 6.

60. Kondō Yūshō, "Hansenbyō ryōyōjo ni okeru taien to shakai fukki ni tsuite," *Shintennōji Daigaku Daiguakuin kenkyū ronshū*, no. 8 (2013): 24.

61. Zenkoku Hansenbyōshi Kanja Kyōgikai, *Zenkankyō undōshi*, 142.

62. Of nine patients profiled in a 2012 exhibit at the National Hansen's Disease Museum on "returning to society," eight were eventually readmitted to a sanitarium.

63. Arakawa Iwao, "Rai ryōyōjo nyūjo kanja no shakai fukki iyoku," *Kōda no suso* 32, no. 11 (December 1962): 2–12; Kobayshi Shigenobu and Matsumura Jō, "Shakai fukki ni kansuru taido chōsa ni tsuite," *Takahara* 17, no. 4 (1965): 1–9.

64. Morita Takeji, "Damin ni ha dare ga shita: shakai fukki wo kobamuru mono," *Aisei* 11, no. 1 (January 1957).

65. Sawada Gorō, "Mori ronbun ni tsuite," *Takahara* 12, no. 8 (August 1957).

66. Sasakawa Makoto, "Hashibyō ha shaikai fukki wo negatte iru," *Kōda no suso* 31, no. 10 (December 1960): 3.

67. Morioka Ryōji, "Sengo ryōyōjo ron: Hitotsu no josetsu toshite," *Tama* 30, no. 1 (January 1958).

68. Sheldon Garon, "Saving for 'My Own Good and the Good of the Nation': Economic Nationalism in Modern Japan," in *Nation and Nationalism in Japan*, ed. Sandra Wilson, 109 (Oxford: Routledge-Curzon, 2013).

69. Mitsuda Kensuke, *Aiseien nikki* (Tokyo: Mainichi Shinbunsha, 1958), 211.

70. "Kanja no seikatsuhi jittai chōsa jisshi suru," *Zenkankyō nyuzu*, no. 72 (October 1, 1956): 1. For wages in this era, see Japan Statistics Association, ed., *Historical Statistics of Japan*, vol. 4, *Labor, Wages, Housing, Prices* (Tokyo: Japan Statistical Association, 1987), 256–257.

71. Tama Zenshōen Kanja Jichikai, *Kue issho*, 175–176; Kuryū Rakusen'en Kanja Jichikai, *Fūsetsu no mon*, 335–339.

72. Tetsuya Fujiwara, "Restoring Honor: Japanese Pacific War Disabled Veterans from 1943 to 1963" (PhD diss., University of Iowa, 2011), 96–101.

73. "Kuryū Rakusen'en: Yokoyama Ishitori," *Amenbo tsūshin* (January 20, 2015), http://terayama2009.blog79.fc2.com/blog-entry-2736.html, accessed August 8, 2016.

74. Yokoyama Ishitori, "Tenkanki no kanja undō ni riron no urazuke wo," *Takahara* 15, no. 4 (April 1960): 5.

75. "Seinenkai shijō zadankai: Shakai fukki genjitsuka no tame ni," *Takahara* 15, no. 4 (April 1960): 25.

76. Yokoyama, "Tenkanki no kanja undō ni riron no urazuke wo," 3.

77. "Seinenkai shijō zadankai: Shakai fukki genjitsuka no tame ni," 27.

78. Sasakawa, "Hashibyō ha shaikai fukki wo negatte iru," 3.
79. Sano Reishin, "Watachi no koronii kōzō: Hikari no machi tanpōki," *Shinsei* 10, no. 2 (1957): 14–17.
80. Mita Ryō, "Shakai fukki undō wo suishin suru tame ni uttaemasu," *Kōda no suso* 27, no. 7 (1956): 2–4.
81. Ishimura Mishiaki (Shima Hiroshi), "Ryōen no koroniika ni tsuite," *Kikuchino* 3, no. 1 (March 1953): 16–19.
82. Shima Hiroshi, "Koronii setchi ni tsuite," *Takahara* 11, no. 12 (1956): 6–11.
83. Jane S. H. Kim, "In Search of Anti-Communist Nation: The World Health Organization and Public Health Planning in Post–war Korea" (unpublished manuscript, consulted July 23, 2018).
84. Zenkoku Hansenshibyō Kanja Kyōgikai, *Zenkankyō undōshi*, 138–139.
85. Kokuritsu Hansenbyō Shiryōkan, *Seinentachi no "shakai fukki,"* 40–42.
86. Yamamoto Yoriko, "Taiengo no watakushi no seikatsu: Hataraku yorokobi to jiyū no yorokobi wo ete," *Tama* 43, no. 7 (1962): 11–12.
87. Tama Zenshōen Kanja Jichikai, *Kue issho*, 237.
88. See, for example, the makeup of the council at Rakusen'en in the 1960s and 1970s. Kuryū Rakusen'en Kanja Jichikai, ed., *Fūsetsu no mon*, 535–536.

Bibliography

Archival Materials
Archives of Akita Prefecture
Archives of the American Episcopal Church
Archives of Gunma Prefecture
Diplomatic Archives of the Japanese Ministry of Foreign Affairs
Fujikawa Yū Bunko, Keiō University Library
Fujikawa Yū Bunko, Kyoto University Library
Kyōu Shoya (Library of the Takeda Science Foundation)
Hawai'i State Archives
Mission to Lepers (UK)
National Archives of Japan
National Diet Library, Rare Books and Old Materials Collection
New York Academy of Medicine
Sōda Hajime Collection, International Research Center of Japanese Studies
Tokyo University Library
US National Archives (College Park, MD)

Newspapers and Periodicals
Aisei
Annals of Hygiene
Asahi shinbun
Chōya shinbun
Chūgai nippō
Dai Nihon shiritsu eiseikai zasshi
Hifuka hinyōkika zasshi
Igaku chūō zasshi
Journal of Cutaneous and Genito-Urinary Diseases
Kaede
Kikuchino

Kōda no suso
Kyōto iji eisei shi
Los Angeles Times
Missionary Review of the World
National Geographic
New York Times
Ōsaka asahi shinbun
Ōsaka igakkai zasshi
Ōsaka mainichi shinbun
Philadelphia Medical Times
Purufuiru
San Francisco Chronicle
San Francisco Municipal Reports
Science
Shinsei
The Spirit of Missions
Tama
Takahara
Tōkyō igakkai zasshi
Tōkyō iji zasshi
Without the Camp
Yamazakura
Yomiuri shinbun
Zenrai kankyō nyūzu
Zenkankyō nyūzu

Primary Sources and Multivolume Document Collections

Asami Megumi and Yasuda Kei, eds. *Kinsei rekishi shiryō shūsei.* Series 3 (6 vols.), *Minkan chiryō.* Tokyo: Kasumigaseki Shuppan, 1990–1996.

Bälz, Erwin von. "Das heisse Bad in physiologischer und therapischer Hinsicht." *Münchener Medizinische Wochenschrift* 40 (1893): 351–352.

———. "Zur Lehre von der Lepra und ihrer Behandlung." *Berliner Klinische Wochenshrift* 34, no. 46 (November 15, 1897): 997–1001, and no. 47 (November 22, 1897): 1031–1034.

Buraku Mondai Kenkyūjo, ed. *Buraku no rekishi: Kinki hen.* Kyoto: Buraku Mondai Kenkyūjo Shuppanbu, 1982.

———, ed. *Burakushi shiryō senshū.* Vol. 1, *Kodai chūsei hen.* Kyoto: Buraku Mondai Kenkyūjo Shuppanbu, 1988.

Chamberlain, Basil Hall. *A Handbook for Travellers in Japan.* London: John Murray, 1891.

Currie, Donald H. "The Second International Conference on Leprosy, Held in Bergen, Norway." *Public Health Reports* 24, no. 38 (September 17, 1909): 1537–1561.

Eiseikyoku Chōsabu. *Kaku chihō ni okeru rai buraku rai shūgōchi ni kansuru gaikyō.* Tokyo: Naimusho Eiseikyoku, 1920.

Fujino Yutaka, ed. *Kingendai Nihon Hansenbyō mondai shiryō shūsei.* 20 vols. Tokyo: Fuji Shuppan, 2003.

Hanejima Tomoyuki, ed. *Shinbun kōkoku bijutsu taikei Meiji hen.* Vol. 1, *Iyaku keshō hen.* Tokyo: Ōzorasha, 1999.

International Congress of Leprosy, ed. *Mittheilungen und Verhandlungen der Internationalen Wissenschaftlichen Lepra-Conferenz zu Berlin im October 1897.* 2 vols. Berlin: A. Hirschwald, 1897.

Kaibara Ekiken. *Yōjōkun.* Edited by Matsuda Michio. Tokyo: Chūō Kōronsha, 1973.

Kaji Jingo and Narita Ryūichi, eds. *Katō Tokijirō senshū.* Tokyo: Kōryūsha, 1981.

Kajiwara Seizen. *Ton'isho.* Tokyo: Kagaku Shoin, 1986.

Kan Osamu. "Honpō ni okeru seishinbyōsha narabi ni kore ni kensetsu suru seishin ijōsha ni kansuru chōsetsu." *Seishin shinkeigaku zasshi* 41, no. 10 (1937): 793–884.

Koremune Tomotoshi. *Idansho.* Edited by Minobe Shigekatsu. Tokyo: Miyai Shoten, 2006.

Kōseisho, ed. *Isei hachijūnenshi.* Tokyo: Insatsu Chōyōkai, 1955.

Kōseishō Imukyoku, ed. *Isei hyakunenshi.* Tokyo: Gyōsei, 1976.

Kure Shūzō. *Seishinbyō no shitaku kanchi no jikkyō.* Tokyo: Naimusho Eisei-kyoku, 1918.

Kuryū Rakusen'en. *Rakusen'en nenpō Showa 8-nen.* Kusatsu: Rakusen'en, 1935.

———. *Rakusen'en nenpō Showa 9-nen.* Kusatsu: Rakusen'en, 1935.

Mabuchi Kazuo, Kunisaki Fumimaro, and Inagaki Taiichi. *Nihon koten bungaku zenshū,* vol. 37; *Konjaku monogatari shū,* vol. 3. Tokyo: Shogakkan, 1973.

Marchoux, Émile, ed. *IIIe conférence international de la lepre: Strasbourg, 28 au 31 juillet 1923: communications et débats.* Paris: J. B. Baillière et Fils, 1924.

Matsuda Takeshi, ed. *Meiji-ki eiseikyoku nenpō.* Vol. 2. Tokyo: Tōyō Shorin, 1992.

Minami Hiroshi, ed. *Kindai shomin seikatsushi.* Vol. 20, *Byōki eisei.* Tokyo: San'ichi Shobō, 1984.

Mitsuda Kensuke. *Aiseien nikki.* Tokyo: Mainichi Shinbunsha, 1958.

———. *Apercu général sur le traitement de la lèpre au Japon, présenté à la troisième Conférence international scientifique de la lèpre réunie à Strasbourg, le 28 juillet 1923.* Paris: Presses Universitaires, 1923.

———. *Kaishun byōshitsu: Kyūrai Gojūnen no kiroku.* Tokyo: Asahi Shinbun, 1950.

München, Gregor N., ed. *Lepra Studien*. Hamburg: Verlag von Leopold Voss, 1885.

Nakayama Yasumasa, *Shinbun shūsei: Meiji-hennenshi*. 15 vols. Tokyo: Honpō Shoseki, 1982.

Naimusho Eiseikyoku, ed. *Hoken eisei chōsakai dai-4 bu (rai) giji sokki roku*. Tokyo: Naimusho Eiseikyoku, 1920.

————, ed. *Raikanja no kokuhaku*. Tokyo: Naimusho Eiseikyoku, 1923.

————, ed. *Rai ryōyōjo shūyū kanja tōkei*. Tokyo: Naimusho Eiseikyoku, 1917.

Nakayama Yasumasa. *Shinbun shūsei: Meiji-hennenshi*. 15 vols. Tokyo: Honpō Shoseki, 1982.

Nihon Shakai Jigyō Daigaku, ed. *Kubota Seitarō ronshū*. Tokyo: Nihon Shakai Jigyō Daigaku, 1980.

Ogawa Masako. *Kojima no haru*. Tokyo: Nagasaki Shoten, 1938.

Ogino Miho, Matsubara Yōkō, and Saitō Hikaru. *Sei to seishoku no jinken mondai shiryō shūsei*. 35 vols. Tokyo: Fuji Shuppan, 2000.

Ōka Makoto, Otani Fujio, Kaga Otohiko, Tsurumi Shunsuke, and Taguchi Mugihiko, eds. *Hansenbyō bungaku zenshū*. 10 vols. Tokyo: Koseisha, 2002–2010.

Okayama-ken Hansenbyō Mondai Kanren Shiryō Chōsa Iinkai, ed. *Nagashima ha kataru: Okayama-ken Hansenbyō kankei shiryōshū*. 2 vols. Okayama: Okayama-ken Hansenbyō Mondai Kanren Shiryō Chōsa Iinkai, 2007–2009.

Otsuka Yoshinori and Yakazu Dōmei, eds. *Kinsei kanpō igakusho shūsei*. 116 vols. Tokyo: Meicho Shuppan, 1979–1984.

Rai Yōbō Kyōkai, ed. *Kanja sakuhin: Eiga sosaishū*. 4 vols. Tokyo: Rai Yōbō Kyōkai, 1933–1937.

Sakurazawa Fusayoshi. *Zensei konjaku*. Tokyo: Miwa Shōhō, 1991.

Takahashi Bonsen, ed. *Nihon jinkōshi no kenkyū*. Tokyo: Sanyūsha, 1941.

Tanba Yasunori. *Ishinpō*. Edited and translated (modern Japanese) by Maki Sachiko. Tokyo: Chikuma Shobō, 2002.

Tōfū Kyōkai, ed. *Mitsuda Kensuke to Nihon no rai yobō jigyō: Rai yobōhō gojūnen kinen*. Tokyo: Tōfū Kyōkai, 1958.

Uchida Mamoru. *Hinoki no kage*. Kumamoto: Kyūshū ryōyōjo hinoki no kage kai, 1926.

————. "Rai kanja to bungei seikatsu." *Shakai jigyō no tomo* 27 (February 1931): 28–55.

Ury, Marian, trans. *Tales of Times Now Past: Sixty-Two Stories from a Medieval Japanese Collection*. Berkeley: University of California Press, 1979.

Yokomitsu Riichi. "Basha." *Kaizō* (January 1932): 1–32.

Secondary Sources

Ackernecht, E. H. "Anti-Contagionism between 1821–1867." *Bulletin of the History of Medicine* 22 (1948): 562–593.

Agamben, Giorgio. *Homo Sacer: Sovereign Power and Bare Life.* Palo Alto, CA: Stanford University Press, 1998.

Aida Nirō. *Nihon no komonjo ge.* Tokyo: Iwanami Shoten, 1954.

Alter, Andrea, A. Grant, L. Abel, A. Alcaïs, and E. Schur. "Leprosy as a Genetic Disease." *Mammalian Genome* 22, no. 1 (2011): 19–31.

Ambaras, David R. *Bad Youth: Juvenile Delinquency and the Politics of Everyday Life in Japan.* Berkeley: University of California Press, 2005.

"Amenbo tsūshin." http://terayama2009.blog79.fc2.com/blog-entry-2736.html. Accessed August 8, 2016.

Amino Yoshihiko. *Chūsei no hinin to yūjo.* Tokyo: Akashi Shoten, 1994.

Amster, Ellen J. *Medicine and the Saints: Science, Islam, and the Colonial Encounter in Morocco, 1877–1956.* Austin: University of Texas Press, 2013.

Anderson, Warwick. *Colonial Pathologies: American Tropical Medicine, Race, and Hygiene in the Philippines.* Durham, NC: Duke University Press, 2006.

———. "States of Hygiene: Race 'Improvement' and Biomedical Citizenship in Australia and the Colonial Philippines." In *Haunted by Intimacy: Geographies of Intimacy in North American History*, edited by Ann Laura Stoler, 94–115. Durham, NC: Duke University Press, 2006.

Aoki Jun'ichi, "Nihon ni okeru kekkaku ryōyōjo no rekishi to jiki kubun ni kansuru kōsatsu." *Senshū Daigaku shakai kagaku nenpō*, no. 50 (2016): 3–22.

Aoki Takaju. "Buraku shi kenkyū no hoshō to dōwa gyōsei: *Nagano-shi shikō* wo megutte." *Buraku* 33, no. 8 (1981): 55–61.

———. "*Nagano-shi shikō* mondai sono ato." *Buraku* 33, no. 14 (1981): 54–67.

Arai Yūki. *Kakuri no bungaku: Hansenbyō ryōyōjo no jiko hyōgenshi.* Tokyo: Shoshiarusu, 2011.

———. "Kakuri suru bungaku: Rai Yōbo Kyōkai no bungaku senryaku." *Shōwa bungaku kenkyū* 50 (March 2005): 15–29.

Bashford, Alison. *Imperial Hygiene: A Critical Study of Colonialism, Nationalism, and Public Health.* Basingstoke: Palgrave MacMillan, 2004.

Bechelli, L. M., and V. Martinez Domingues. "The Leprosy Problem in the World." *Bulletin of the World Health Organization* 34, no. 6 (1966): 811–826.

Botsman, Daniel. *Punishment and Power in the Making of Modern Japan.* Princeton, NJ: Princeton University Press, 2005.

Boyd, Julia. *Hannah Riddell: An Englishwoman in Japan.* Rutland, VT: Charles E. Tuttle, 1996.

Brubaker, M. L. "Leprosy in Children One Year of Age and Under." *International*

Journal of Leprosy and Other Mycobacterium Diseases 53, no. 4 (1985): 517–523.

Buckley, I. Thomas, and Meg B. Springer. *Penikese: Island of Hope.* Brewster, MA: Stoney Brook Publishing, 1997.

Buraku Kaihō Dōmei Nagano-ken Rengōkai, ed. *Nagano-shi shikō to buraku kaihō no kadai.* Nagano-shi: Buraku Kaihō Dōmei Nagano-ken Rengōkai, 1981.

Burns, Susan L. "The Body as Text: Confucianism, Reproduction, and Gender in Tokugawa Japan." In *Rethinking Confucianism: Past and Present in China, Japan, Korea and Vietnam,* edited by B. A. Elman, J. B. Duncan, and H. Ooms, 178–219. Los Angeles: UCLA Asia Pacific Monograph Series, 2002.

———. "From 'Leper Villages' to Leprosara: Public Health, Medicine, and the Culture of Exclusion in Japan." In *Isolation: Policies and Practices of Exclusion,* edited by Alison Bashford and Carolyn Strange, 97–110. London: Routledge, 2003.

———. "History, Testimony, and the Afterlife of Quarantine: The National Hansen's Disease Museum of Japan." In *Quarantine: Local and Global Histories,* edited by Alison Ashford, 120–129. London: Palgrave, 2016.

———. "Nanayama Jundō at Work: A Village Doctor and Medical Knowledge in Nineteenth-Century Japan." *East Asian Science, Technology, and Medicine* 29 (2008): 62–83.

———. "Reinvented Places: Tradition, Family Care, and Psychiatric Institutions in Japan." *Social History of Medicine,* September 25, 2017. https://doi.org/10.1093/shm/hkx066.

Bynum, Caroline Walker. *Fragmentation and Redemption: Essays on Gender and the Human Body in Medieval Religion.* New York: Zone Books, 1991.

Bynum, W. F. "Policing Hearts of Darkness: Aspects of the International Sanitary Conferences." *History and Philosophy of the Life Sciences* 15, no. 3 (1993): 421–434.

Chen Wei-ti. "Cosmopolitan Medicine Nationalized: The Making of Japanese State-Empire and Migrant Physicians in a Global World." PhD diss., University of Chicago, 2016.

Chichiwa Itaru. "Kishōmon nōto: Keiyaku no sahō." *Jinmin no rekishigaku* 78 (1984): 1–7.

Chimoto Hideshi. "'Katai' kō: Setsuwa ni okeru raisha no mondai." *Ōsaka Kyōiku Daigaku kiyō,* ser. 1, 36, no. 1 (1987): 35–45.

Comelles, J. M. "The Role of Local Knowledge in Medical Practice: A Trans-historical Perspective." *Culture, Medicine, Psychiatry* 24, no. 1 (2000): 41–75.

Cryns, Frederik. "Ranpō-i ga juyō shita jūhasseiki no seiyō iryō: chiryō no konkyo to riron tenkai." In *Jūhasseiki Nihon no bunka jōkyō to kokusai kankyō,* edited by Kasaya Kazuhiko, 103–119. Kyoto: Shibunkaku Shuppan, 2011.

Demaitre, Luke. *Leprosy in Premodern Medicine: A Malady of the Whole Body.* Baltimore, MD: Johns Hopkins University Press, 2007.

Duara, Prasenjit. *Rescuing History from the Nation: Questioning Narratives of Modern China.* Chicago: University of Chicago Press, 1996.

Duncan, M. E. "An Historical and Clinical Review of Leprosy and Pregnancy: A Cycle to Be Broken." *Social Science Medicine* 37, no. 4 (1993): 457–472.

Durrheim, D. N., and R. Speare. "Global Leprosy Elimination: Time to Change More than the Elimination Date." *Journal of Epidemiology and Community Health* 57, no. 5 (2003): 316–317.

Edmond, Rod. *Leprosy and Empire: A Medical and Cultural History.* Cambridge: Cambridge University Press, 2006.

Erickson, P. T. "Relapse Following Apparent Arrest of Leprosy by Sulfone Therapy." *Public Health Report* 65 (1950): 1147–1157.

Faget, Guy Henry, R. C. Pogge, F. A. Johansen, J. F. Dinan, and C. G. Eccles. "The Promin Treatment of Leprosy: A Progress Report." *Public Health Reports* 58, no. 48 (1943): 1729–1741.

Fitness, J., K. Tosh, and A. V. Hill. "Genetics of Susceptibility to Leprosy." *Genes and Immunity* 3 (2002): 441–453.

Fujino Yutaka. "Eugenics and Hansen's Disease Patients." In *Eugenics in Japan,* edited by Karen J. Schafner. Fukuoka: Kyūshū University Press, 2014.

———. *"Inochi" no kindaishi: "Minzoku jōka" no na no motoni hakugai sareta Hansenbyō kanja.* Kyoto: Kamogawa Shuppan, 2001.

———. *Nihon fashizumu to iryō: Hansenbyō wo meguru jisshōteki kenkyū.* Tokyo: Iwanami Shoten, 1993.

———, ed. *Rekishi no naka no raisha.* Tokyo: Yumiru Shuppan, 1996.

Fujiwara, Tetsuya. "Restoring Honor: Japanese Pacific War Disabled Veterans from 1943 to 1963." PhD diss., University of Iowa, 2011.

Fujiwara Yoshiaki. "Chūsei zenki no byōsha to kyūsai." *Rettō no bunkashi* 3 (1986): 79–114.

Fukumoto Ichirō. *Haiku no hakken: Masaoka Shiki to sono jidai.* Tokyo: Nihon Hōsoku Shuppan Kyōkai, 2007.

Furth, Charlotte. *A Flourishing Yin: Gender in China's Medical History, 960–1665.* Berkeley: University of California Press, 1999.

Garon, Sheldon. *Molding Japanese Minds: The State in Everyday Life.* Princeton, NJ: Princeton University Press, 1997.

———. "Saving for 'My Own Good and the Good of the Nation': Economic Nationalism in Modern Japan." In *Nation and Nationalism in Japan,* edited by Sandra Wilson, 97–114. Oxford: Routledge-Curzon, 2013.

Gelder, Robert H., and Jacques Grosset. "The Chemotherapy of Leprosy: An Interpretive History." *Leprosy Review,* no. 83 (2012): 221–240.

George, D. Joseph. "'Essentially Christian, Eminently Philanthropic': The Mission to Lepers in India." *História, Ciências, Saúde-Manguinhos* 10, supp. 1 (2003): 247–275.

Goble, Andrew Edmund. "Song Printed Medical Works and Medieval Japanese Medicine." In *Chinese Medicine and Healing: An Illustrated History,* edited by T. J. Hinrichs and Linda Barnes, 123–127. Cambridge, MA: Belknap Press, 2013.

Goffman, Erving. *Asylums: Essays on the Social Situation of Mental Patients and Other Inmates.* Garden City, NY: Anchor Books, 1961.

Goodwin, Janet R. *Alms and Vagabonds: Buddhist Temples and Popular Patronage in Medieval Japan.* Honolulu: University of Hawai'i Press, 1994.

———. "Outcasts and Marginals in Medieval Japan." In *The Routledge Handbook of Premodern Japanese History,* edited by Karl F. Friday, 296–309. London: Routledge, 2017.

Gordon, Andrew. *Labor and Imperial Democracy in Prewar Japan.* Berkeley: University of California Press, 1991.

Gussow, Zachary. *Leprosy, Racism, and Public Health: Social Policy in Chronic Disease Control.* Boulder, CO: Westview Press, 1989.

Hansenbyō Iken Kokubai Soshō Bengodan, ed. *Hirakareta tobira: Hansenbyō saiban wo tatakatta hitotachi.* Tokyo: Kōdansha, 2003.

Harata Nobuo. "Tategaki de yonda rai." *Aisei,* nos. 387–415 (1972–1975).

Higashi Eizō. "Nagano-shi shikō no mondai wo meguru shaken." *Shin Nihon bungaku* 36, no. 9 (1981): 84–97 and no. 10 (1981): 92–96.

Higashimurayama-shi hensan iinkai, ed. *Higashimurayama-shi shi.* Vol. 2. Tokyo: Higashimurayama, 1981.

Hirai Yuichirō. "Yōikuen kara Ihaien he: Hansenbyō seisaku zenya no issōwa." *Shibusawa kenkyū* 13 (2000): 65–82.

Hirokawa Waka. *Kindai Nihon no Hansenbyō mondai to chiiki shakai.* Osaka: Osaka Daigaku Shuppankai, 2011.

Hosokawa Ryōichi. *Chūsei mibunsei to hinin.* Tokyo: Nihon Editā Sukūru, 1994.

Howell, David L. *Geographies of Identity in Nineteenth-Century Japan.* Berkeley: University of California Press, 2005.

Howland, Douglas R. *Translating the West: Language and Political Reason in Nineteenth-Century Japan.* Honolulu: University of Hawai'i Press, 2001.

Hundeiker, M., and H. Brömmelhaus. "Leprakranke in Deutchland und Einführung industriell hergestellter Lepramedikamente von 100 Jahnen." *Dermatologie in Kunst und Geschichte* 58 (2007): 899–903.

Igarashi Masahiro. "Nihon no 'sengo hoshō saiban' to kokusaihō." *Kokusaihō gaikō zasshi* 1, no. 12 (2006): 1–28.

Ikai Takaaki. *Hanna Rideru to Kaishun Byōin.* Tokyo: Sōryū Shuppan, 2005.

Irgens, Lorentz M., and Tor Bjerkedal. "Epidemiology of Leprosy in Norway: The History of the National Leprosy Registry of Norway from 1856 until Today." *International Journal of Epidemiology* 2, no. 1 (1973): 81–89.

Itakura Kazuko. "Shiritsu rai ryōyōjo Biwasaki Tairōin no rekishi." *Nihon Hansenbyō gakkai zasshi* 61, no. 2 (1992): 112–116.

Japan Statistical Association, ed. *Historical Statistics of Japan.* Vol. 4, *Labor, Wages, Housing, Prices.* Tokyo: Japan Statistical Association, 1987.

Jennings, Eric T. *Curing the Colonizers: Hydrotherapy, Climatology, and French Colonial Spas.* Durham, NC: Duke University Press, 2006.

Johnston, William. *The Modern Epidemic: A History of Tuberculosis in Japan.* Cambridge, MA: Harvard East Asian Monographs, 1995.

Kaihō Shuppansha, ed. *Hansenbyō kokubai soshō hanketsu: Kumamoto chisai dai ichiji daiyoji.* Osaka: Kaihō Shuppansha, 2001.

Kakar, Sanjiv. "Leprosy in British India, 1860–1940: Colonial Politics and Missionary Medicine." *Medical History* 40 (1996): 215–230.

Kaneko Junji. *Nihon seishin igaku nenpyō.* Tokyo: Nihon Seishinbyōin Kyōkai, 1973.

Katō Naoko. *Moto Minobu Jinkyōenchō Tsunawaki Michi-san ni kiku: Yama no naka no chiisana en ni te: Mōhitotsu no Hansenbyō shi.* Tokyo: Iryō Bunkashi, 2005.

Kawata Mitsuo. "Chūsei hisabetsunin no yosoi." Vol. 2, *Kawata Mitsuo Chosakushū.* Tokyo: Akashi Shoten, 1995.

Keene, Dennis, trans. *Love and Other Stories of Yokomitsu Riichi.* Tokyo: Tokyo University Press, 1979.

Kierstead, Thomas. "Outcasts before the Law: Pollution and Purification in Medieval Japan. In *Currents in Medieval Japanese History: Essays in Honor of Jeffrey P. Mass*, edited by Gordon M. Berger, Andrew Edmund Goble, Lorraine F. Harrington, and G. Cameron Hurst III, 267–298. Los Angeles: Figueroa Press, 2009.

Kikuchi Keifūen Jichikai, ed. *Jichikai Gojūnenshi.* Kumamoto: Kokuritsu Ryōyōjo Kikuchi Keifūen, 1977.

Kim, Hoi-eun. *Doctors of Empire: Medical and Cultural Encounters between Imperial Germany and Meiji Japan.* Toronto: University of Toronto, 2014.

Kim, Jane S. H. "In Search of Anti-Communist Nation: The World Health Organization and Public Health Planning in Post-war Korea." Unpublished manuscript, consulted July 23, 2018.

Kobayashi Keiichirō. *Nagano-shi shikō: Zenkōji machi no kenkyū.* Tokyo: Yoshikawa Kōbunkan, 1969.

———. "Raibyōnin no shiyaku chōshūken." *Nihon rekishi* 115 (1958): 49–50.

———. "Watakushi no tachiba wo kangae." *Buraku* 36, no. 9 (1984): 41–46.

————. "Zenkōji no raibyōnin buraku." *Nihon rekishi* 233 (1967): 64–72.

Koch, Robert. *Die Lepra-Erkrankungen in Kreise Memel*. Jena: Verlag von Gustav Fischer, 1897.

Kokuritsu Hansenbyō Shiryōkan, ed. *Hyakunen no kakuri: Kōritsu rai ryōyōjo no tanjō*. Higashiyama: Kokuritsu Hansenbyō Shiryōkan, 2009.

————, ed. *Kimono ni miru ryōyōjo no kurashi*. Higashiyama: Kokuritsu Hansenbyō Shiryōkan, 2010.

————, ed. *Shiritsu Hansenbyō ryōyōjo Tairōin no arumi: Sōritsu kara heiin made no 115-nen*. Higashimurayama: Kokuritsu Hansenbyō Shiryōkan, 2015.

————, ed. *Zensei Byōin wo aruku—Utsusareta 20-seiki zenhan no ryōyōjo*. Higashiyamamura: Kokuritsu Hansenbyō Shiryōkan, 2010.

"Kokuritsu Hansenbyō Shiryōkan saikaikan." *Shiryōkan tayori* 55 (April 2007): 1.

Kokuritsu Ryōyōjo Kikuchi Keifūen, ed. *Kikuchi Keifūen 50-nen shi*. Kumamoto: Kokuritsu Ryōyōjo Kikuchi Keifūen, 1960.

Komatsu Yoshio. *Kekkaku: Nihon kindaishi no uragawa*. Osaka: Seifūdō, 2000.

Kondō Yūshō. "Hansenbyō ryōyōjo ni okeru taien to shakai fukki ni tsuite." *Shintennōji Daigaku Daigakuin kenkyū ronshū*, no. 8 (2013): 23–37.

Kosoto Hiroshi. *Nihon kanpō tenseki jiten*. Tokyo: Taishūkan, 1999.

Koyama Fūkusei Byōin Hyakunen Henshū Iinkai, ed. *Koyama Fūkusei Byōin Hyakunen shi*. Tokyo: Shunjusha, 1989.

Kōzensha, ed. *Aru gunzō: Kōzensha no hyakunen no ayumi*. Tokyo: Nihon Kirisutokyōdan Shuppankyoku, 1978.

Krämer, Hans Martin. " 'Not Befitting Our Divine Country': Eating Meat in Japanese Discourses of Self and Other from the Seventeenth Century to the Present." *Food and Foodways* 16 (2008): 33–62.

Kujirai Chisato. *Kyōkai no genba: Fōkuroa no rekishigaku*. Ibaragi: Henkyōsha, 2006.

Kuryū Rakusen'en Kanja Jichikai, ed. *Fūsetsu no mon: Kuryū Rakusen'en kanja gojūnenshi*. Gumma: Kuryū Rakusen'en Kanja Jichikai, 1982.

Kuroda Hideo. *Kyōkai no chūsei shōchō no chūsei*. Tokyo: Tōkyō Daigaku Shuppankai, 1986.

Kuroda Toshio. *Nihon chūsei kokka to shūkyō*. Tokyo: Iwanami Shoten, 1975.

Lara, C. B., and C. A. Palafox. "The Care of Culion-Born Children." In *Culion: A Record of Fifty Years Work with the Victims of Leprosy at the Culion Sanitarium, Prepared by Members of the Staff and Patient Body*. Manila: Bureau of Printing, 1956.

Latour, Bruno. *The Pasteurization of France*. Translated by Allen Sheridan and John Law. Cambridge, MA: Harvard University Press, 1993.

Law, Anwei Skinsnes. *Kalaupapa: A Collective Memory*. Honolulu: University of Hawai'i Press, 2012.

Leung, Angela Ki Che. *Leprosy in China: A History.* New York: Columbia University Press, 2009.

Macé, Mieko. "Dissection, Blood-Letting and Medicine as per Yamawaki Tōmon and Ogino Gengai." In *East Asian Science: Tradition and Beyond. Papers from the Seventh International Conference on the History of Science in East Asia, Kyoto, 2–7 August 1993.* Edited by Hashimoto Keizō, Catherine Jami, and Lowell Skar, 353–357. Osaka: Kansai University Press, 1995.

Matsubara Yōko. "Minzoku yūsei hogohō to Nihon no yūseihō no keifu." *Nihon kagakushi gakkai zasshi* 36, no. 201 (1997): 42–50.

———. "Nihon no yūseihō no rekishi." In *Yūsei hogohō ga okashita tsumi.* Edited by Yūsei shujutsu ni taisuru shazai wo motomeru kai, 104–115. Tokyo: Gendai Shokan, 2003.

Matsuda Yoshinori. "Kitayama Jūhachikenko wo chūshin ni shita jinken no machizukuri." *Buraku kaihō* 542 (2003): 76–83.

Matsuoka Hiroyuki. "Hansenbyō ryōyōjo ni okeru kanja jichi no mosaku: Daisan fukenritsu no ryōyōjo Sotojima Hoyōin ni tsuite." *Buraku mondai kenkyū,* no. 173 (2005): 2–21.

———. *Kakuri no shima ni ikiru: Okayama Hansenbyō mondai kiroku.* Okayama: Fukuro Shuppan, 2011.

Matsuoka Hōyōen 70-nen Kinenshi Kankō Iinkai. *Hikkyō wo hiraku.* Aomori: Aomori Kyūrai Kyōkai, 1979.

Matsushita Shirō. *Kyūshū hisabestsu burakushi kenkyū.* Tokyo: Akashi Shoten, 1985.

Meguro-ku Kyōdo Kenkyūkai, ed. *Meguro-ku no rekishi.* Tokyo: Meicho Shuppan, 1978.

Misch, Elizabeth A., W. R. Berrington, J. C. Vary Jr., and T. R. Hawn. "Leprosy and the Human Genome." *Microbiology and Molecular Biology Review* 74, no. 4 (2010): 589–620.

Miyagawa Ryō. "Kyūrai shiseki Nishiyama Kōmyōin ni tsuite." *Lepura* 6, no. 2 (1935): 81–103.

Miyagi kenshi hensan iinkai, ed. *Miyagi kenshi.* Vol. 18, *Iyaku taiiku.* Sendai: Miyagi Kenshi Kankōkai, 1959.

Miyamae Chikako. "'Raijin koya' no kanshin to chiiki shakai." *Buraku kaihō kenkyū* 197 (2013): 16–29.

———. "Zen-kindai ni okeru raisha no sonzai keitai ni tsuite, ge." *Buraku kaihō kenkyū* 167 (2005): 71–84.

Monot, Marc, N. Honoré, T. Garnier, R. Araoz, J. Y. Coppée, C. Lacroix, S. Sow, et al. "On the Origin of Leprosy." *Science* 308, no. 5724 (2005): 1040–1042.

Moran, Michelle. *Colonizing Leprosy: Imperialism and Public Health in the United States.* Chapel Hill: University of North Carolina Press, 2007.

Mori Shūichi and Ishii Norihisa. "Hansenbyō to igaku 1: Kakuri seisaku no teishō to sono haikei." *Japanese Journal of Leprosy* 75, no. 1 (2006): 22–28.

Murakami Kimiko. "Kekkaku yobōhō no seiritsu yōin ni kansuru kōsatsu." *Kansai Fukushi Daigaku shakai fukushi gakubu kiyō* 17, no. 1 (2013): 27–36.

Nagashima Aiseien Nyūensha Jichikai, ed. *Kakuzetsu no ritei: Nagashima Aiseien nyūensha 50-nenshi.* Okayama: Nagashima Aiseien Nyūensha Jichikai, 1982.

Nagashima Aiseien Nyūjosha Jichikai, ed. *Akebono no shiokaze.* Okayama: Nihon Bunkyō Shuppan, 1998.

Nara Daigaku Sōgō Kenkyūjo, ed. *Nara Daibutsumae ezuya Tsutsui-ke kokusei ezu shūsei.* Nara: Nara Daigaku Sōgō Kenkyūjo, 2002.

Narusawa Hiroyuki. "Kankō bunka to kindai onsen ryōyō: Kusatsu onsen to Eruvuin Berutsu." *Keizaigaku ronsō* 13, no. 1 (2004): 85–112.

Nichibenren Hōmu Kenkyū Zaidan. *Hansenbyō mondai ni kansuru kenshō kaigi saishū hōkokusho.* 2 vols. Tokyo: Akashi Shoten, 2007.

Niunoya Tetsuichi. *Kebiishi: Chūsei no kegare to kenryoku.* Tokyo: Heibonsha, 1986.

Norgen, Christina. *Abortion before Contraception: The Politics of Reproduction in Postwar Japan.* Princeton, NJ: Princeton University Press, 2001.

Obregón, Diana. "The State, Physicians, and Leprosy in Modern Colombia." In *Disease in the History of Modern Latin America,* edited by Diego Armus and Nancy Lews Stepan, 130–157. Durham, NC: Duke University Press, 2003.

Okada Yasuo. *Shisetsu Matsuzawa Byōin shi, 1879–1980.* Tokyo: Iwasaki Gakujutsu Shuppankai, 1981.

Okamoto Takehiro. "Sono ato no Kitayama Jūhachikenko." *Nara kenritsu dōwa mondai kankei shiryō sentā kenkyū kiyō* 19 (2015): 41–60.

Okiura Kazuteru and Tokunaga Susumu, eds. *Hansenbyō: Haijo, sabetsu, kakuri no rekishi.* Tokyo: Iwanami Shoten, 2001.

Ōshima Seishōen Nyūensha Jichikai, ed. *Tōzasareta shima no Shōwashi.* Ajichō, Kagawa-ken: Ōshima Seishōen Nyūensha Jichikai, 1981.

Ōuchi Hirotaka. "Kinsei Mutsu no kuni nanbu ni okeru hisabetsu mibun no jittai." *Bessatsu Tōhokugaku* 5 (2003): 216–249.

———. "Kinsei ni okeru hisabestu mibun no jittai." In *Higashi Nihon no kinsei buraku no gutaizō,* edited by Higashi Nihon Buraku Kaihō Kenkyūjo, 367–400. Tokyo: Akashi Shoten, 1992.

Ōyama Kyōhei. *Nihon chūsei nōsonshi no kenkyū.* Tokyo: Iwanami Shoten.

Pandya, Shubhada S. "The First International Leprosy Conference, Berlin, 1897: The Politics of Segregation." *História, Ciências, Saúde-Manguinhos* 10, supp. 1 (2003): 161–177.

Parascandola, J. "Chaulmoogra Oil and the Treatment of Leprosy." *Pharmaceutical History* 45, no. 2 (2003): 47–57.

———. "Miracle at Carville: The Introduction of the Sulfones for the Treatment of Leprosy." *Pharmacy in History* 40, nos. 2–3 (1998): 59–66.

Pennington, Lee. *Casualties of History: Wounded Japanese Servicemen and the Second World War.* Ithaca, NY: Cornell University Press, 2015.

Petryna, Adriana. *Life Exposed: Biological Citizenship after Chernobyl.* Princeton, NJ: Princeton University Press, 2002.

Ra, Charo. "Body of Research: Ownership and Use of Human Tissue." *New England Journal of Medicine* 355 (2005): 1517–1519.

Reibel, F., E. Cambeau, and A. Aubry. "Update on the Epidemiology, Diagnosis, and Treatment of Leprosy." *Médecine et maladies infectieuses* 45 (2015): 383–393.

Reilly, Philip R. *The Surgical Solution: A History of Involuntary Sterilization in the United States.* Baltimore, MD: Johns Hopkins University Press, 1991.

Richards, Peter. "Leprosy: Myth, Melodrama, and Mediaevalism." *Journal of the Royal College of Physicians* 24, no. 1 (1990): 55–62.

———. *The Medieval Leper and His Northern Heirs.* Totowa, NJ: Rowman and Littlefield, 1977.

Riddel [*sic*], H. "Rai no kyūsai oyobi yobō mondai." *Nihon no ikai,* no. 124 (February 1914): 4–5.

Robertson, Jo. "Leprosy and the Elusive *M. leprae*: Colonial and Imperial Medical Exchanges in the Nineteenth Century." *História, Ciências, Saúde-Manguinhos* 10, supp. 1 (2003): 13–40.

Rose, Nikolas. *The Politics of Life Itself: Biomedicine, Power, and Subjectivity in the Twenty-First Century.* Princeton, NJ: Princeton University Press, 2007.

Rose, Nikolas, and Carlos Nova. "Biological Citizenship." In *Global Assemblages: Technology, Politics, and Ethics as Anthropological Problems,* edited by Aihwa Ong and Stephen J. Collier, 439–463. Malden, MA: Blackwell Publishing, 2005.

Rotermund, Hartmut. "Demonic Affliction or Contagious Disease? Changing Perceptions of Smallpox in the Late Edo Period." *Japanese Journal of Religious Studies* 28, nos. 3–4 (2001): 373–398.

Sato, Hajime, and Janet E. Frantz, "Termination of the Leprosy isolation Policy in the US and Japan: Science, Policy Changes, and the Garbage Can Model." *BMC International Health and Human Rights* 5 (2005).

Satō Tsutomu. "Hansenbyō 'muraiken undō' no hatten ni tsuite." *Hansenbyō shimin gakkai nenpō,* no. 3 (2007): 44–53.

Satomichi Tokuo. "Suzuki Shosan 'Inga monogatari' ni miru bukkyō shinkō no kitei." In *Kinsei no seishin seikatsu,* edited by Ōkura Seishin Bunka Kenkyūjo, 371–418. Tokyo: Zoku Gunsho Ruiju Kanseikai, 1996.

Saunderson, P. R. "Drug Resistant *M. leprae.*" *Clinical Dermatology* 34, no. 1 (2016): 79–81.

Sawano Masaki. *Raisha no sei: Bunmei kaika no jōken toshite no.* Tokyo: Seikyūsha, 1994.

Schuenemann, Verena J., P. Singh, T. A. Mendum, B. Krause-Kyora, G. Jäger, K. I. Bos, A. Herbig, et al. "Genome-Wide Comparison of Medieval and Modern *Mycobacterium leprae.*" *Science* 341, no. 6142 (2013): 179–183.

Screech, Timon. *The Lens within the Heart: The Western Scientific Gaze and Popular Imagery in Later Edo Japan.* Cambridge: Cambridge University Press, 1996.

Serizawa Ryōko. "Hansenbyō iryō wo meguru seisaku to dendō: Nihon tōchiki Taiwan ni okeru jirei kara." *Rekishigaku kenkyū,* no. 834 (2007): 27–36.

Shimizu Kairyu. "Shūkyō Byōin DaiNihon Kyūsekan wo meguru jinbutsuzō: Ota Kōsaku." In *Indo bukkyōshi bukkyōgaku ronsō: Nakazawa Kōyū Hakushi koki kinen ronbunshū,* edited by Nakazawa Kōyū Hakushi koki kinen ronbunshū kankōkai. Tokyo: Sankibō Busshorin, 2011.

Shimosaka Mamoru. "Chūsei hinin no sonzai keitai: Kiyomizu-zaka 'Chōtōdō' kō." *Geinōshi kenkyū* 110 (1990), 1–22.

Shinmura Taku. *Nihon iryō shakaishi no kenkyū.* Tokyo: Hōsei Daigaku Shuppankyoku, 1985.

Shiomi Sen'ichirō. *Binmin no teito.* Tokyo: Bungei Shinsho, 2008.

Sontag, Susan. *Illness as Metaphor and AIDS and Its Metaphors.* New York: Anchor Books, 1990.

Sugiyama Hiroaki. "Yamaguchi-ken ni okeru Hansenbyō taisaku no tenkai: Murai-ken undōki wo chūshin ni." *Yamaguchi kenshi kenkyū* 14 (2006). http://takaamami.fc2web.com/sugiyama_yamaguchiken.html. Accessed November 9, 2017.

"Summary of Vital Statistics." Ministry of Health, Labour, and Welfare website. http://www.mhlw.go.jp/english/database/db-hw/populate/xls/inter2.xls. Accessed November 14, 2017.

Suzuki Motozo. "Nara, Kitayama Jūhachikenko." *Jinsen* 7 (1936): 105–136.

Tabuteau, Bruno. "Combien de lépreux au Moyen Âge? Essai d'étude quantitative appliquée à la lèpre. Les exemples de Rouen et de Bellencombre au XIIIe siècle." *Sources: Travaux historiques* 13 (1988): 19–24.

Tachibana Terumasa. *Nihon igaku senjin den: Kodai kara Bakumatsu made.* Tokyo: Ijiyakugyō Shinpōsha, 1969.

Takayanagi Shinobu. "Nakamura Masanao to Yan Fu ni okeru J. S. Miru 'Jiyūron' honyaku no imi." Kyoto University, Institute for Research on the Humanities. http://www.zinbun.kyoto-u.ac.jp/~rcmcc/h2-takayanagi.pdf. Accessed November 15, 2017.

Takio Eiji. *Chōsen Hansenbyō shi: Nihon shokuminchika no Sorokuto.* Tokyo: Miraisha, 2001.

Tama Zenshōen Kanja Jichikai, ed. *Kue issho: Kanja ga tsuzuru Zenshōen no nanajūnen.* Tokyo: Ikkōsha, 1979.

Tamamura Kōzō and Yajima Ryōichi. "Rai kanja ni taisuru danshu shujutsu ni tsuite." *Kōshū eisei hoken kyōkai zasshi* 17, no. 11 (1942): 554–566.

Tanaka, Katherine. "Through the Hospital Gates: Hansen's Disease and Modern Japanese Literature." PhD diss., University of Chicago, 2012.

Tanaka Sukeichi. *Hagi no unda kindai Nihon no iseika Yamane Masatsugu.* Hagi: Daiaikai, 1967.

Tobimatsu Jingo. *Hannah Riddell: Known in Japan as "The Mother of Lepers."* Kumamoto: Kaishun Byōin Jimusho, 1937.

Tōkyō Toritsu Daigaku Gakujutsu Kenkyūkai, ed. *Meguro-ku shi.* 3 vols. Tokyo: Meguro-ku, 1961.

Tottori-ken Sōmubu Sōmuka Kenshi Hensanshitsu. *Tottori-ken no muraiken undō: Hansenbyō no kindaishi.* Tottori-shi: Tottori Heibonsha, 2008.

Trambaiolo, Daniel. "Writing, Authority, and Practice in Tokugawa Medicine, 1650–1850." PhD diss., Princeton University, 2014.

Usami Hideki. "Kyō rakuchū rakugai bachō: Kinsei Kyōto raisha no kanshinba zu." Pt. 1, *Buraku mondai kenkyū* 114 (1991): 64–77; pt. 2, *Buraku mondai kenkyū* 115 (1992): 100–114.

Utsunomiya Minori. "Taisho 8-nen Seishin Byōinhō no rippō teian to sono giron." *Kinjō Gakuin Daigaku ronshū shakaigakuhen* 8, no. 1 (2011): 6.

Wakita Osamu. *Kawara makimono no sekai.* Tokyo: Tōkyō Daigaku Shuppankai, 1991.

Watson, Burton, trans. *The Lotus Sutra.* New York: Columbia University Press, 1993.

Williams, Diana L., and Thomas P. Gillis. "Drug-Resistant Leprosy: Monitoring and Current Status." *Leprosy Review* 83 (2012): 269–281.

Williams, Duncan Ryūken. *The Other Side of Zen: A Social History of Sōtō Zen Buddhism in Tokugawa Japan.* Princeton, NJ: Princeton University Press, 2009.

Wingfield, Lewis Strange. *Wanderings of a Globe-Trotter in the Far East.* London: R. Bentley and Sons, 1889.

Wyman, Walter. "National Control of Leprosy." *Transactions of the Congress of American Physicians and Surgeons.* New Haven, CT: Congress of American Physicians and Surgeons, 1894.

Yamaguchi Junko. "Gotō Masafumi Masanao fushi to Kihai Byōin no jiseki ni tsuite." *Hansenbyō shimin gakkai nenpō* (2005): 115–132.

Yamamoto Masanori, ed. *Kakunshū*. Tokyo: Heibonsha, 2001.

Yamamoto Shun'ichi. *Nihon raishi*. Tokyo: Tokyo Daigaku Shuppankai, 1993.

———. *Zōhō Nihon raishi*. Tokyo: Tokyo Daigaku Shuppankai, 1997.

Yamamoto Sumiko and Katō Naoko. *Hansenbyō ryōyōjo no esunogurafi: Kakuri no naka no kekkon to kodomo*. Tokyo: Iryō Bunkasha, 2008.

Yamashita Michisuke and Arai Yūki, eds. *Hansenbyō bungaku shiryō shūi*. 2 vols. Higashimurayama: Kokuritsu Ryōyōjo Tama Zenshōen Jichikai Hansenbyō Toshokan, 2004.

Yamashita Takaaki. "Kinsei Sanuki ni okeru hisabetsumin no kenkyū." *Buraku kaihō kenkyū* 124 (1998): 42–61.

Yamazaki Teijirō. *Kinsei Nihon no iyaku bunka: miira, ahen, kōhī*. Tokyo: Heibonsha, 1995.

Yanagiya Keiko. *Kinsei no josei sōzoku to kaigo*. Tokyo: Yoshikawa Kōbunkan, 2007.

Yokoi Kiyoshi. *Chūsei minshū no seikatsu bunka*. Tokyo: Tōkyō Daigaku Shuppankai, 1975.

———. "Raisha." In *Chūsei no minshū to geinō,* edited by Kyōto Burakushi Kenkyūjo, 128–132. Kyoto: Aunsha, 1986.

Yokota Noriko. "'Monoyoshi' kō: Kinsei Kyōto no raisha ni tsuite." *Nihonshi kenkyū* 352 (1991): 1–29.

Yokoyama Takashi. *Nihon ga yūsei shakai ni naru made: Kagaku keimō, media, seishoku no seiji*. Tokyo: Keisō Shobō, 2015.

Yoshida Eijirō. "Kyūrai shisetsu Kitayama Jūhachikendo itenron no airo wo megutte." *Regional* 3 (2006): 61–96.

———. "Yakushiji saikō no shuku mura to kyūrai shisetsu Nishiyama Kōmyōin." *Regional* 4 (2006): 1–13.

Yoshida Fumio. "Ninshō no shakai jigyō ni tsuite." In *Nihon ni okeru shakai to shūkyō,* edited by Kasahara Kazuo, 99–144. Tokyo: Yoshikawa Kōbunkan, 1969.

Yuasa Yō. "Nihon de puromin no gassei to sekai no Hansenbyō seiatsu." *Yakugaku zasshi,* no. 117 (1997): 957–962.

Zenkoku Hansenshibyō Kanja Kyōgikai, ed. *Zenkankyō undōshi*. Tokyo: Ikkōsha, 1977.

Zimmerman, Susan. "Leprosy in the Medieval Imagination." *Journal of Medieval and Early Modern Studies* 38 (2008): 559–587.

Index

Page numbers followed by letters *f*, *m*, and *t* refer to figures, maps, and tables, respectively.

About the Author

SUSAN L. BURNS is professor of Japanese history and East Asian languages and civilizations at the University of Chicago. She is the author of *Before the Nation:* Kokugaku *and the Imagining of Community in Early Modern Japan* and coeditor (with Barbara J. Brooks) of *Gender and Law in the Japanese Imperium.* Her research interests include medicine, public health, gender, sexuality, law, and the family in early modern and modern Japan.